Treatment and Management of Bladder Cancer

Edited by

Seth P Lerner MD FACS
Professor, Beth and Dave Swalm
Chair of Urologic Oncology
Scott Department of Urology
Baylor College of Medicine
Houston, TX
USA

Mark P Schoenberg MD
Professor of Urology and Oncology
Director of Urologic Oncology
James Buchanan Brady Urological Institute
The Johns Hopkins Medical Institutions
Baltimore, MD
USA

Cora N Sternberg MD FACP
Chief, Department of Medical Oncology
San Camillo Forlanini Hospital
Rome
Italy

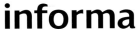

informa
healthcare

First published in the United Kingdom in 2008 by Informa Healthcare, Telephone House, 69-77 Paul Street, London EC2A 4LQ. Informa Healthcare is a trading division of Informa UK Ltd. Registered Office: 37/41 Mortimer Street, London W1T 3JH. Registered in England and Wales number 1072954.

Tel: +44 (0)20 7017 5000
Fax: +44 (0)20 7017 6699
Website: www.informahealthcare.com

A CIP record for this book is available from the British Library.
Library of Congress Cataloging-in-Publication Data

Data available on application

ISBN-10: 0 415 46217 7
ISBN-13: 978 0 415 46217 4

Distributed in North and South America by
Taylor & Francis
6000 Broken Sound Parkway, NW, (Suite 300)
Boca Raton, FL 33487, USA

Within Continental USA
Tel: 1 (800) 272 7737; Fax: 1 (800) 374 3401
Outside Continental USA
Tel: (561) 994 0555; Fax: (561) 361 6018
Email: orders@crcpress.com

Book orders in the rest of the world

Paul Abrahams
Tel: +44(0)20 7017 4036
Email: bookorders@informa.com

Composition by Exeter Premedia Services Private Ltd., Chennai, India
Printed and bound in India by Replika Press Pvt Ltd

Treatment and Management of Bladder Cancer

Dedication

With deep sorrow and a sense of tremendous loss to our community, the editors dedicate *Treatment and Management of Bladder Cancer* to the memory of Dr. John Stein, Chairman of Urology, The University of Southern California. John was an outstanding surgeon and scholar; throughout his professional life, he dedicated himself to the advancement of our collective understanding of bladder cancer. John made many seminal contributions to our scientific knowledge of this disease. We mourn the loss of a genuine talent and a true friend taken away from us in an untimely and tragic fashion. The work reflected in this text should serve as a testimony to our affection for John and our commitment to a cause to which he had devoted himself.

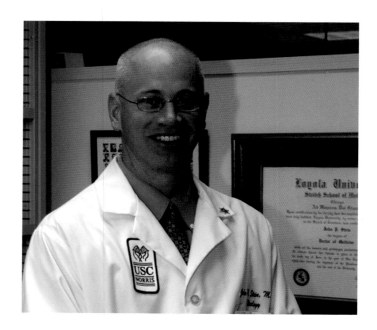

Contents

Contributors

Alex F Althausen MD
Clinical Professor of Urology
Harvard Medical School, Department of Urology
Massachusetts General Hospital
Boston, MA
USA

Aristotelis G Anastasiadis MD
Assistant Professor and Chairman
Department of Urology
Krankenhaus Großburgwedel der Region Hannover
Burgwedel
Germany

Jessie L-S Au PharmD PhD
Distinguished University Professor
College of Pharmacy
The Ohio State University
Columbus, OH
USA

Joaquim Bellmunt MD PhD
Section Chief, Solid Tumor Oncology (GU & GI)
Medical Oncology Service
Hospital del Mar
Barcelona
Spain

Bernard H Bochner MD FACS
Associate Attending Physician
Department of Urology
Memorial Sloan-Kettering Cancer Center
New York, NY
USA

Michelle Boyar MD
Clinical Fellow in Medical Oncology and Hematology
Columbia University Medical Center
New York, NY
USA

Robert Bristow MD PhD FRCP(C)
Associate Professor
Departments of Radiation Oncology and Medical Biophysics
University of Toronto; Clinician-Scientist
Radiation Oncology and Applied Molecular Oncology
Princess Margaret Hospital/University Health Network
Toronto, ON
Canada

Marc S Chuang MD
Chief Resident in Urology
The University of Chicago
Chicago, IL
USA

John J Coen MD
Assistant Professor of Radiation Oncology
Harvard Medical School; Genitourinary Oncology Unit
Department of Radiation Oncology
Massachusetts General Hospital
Boston, MA
USA

Roland Dahlem MD
Asklepios Clinic Harburg
Hamburg
Germany

Guido Dalbagni MD FACS
Associate Attending Surgeon
Department of Urology
Memoral Sloan-Kettering Cancer Center
New York, NY
USA

S Machele Donat MD FACS
Associate Attending Urology
Memorial Sloan-Kettering Cancer Center
Cornell-Weill Medical College
New York, NY
USA

Paolo Emiliozzi
San Giovanni Hospital
Rome
Italy

Susan Feyerabend MD
Department of Urology
University Hospital
University of Tuebingen
Tuebingen
Germany

Margit Fisch MD
Professor of Urology
Director of the Center of Urology and Pediatric Urology
Asklepios Clinic Harburg
Hamburg
Germany

Inderbir S Gill MD MCh
Professor of Surgery
Head
Section of Laparoscopic and Robotic Urology
Glickman Urological Institute
Cleveland, OH
USA

Mary K Gospodarowicz MD FRCPC FRCR(Hon)
Professor and Chair
Deparment of Radiation Oncology
University of Toronto
Medical Director
Princess Margaret Hospital/University Health Network
Cancer Program
Toronto, ON
Canada

Richard E Hautmann MD MDHon
Professor of Urology
Chairman Department of Urology
University of Ulm, Ulm
Germany

Niall M Heney MD
Clinical Professor of Urology
Harvard Medical School
Departmentof Urology
Massachusetts General Hospital
Boston, MA
USA

Harry W Herr MD
Attending Surgeon
Department of Urology
Memorial Sloan-Kettering Cancer Center
Professor of Urology
Cornell University of Medical College
New York, NY
USA

James O Jin MD PhD
Elkhart Clinic
Elkhart, IN
USA

Donald S Kaufman MD
Clinical Professor of Medicine, Harvard Medical School
Director, The Claire and John Bertucci Center for
Genitourinary Cancers
Massachusetts General Hospital
Boston, MA
USA

Melissa R Kaufman MD
Instructor
Department of Urologic Surgery
Vanderbilt University Medical Center
Nashville, TN
USA

Markus A Kuczyk MD
Professor and Chairman
Medizinische Hochschule Hannover
Urologie
Hannover
Germany

Donald L Lamm MD FACS
Clinical Professor
University of Arizona
Directory, BCG Oncology
Phoenix, AZ
USA

Seth P Lerner MD FACS
Associate Professor of Urology
Beth and Dave Swalm Chair in Urologic Oncology
Scott Department of Urology
Baylor College of Medicine
Houston, TX
USA

Frederik Liedberg MD
Senior Registrar
Department of Urology
University Hospital
Lund
Sweden

Yair Lotan MD
Assistant Professor of Urology
Department of Urology
University of Texas Southwestern Medical Center
Dallas, TX
USA

S Bruce Malkowicz MD
Professor of Urology
University of Pennsylvania
School of Medicine
Philadelphia, PA
USA

Åsa Månsson RN PhD
Senior Lecturer
Department of Health Sciences
Medical Faculty
Lund University
Sweden

Michael F Milosevic MD FRCP(C)
Associate Professor
Department of Radiation Oncology
University of Toronto; Clinician-Scientist
Radiation Medicine Program
Princess Margaret Hospital/University Health Network
Toronto, ON
Canada

Willem Oosterlinck PhD MD
Professor of Urology
Head of the Department of Urology
Ghent University Hospital
Ghent
Belgium

Vito Pansadoro MD
President
Vincenzo Pansadoro Foundation
Rome
Italy

Daniel P Petrylak MD
Associate Professor of Medicine
Director
Genitourinary Oncology Program
College of Physicians and Surgeons
Columbia Presbyterian Medical Center
New York, NY
USA

Lori A Pinke MD
Urologist
Urology Associates Ltd.
Phoenix, AZ
USA

Randall G Rowland MD PhD
Professor and James F Glenn Chair of Urology
Division of Urology
University of Kentucky
Lexington, KY
USA

Arthur I Sagalowsky MD
Professor and Chief of Urologic Oncology
Dr. Paul Peters Chair in Urology in Memory of Rumsey and
Louis Strickland
Department of Urology
University of Texas Southwestern Medical Center
Dallas, TX
USA

Mark P Schoenberg MD
Professor of Urology and Oncology
Director of Urologic Oncology
James Buchanan Brady Urological Institute
The Johns Hopkins Medical Institutions
Baltimore, MD
USA

Avishay Sella MD
Professor
Head
Department of Oncology
Asaf Harofeh Medical Center
Zerifin
Tel-Aviv University
Israel

William U Shipley MD
Andres Soriano Professor of Radiation Oncology
Harvard Medical School
Head
Genitourinary Oncology Unit
Department of Radiation Oncology
Massachusetts General Hospital
Boston, MA
USA

Donald G Skinner MD
Professor and Chairman of Urology
Department of Urology
University of Southern California Keck School of Medicine
Norris Comprehensive Cancer Center
Los Angeles, CA
USA

Joseph A Smith Jr MD
Professor and Chairman
Department of Urologic Surgery
Vanderbilt University Medical Center
Nashville, TN
USA

Eduardo Solsona MD
Chief of Urology
Valencia Oncology Institute
Valencia
Spain

Walter M Stadler MD FACP
Fred C Buffett Professor
Associate Dean of Clinical Research
Departments of Medicine and Surgery
Sections of Hematology-Oncology and Urology
University of Chicago
Chicago, IL
USA

John P Stein MD FACS
Associate Professor of Urology
Department of Urology
University of Southern California Keck School of Medicine
Norris Comprehensive Cancer Center
Los Angeles, CA
USA

Gary D Steinberg MD FACS
Professor and Vice Chairman of Urology
Director of Urologic Oncology
University of Chicago
Section of Urology
Chicago, IL
USA

Arnulf Stenzl MD
Professor and Chairman
Department of Urology
University Hospital
University of Tuebingen
Tuebingen
Germany

Cora N Sternberg MD FACP
Chairman
Department of Medical Oncology
San Camillo and Forlanini Hospitals
Rome
Italy

David A Swanson MD
Clinical Professor of Urology
The University of Texas MD Anderson Cancer Center
Houston, TX
USA

Richard J Sylvester ScD
Assistant Director
Head of Biostatistics
European Organisation for Research and Treatment of Cancer
Brussels
Belgium

Joachim W Thüroff MD
Professor and Chairman
Department of Urology and Paediatric Urology
Johannes Gutenberg-University Medical School
Mainz
Germany

Ingolf Tuerk MD PhD
Professor of Urology
Tufts University, School of Medicine
Vice Chair
Director for Minimal Invasive Laparoscopic Urology
Institute of Urology
Lahey Clinic Medical Center
Burlington, MA
USA

Hendrik van Poppel MD PhD FEBU
Professor and Chairman of Urology
Department of Urology
University Hospital of the Catholic University of Leuven
Leuven
Belgium

M Guillaume Wientjes PhD
Professor
College of Pharmacy
James Cancer Hospital and Solove Research Institute
The Ohio State University
Columbus, OH
USA

Christoph Wiesner MD
Department of Urology and Pediatric Urology
Johannes Gutenberg-University Medical School
Mainz
Germany

Anthony L Zietman MD
Jenot and William Shipley Professor of Radiation Oncology
Harvard Medical School
Massachusetts General Hospital
Boston, MA
USA

Section 1

Treatment

1

Transurethral resection of bladder tumors

Harry W Herr

Introduction

More than 60,000 new cases of bladder cancer are diagnosed each year in the United States.[1] Another 600,000 men and women are under surveillance for recurrent bladder tumors.[2] About 70% of bladder tumors are superficial, i.e. nonmuscle invasive (stage Ta, Tis, T1), and 30% invade the bladder muscle (stage T2) or perivesical fat (stage T3). Transurethral resection (TUR) is the essential surgical procedure used to diagnose, stage, and treat the majority of primary and recurrent bladder tumors.

TUR of bladder tumors is both a diagnostic and a therapeutic procedure. The initial TUR of a bladder tumor has three main goals:

1. to provide pathologic material to determine the histologic type and grade of bladder tumor
2. to determine the presence, depth, and type of tumor invasion (broad front or tentacular); such information is critical because tumor stage, grade, extent, and pattern of tumor growth direct additional therapy, determine the frequency of follow-up examinations and influence prognosis
3. to remove all visible and microscopic superficial and invasive tumor(s).

This chapter discusses the surgical technique, staging accuracy, and therapeutic efficacy of transurethral resection of bladder tumors.

Surgical technique

A TUR coupled with bimanual examination is best performed under general anesthesia. Anesthesia is induced with propathol (sedative) and fentanyl (narcotic) and maintained during the procedure using inhalational sevofluorane delivered through a laryngeal mask airway (LMA). The LMA is used for both spontaneous and controlled ventilation, and avoids the trauma and discomfort of endotracheal intubation. Such anesthesia is rapid, provides excellent general relaxation for procedures lasting up to an hour, and permits full recovery within 30 minutes.

When fully relaxed, the patient is placed in a low lithotomy position using adjustable stirrups. A bimanual examination is performed both before and after resection. A 24 Fr. resectoscope sheath is introduced into the bladder using the visual obturator, facilitated by a video camera. Urine is collected for cytology. An Iglesias resectoscope is inserted with the video camera attached to a 30° lens. All regions of the bladder are easily visualized using this one lens. Changing the angle of the scope and position of the table facilitates

resection. Glycine 1.5% (3000 cc bag) serves as irrigation. A pure monopolar point electrocautery current is used. The cutting current is set at 120 watts and the coagulation current at 60 watts. An Ellik evacuator filled with sterile water retrieves bladder and tumor specimens. The entire procedure is visually performed on a magnified screen using the video camera. Resection of tumors is best performed with the bladder half full.

Box 1.1 illustrates the information desired from a TUR of bladder tumor. Tumors involving the bladder, bladder neck, urethra and prostate should be noted as to their individual characteristics. All visible tumors are systematically resected and submitted separately for histology. It is helpful to record the type, size and location of each tumor on a bladder map, including areas of carcinoma in situ (CIS). At the end of the procedure, the urologist should state whether the TUR is complete or incomplete. The urologist (not the pathologist) is responsible for assigning a primary tumor stage based on assessment of the tumor during cystoscopy and resection coupled with the pathologic findings.

At the initial evaluation, a complete resection of all gross and suspected tumor(s) is attempted, including all areas involved with CIS. This may take more than one procedure, but with due diligence and patience, it is rare that a bladder cannot be cleared of all visible tumors. The bladder neck and prostate are biopsied to detect tumor spread within the bladder neck musculature, prostatic urethra, ducts, and stroma. Biopsies at 4- and 8-o'clock are obtained, extending from the bladder neck to the verumontanum. Selected site loop or cold-cup biopsies of suspicious mucosal lesions are performed,[3] but random biopsies of normal-appearing mucosa rarely show tumor, and urine cytology is more accurate in detecting diffuse mucosal abnormalities. A variety of resectoscope loops are available, but finer diameter loops project a more concentrated current and cut more easily. Figure 1.1 illustrates the loop preferred by the author. The attached 'runner' projecting in front of the right-angled loop allows resection of tumors on a flat surface, even in concave regions of the bladder, reduces cautery artifact, and helps to control a uniform and safe depth of resection.[4] The loop has a cross-width of 8 mm, permitting most tumors 1.0–1.5 cm in size to be resected completely as one specimen (Figure 1.2). Others have also developed innovative methods for en bloc removal of bladder tumors using flat loop, knife, or needle electrodes.[5–7]

Each tumor should be resected completely, if possible, and delivered to pathology as one contiguous specimen oriented so that a longitudinal histologic section through the tumor shows intact overlying and surrounding mucosa, and underlying lamina propria and deep muscle. Figure 1.2 shows the position of the loop prepared to resect a 1.5 cm papillary tumor toward the operator, removing the tumor as one specimen with a single broad sweep of the loop. Larger tumors are resected in multiple pieces, progressing in an orderly fashion from one side of the tumor to the other, until the entire base is reached and excised. The muscle fibers of the detrusor should be readily distinguished from the granular appearance of tumor. Figures 1.3 and 1.4, respectively, show complete resections of solid and papillary tumors. In each case, muscle deep to the tumor bed appears normal, indicating a complete visible resection. In cases of multiple, low-grade papillary tumors, it is not necessary to obtain muscle in each individual specimen if

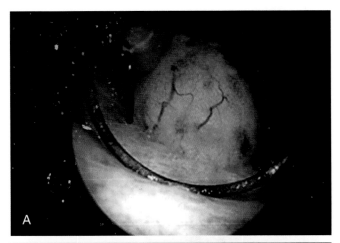
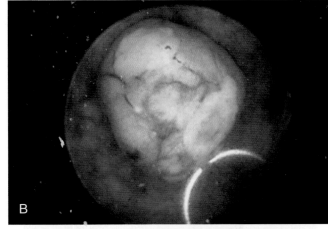
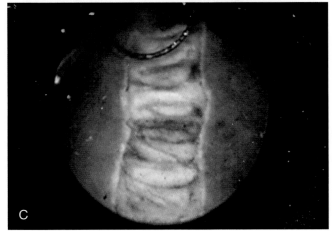

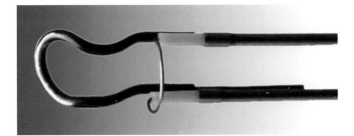

Figure 1.1
Resectoscope loop.

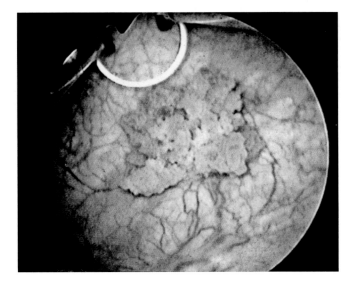

Figure 1.2
Transurethral resection of a papillary tumor.

Figure 1.3
Complete transurethral resection of a solid bladder tumor.

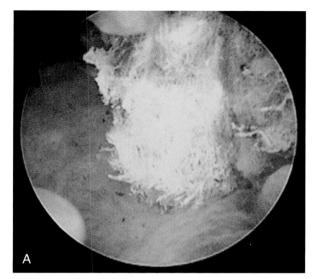

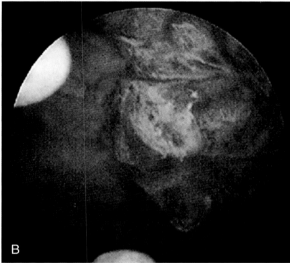

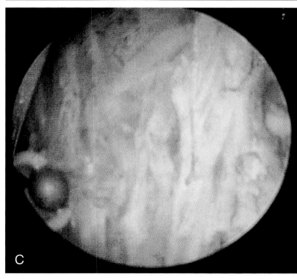

Figure 1.4
Complete transurethral resection of a papillonodular bladder tumor.

contiguous normal-appearing lamina propria beneath the tumor is provided. For bulky, invasive tumors likely to require cystectomy, biopsies of the margin of the lesion containing muscle suffice. Biopsy of the central portion of such tumors may reveal only necrotic tissue and risks unnecessary bleeding that may prove difficult to control.

Tumors located in the dome or anterior wall can be difficult to reach and resect, especially if the prostate is enlarged. Placing the patient in Trendelenburg position, avoiding overdistension of the bladder, and applying gentle suprapubic pressure brings upper regions of the bladder into sharp focus and permits resection of anterior tumors on a flat surface. An extra long resectoscope sheath can also be used to resect difficult-to-reach tumors. An inferior lateral wall tumor can be difficult to resect because of the stimulated 'obturator nerve reflex' and the risk of bladder wall perforation. Reducing the cutting current and repeatedly tapping the cut peddle during resection of tumors from the lateral walls of the bladder greatly facilitates a controlled and complete resection of even deeply invasive tumors. Moving the entire sheath during resection (in a fashion similar to scooping ice cream with a spoon), rather than using the Iglesias working element, permits a more controlled, smoother, and better resection. Tumor and bladder wall specimens should be at least 1–2 cm in length or longer.

Retrograde resection is usually avoided because it may cause a perforation, but this method may be preferred to separate a papillary tumor from the mucosa if a narrow stalk is clearly visible rather than extending the loop behind a bulky tumor and resecting blindly in the usual manner with the spring-loaded working element. The ureteral orifice can be resected, if necessary, to completely remove a tumor overlying this structure.

In cases of multiple papillary tumors, the larger tumors are resected completely for histology, but smaller tumors (≤5 mm) and adjacent mucosa that may harbor CIS can be fulgurated using a roller ball electrode. An experienced urologist can usually distinguish low-grade papillary tumors from high-grade invasive tumors to permit fulguration of multiple, especially recurrent, tumors.[8] To ensure adequate visibility, bleeding is controlled at each resection site before moving on to another lesion. After all tumors have been resected, the margins and base of each tumor site are fulgurated using a roller ball electrode (see Figure 1.4).

Bladder tumors arising within a bladder diverticulum pose a unique diagnostic and therapeutic challenge. The paucity of muscle in a diverticulum renders TUR of diverticular tumors difficult, entailing an increased risk of incomplete resection and bladder perforation. Cystoscopic access and complete visualization of the entire diverticular mucosa is necessary to resect tumors safely and completely within a diverticulum. A narrow-mouthed ostium may be resected to gain access to a capacious diverticulum. A careful TUR of tumors confined to a diverticulum in 39 patients controlled 83% of non-invasive (Ta, Tis) or minimally invasive (T1) diverticular tumors. Our data support a conservative approach for superficial tumors confined to a bladder diverticulum, provided a complete transurethral resection is feasible.[9]

Sessile, nodular, and papillonodular tumors are more likely than papillary tumors to be high grade and invasive. In order to remove and accurately stage such tumors, they must be resected wide and deep. How wide and how deep has practical implications for tumor staging and treatment, and requires considerable judgment, experience, and skill. For example, Figure 1.5 shows a sessile tumor resected at its peripheral margin A. The resection is then extended laterally into normal mucosa for 2 cm to margin B, to ensure complete wide excision of the lesion and to detect adjacent CIS. Figure 1.6 shows how different patterns of invasion of T1 tumors

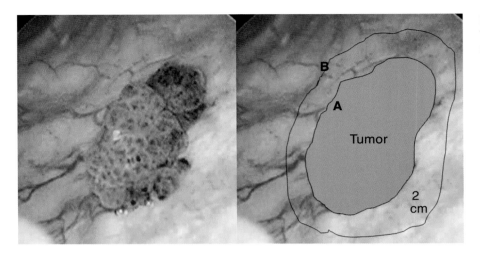

Figure 1.5
Transurethral resection of bladder tumor:
margins of resection.

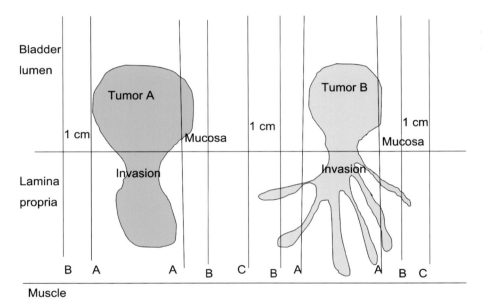

Figure 1.6
Transurethral resection of T1 bladder
tumors.

affect margins of resection. Tumor A has broad-front invasion and tumor B displays tentacular invasion. Resection of tumor A around its A margins results in complete resection of all exophytic and invasive components of the tumor. Resecting out to margin B verifies complete resection and may detect adjacent CIS. For tumor B, resection from margin A to A or margin B leaves tumor behind because of finger-like submucosal invasion extending laterally beyond the visible limits of the tumor. Complete resection of tumor B requires extending the resection another 1 or 2 cm out to margin C. Figure 1.7 shows a sagittal view of a tumor invading the deep lamina propria. The tumor is resected at margin A, to include much or all of the lamina propria with the tumor. Lateral resection out to margin B includes an ample portion of bladder muscle (that may not be included in the resection margins A to A) to verify complete tumor resection. Transurethral resection performed in this manner is more likely to remove the tumor completely and provides sufficient material to pathology to determine depth of invasion and centripetal extension of bladder tumor. Proof of this concept is illustrated by a study in which 35% of 462 TURs had residual tumor on extended deep resection of the tumor base and at least 2 cm lateral to visible tumor.[10] The extended TUR found incomplete initial resections of 13% of Ta, 36% of T1, 56% of T2, and 83% of T3 tumors.

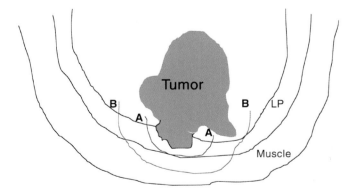

Figure 1.7
Transurethral resection of invasive bladder tumor. (LP, lamina propria.)

In cases of muscle-invasive tumors considered for bladder-sparing, a maximum, aggressive transurethral resection is required and is an integral component of multimodality therapy of locally advanced tumors. Deep resection of the detrusor is commenced only after all exophytic tumor has been removed. Tumor deep in the bladder wall is resected one layer at a time, avoiding deep excavation in one place, to maintain a clear view of the whole resection area. Deep resection is considered complete when normal glistening yellow fat is seen between the deep muscle bundles or perivesical tissues. Invasive tumor is usually firm and easy to resect whereas uninvolved 'normal' fat is difficult to cut or cauterize with the resectoscope. This is a useful finding indicating a complete tumor resection when corroborated by negative histologic examination of separate deep muscle specimens.

At the end of the procedure, a belladonna and opium (B&O) rectal suppository is inserted (may be repeated in 4–6 hours as needed) to reduce bladder spasms. Intravenous diazepam (2.5 mg) also relaxes the bladder and helps to stem bleeding caused by bladder spasms. Intravenous fentanyl (25 mcg) effectively controls postoperative discomfort. Rarely, continuous bladder irrigation through a three-way catheter is necessary to control postoperative hemorrhage. The patient may be safely discharged with or without a Foley catheter (depending on the extent of resection) an hour or two after the operation. In cases of an enlarged prostate, or after vigorous resection of tumor, especially around the bladder neck or prostatic urethra, it is best to leave a catheter overnight to prevent delayed acute urinary retention owing to edema or blood clots.

Complications of TUR of bladder tumors

Transurethral resection of bladder tumors is associated with a low (5%) overall complication rate.[11] The frequency of complications is higher with large (>5 cm) tumors, multiple tumors, and tumors located in the dome of the bladder. The most common complication, occurring in 1% to 3% of cases, is postresection bleeding, requiring return to the operating room to evacuate retained blood clots and fulgurate bleeders. On occasion, although the urine is crystal clear at the end of the procedure, bleeding may erupt in the recovery room if the patient coughs or suffers postanesthetic rigors. Vigilant nursing care to maintain a patent catheter (and a collapsed bladder) by gentle bladder irrigation may avert this problem. It is also not uncommon for patients to report passing blood clots and pieces of tissue 7–10 days after the procedure when necrotic tissue sloughs from resection sites. Such blood clots usually pass spontaneously and do not require intervention.

The second most serious complication, occurring in 1% of cases of TUR of bladder tumors, is bladder perforation. The majority (80%) are extraperitoneal perforations (managed with catheter drainage); in 20% of cases they are intraperitoneal (requiring open surgical repair if gaping and associated with significant extravasation of fluid and urine despite bladder drainage). Although tumor seeding is of concern when the bladder is perforated, documented cases of extravesical pelvic disease after resection of invasive tumors have not been reported. TUR of invasive tumors does not appear to disseminate urothelial cells in the peripheral circulation.[12] Clinically silent extravasation probably occurs during many procedures.

Ureteral obstruction owing to resection of a ureteral orifice may occur, but it is unlikely if only the cutting current is used across the orifice. Cautery is used sparingly around the orifices. Obstruction usually is caused by temporary edema and will resolve without stenting. On occasion, a scarred ureteral orifice requires operative intervention to relieve hydronephrosis.

Staging accuracy and restaging TUR

Incomplete resection and understaging of bladder tumors is well known owing to the stochastic nature of transurethral resection. Tumors recur at the same site of resection in 20% to 40% of cases and they may progress to invade the muscle layers of the bladder.[13,14] Among patients undergoing cystectomy for nonmuscle-invasive bladder cancer, 25% to 40% are upstaged to muscle invasion,[15] and about half of muscle-invasive tumors are found to have tumor spread outside the bladder or positive pelvic lymph nodes.[16] Accuracy in determining pathologic stage is largely related to the completeness of TUR.

Although most urologists agree that ideally initial TUR of bladder tumors should be thorough and complete, many factors confound the adequacy of resection, including multiplicity and extent of disease, capability and perseverance of the resectionist, quality of specimens provided, and pathologic analysis. The fact that local tumor control and accurate tumor staging depend on a complete TUR suggests that a second, restaging TUR may be of value in evaluating patients with bladder tumors. Another TUR reduces the uncertainty of depth of tumor invasion, better controls the primary tumor, and provides additional pathologic information that may help select appropriate treatment.[17]

Table 1.1 shows results of a second TUR performed 2–6 weeks after an initial TUR in 150 consecutive patients evaluated with

Table 1.1 Comparison of bladder tumor stage after first and second transurethral resections

Stage at first TUR	No. pts	No. stage at second TUR (%)				
		T0	Ta/Tis	T1	T2	T3–4
Tis	20	6 (30)	8 (40)	4 (20)	2 (10)	
Ta	18	5 (28)	7 (39)	5 (28)	1 (5)	
T1	58	13 (22)	15 (26)	14 (24)	16 (28)	
Muscle	35	9 (26)	11 (31)	10 (29)	5 (14)	
No muscle	23	4 (17)	4 (17)	4 (17)	11 (49)	
T2	54	12 (22)	7 (13)	3 (6)	30 (55)	2 (4)
Totals	150			114 (76)		

Table 1.2 Bladder tumor stage after second transurethral resection of T1 tumors

Series	Year	No. pts	Stage at second TUR (%)			
			T0	Ta/Tis	T1	T2
Klan et al[20]	1991	46		15	26	2
Herr[18]	1999	58	22	26	24	28
Schwaibold et al[21]	2000	60		17	24	5
Brauers et al[22]	2001	42	35	17	24	24
Ozen et al[23]	2001	28		18	53	29
Schips et al[24]	2002	76	67	11	15	8
Rigaud et al[25]	2002	52		16	17	4
Grimm et al[26]	2003	19		37	43	19

Table 1.3 Recurrent bladder tumors after one versus two TURs and BCG therapy

TUR	No. cases	No. recurrent tumor present at			
		3 months	6 months	12 months	Progression
Initial TUR	96	57 (59%)	58 (60%)	57 (59%)	31 (32%)
Repeat TUR	154	45 (29%)	34 (22%)	25 (16%)	11 (7%)

All differences are p = 0.000 by Pearson's chi-square and Fisher's exact test.

localized bladder tumor.[18] A significant proportion (76%) was found on a second TUR to have residual tumor. Of 96 patients with superficial (stage Ta, Tis, T1) tumors, only 25% had no tumor left; 31% had residual non-invasive tumor; 15% had persistent submucosal invasion; and 29% were upstaged to muscle invasion. An incomplete initial resection (and clinical understaging) was observed in 49% of stage T1 tumors with no muscle submitted in the first TUR specimen compared to 14% when muscle was identified. Of 54 patients with muscle-invasive tumors (confirmed by review of initial pathology), 22% had no residual tumor found on a restaging TUR, leading to changes in treatment.

A recent pathology review found that muscularis propria was missing in up to 51% of TUR specimens submitted by urologists.[19] Many of these were papillary low-grade tumors and the absence of muscle can be justified, but in 26% of invasive tumors, a muscle specimen was not submitted. Proper execution of TUR is critical for primary tumor staging and definitive treatment. The pathologist can only evaluate what the urologist submits!

Table 1.2[18–26] shows recently reported series of repeat TUR of stage T1 bladder tumors. Residual invasive T1 tumor was present in 15% to 53% of cases, and another 4% to 29% were upstaged to muscle invasion. The collective data suggest that a restaging TUR improves staging, but can it improve local control of T1 bladder tumors? We addressed this question in a recent cohort of 71 patients with T1 bladder tumors that underwent immediate cystectomy after we performed two sequential resections (same surgeon for both TURs) inclusive of muscle in the specimen.[27] Thirteen percent of the patients had muscle-invasive tumor in the cystectomy specimen, 24% had residual T1 tumor, and the others had either no or non-invasive tumors. All but two of these tumors were correctly identified and staged by the restaging TUR. We concluded from this small study that a restaging TUR of our own previously resected patients markedly improves both staging accuracy and local control of T1 bladder tumors.

Can a second TUR improve the outcome of patients with superficial bladder cancer?

A recent long-term observational study[26] showed that among a cohort of 124 consecutive patients, a restaging TUR found residual tumor in 33% of cases, including 27% of those with Ta and 53% of those with T1 disease. Residual tumor was found at the original resection site in 81% of cases. After 5 years follow-up, 63% of the patients undergoing a second TUR had disease-free bladders compared to 40% after one TUR. Progression to muscle invasion was observed in only two (3%) patients undergoing a restaging TUR. A second therapeutic TUR also appears to improve the short-term response to bacillus Calmette–Guérin (BCG) therapy.[28] Of 250 consecutive cases of nonmuscle-invasive bladder tumors treated with BCG (with or without maintenance BCG), 96 had one initial TUR before BCG and 154 had two TURs 2–6 weeks apart before starting BCG therapy. Table 1.3 shows that response rates were better after two TURs, and responses improved over time. Further, tumor progression to muscle invasion was more common in patients having only one TUR before BCG therapy. A second TUR appears to provide better local control of superficial bladder tumors and, by reducing tumor volume, contributes to earlier and more complete responses to intravesical therapy against minimal residual disease.

TUR of superficial bladder tumors

Although a thorough TUR is capable of ablating all visible nonmuscle-invasive tumors, subsequent tumor recurrence is common. Many studies show that the presence of tumor within 3 or 6 months after initial TUR is a significant predictor of tumor recurrence and progression, suggesting that an inadequate first resection is partly to blame for the high recurrence rate.[29,30] The 5- and 10-year recurrence rates after TUR exceed 70% and 85%, respectively. The 10-year survival rate after TUR for Ta tumors is 85% and is 70% for T1 tumors. These data argue persuasively for a restaging TUR, especially in high-risk tumors, for which TUR (with and without intravesical therapy) to preserve the bladder is the mainstay of treatment.

A review of the literature reporting more than 600 cases of T1 bladder tumors treated only by TUR shows that 75% to 90% recurred during follow-up of 5–10 years. In a third of patients disease progressed to muscle invasion in 5 years, and in 39% to 53% it had progressed by 10 years.[31] T1 tumors most likely to be cured by TUR are solitary low-grade papillary T1 tumors, superficially invading the lamina propria (stage T1a) and unassociated with diffuse CIS. Such tumors represent only 10% of all T1 bladder tumors. Tumor recurrence and increased risk of tumor progression are significantly associated with high-grade, multiple, solid T1 tumors displaying vascular invasion, surrounding CIS, and invading the deep portion of the lamina propria (T1b).

Whether subdividing T1 tumors according to depth of invasion, above (T1a) or below (T1b), the muscularis mucosa truly distinguishes different outcomes of T1 tumors is problematic owing to a discontinuous muscularis mucosa layer within the bladder wall and the difficulty pathologists face in evaluating tumor invasion in multiple fragmented pieces of tissue.[32] Most studies are based only on single TURs.[33] Common problems in T1 staging evaluation include tangential sectioning, due to an inability to orient the specimens, crush and cautery artifacts, and a streaking inflammatory infiltrate. All of these inherent pathologic difficulties can be largely eliminated if the urologist resects and submits suspected T1 tumors in a single specimen containing contiguous deep muscle. In one study,[34] substaging T1 tumors did not affect response to BCG therapy in regard to recurrence or progression, suggesting that completeness of the TUR was more important than distinguishing histologic subtypes of T1 tumor.

Radical TUR of invasive bladder cancer

A radical TUR may cure some muscle-invasive bladder cancers. Evidence for this is two-fold. From the early 1950s until 1977, before the widespread use of radical cystectomy, several series reported 5-year survival rates of 40% to 60% following TUR alone for stage T2 bladder tumors.[35–38] About 10% to 15% of patients having cystectomy for stage T2 bladder tumors will have no tumor (P0) found within the cystectomy specimen, indicating that the initial 'diagnostic' TUR had completely removed the invasive cancer.[29]

Several recent prospective studies confirm these results. In the first study,[39] of 432 evaluated patients with locally advanced bladder cancer, 99 (23%) were treated by definitive TUR if a restaging TUR of the primary tumor site showed no residual muscle invasion. The 10-year disease-specific survival was 76% (57% with bladder preserved). Of the 99 patients treated by TUR, 82% of 73 that had no tumor on restaging TUR survived, versus 57% of 26 that had residual T1 tumor on restaging TUR. Of the 34 patients (34%) that had recurrence in the bladder with a new invasive cancer, 18 (53%) were successfully treated by salvage cystectomy, and 16 patients (16%)

died of disease. In a second study,[40] 133 patients with invasive bladder cancer were treated by radical TUR if they had negative biopsies of the periphery and muscle layer of the tumor bed. At 5 and 10 years follow-up, the cause-specific survival rates were 80% and 75%, respectively. Both of these mature prospective studies justify radical TUR as a successful bladder-sparing therapeutic strategy in selected patients that have their primary muscle-invasive cancers completely and verifiably removed by negative re-resection biopsies of the primary tumor site.

Muscle-invasive bladder neoplasms successfully treated by radical TUR are usually solitary papillary tumors, <5 cm in size, that invade only the superficial layer of muscularis propria (stage T2a). A TUR may be curative only if the margins and base of the tumor site show no residual disease. Radical TUR cures only 20% or fewer bladder tumors that invade the deep muscle (stage T2b) or perivesical fat (stage T3a).

A radical TUR is also the essential first step in any combined modality strategy designed to spare the bladder.[41–45] Debulking the primary tumor, and indeed a visibly complete TUR, is required to select patients with invasive cancers for bladder preservation. In all such cases, biopsies of the tumor base, periphery of the tumor, and adjacent mucosa should verify a microscopically complete (R0) resection. Complete TUR of invasive bladder cancer is the most significant predictor of local control and survival after combined modality therapy. Response to chemotherapy, radiation, bladder preservation, and survival is improved after a maximum TUR. In one study, patients that had a radical TUR (R0) before chemotherapy and radiation had a 69% survival rate at 10 years, with 85% preserving their bladders, compared with only a 40% survival rate with incomplete tumor resection.[46] Cure and survival rates after conservative therapy decline substantially when the primary invasive tumor is incompletely resected.

A TUR also determines the response to induction chemotherapy. Neoadjuvant chemotherapy induces significant responses of invasive bladder cancer. A recently published randomized study showed that compared to radical cystectomy alone, neoadjuvant chemotherapy increases the likelihood of eliminating residual cancer in the cystectomy specimen and improved survival among patients with locally advanced bladder cancer.[47] Significantly more patients in the combination-therapy group had no residual disease (38%) than patients in the cystectomy group (15%). At 5 years, 85% of the patients with a pT0 surgical specimen were alive. This suggests that clinically 'complete responders' that have no tumor (P0) on a postchemotherapy TUR may be candidates for bladder preservation. Such approaches depend entirely on the accuracy of repeat TUR staging.[48] After chemotherapy, the tumor site often shows only a scar. This scar must be re-resected wide and deep in a determined effort to detect residual tumor. Successful bladder preservation requires an initial, visibly complete TUR of invasive tumor, response to chemotherapy, and a skillful re-resection of the primary tumor site.

We evaluated the 10-year outcome of patients with invasive (T2–3N0M0) bladder cancer that responded completely to neoadjuvant chemotherapy followed by bladder-sparing surgery.[49] All patients had residual muscle invasion on a restaging TUR. Of 111 surgical candidates, 60 (54%) achieved a complete clinical response (T0) on postchemotherapy TUR of the primary tumor site. Of 43 patients that elected treatment by chemotherapy plus TUR alone, 32 (74%) survived from 8 to 13 years, including 25 (58%) with an intact functioning bladder. Thirteen patients required salvage cystectomy. A similar study in 87 patients reported that 40 (51%) were T0 on TUR after neoadjuvant chemotherapy.[50] Thirty patients (71%) that had chemotherapy and TUR alone were alive after median follow-up of 54+ months, and 24 (57%) maintained an intact bladder. These two studies suggest that the majority of patients with invasive bladder cancer that achieve T0 status after neoadjuvant chemotherapy may preserve their bladders. Selection of such patients requires an aggressive, radical, postchemotherapy TUR of the primary tumor site to document absence of residual bladder cancer. The retained bladder remains at risk for new tumors, mandating frequent cystoscopies and repeated TURs to detect any sign of recurrent disease.

Conclusion

Transurethral resection of bladder tumor is both diagnostic and therapeutic for nonmuscle-invasive bladder tumors. A restaging TUR improves staging accuracy and improves local control of superficial and minimally invasive bladder tumors. A restaging TUR is recommended for all T1 tumors, multiple high-grade Ta tumors, and in all cases in which an initial TUR fails to clear the bladder of visible tumor. It is not necessary for TaG1 tumors. A radical TUR is curative for some patients with minimal muscle-invasive cancers if a verifiably complete resection is performed, and is an essential component of multimodality bladder-sparing strategies. Such cases usually require a restaging TUR.

Although TUR of bladder tumors is an essential procedure familiar to most urologists, it is difficult to perform well and may not achieve its desired goals. Although treatment outcome is often determined by tumor biology, a complete TUR identifies characteristics and extent of bladder tumors, providing the best method currently available to define individual tumor biology. In the present era of molecular medicine, high tech imaging, better drugs, and advanced surgical techniques, TUR has become a 'lost art'. However, a properly performed and aggressive TUR is one of the most successful and powerful procedures available to the urologist if it is appropriately applied with full knowledge of its inherent limitations. The TUR alone is the most important diagnostic, staging, and treatment modality for the vast majority of bladder tumors. Its success or failure, as well as that of subsequent treatments of non-invasive and invasive tumors localized to the bladder, are directly dependent on the information provided by a well-executed transurethral resection providing quality tumor specimens to permit accurate pathologic evaluation.

References

1. Jemal A, Tiwari RC, Murray T, et al. Cancer statistics, 2004. CA Cancer J Clin 2004; 54(1): 8–29.
2. Schrag D, Rabbani F, Herr HW, et al. Adherence to surveillance among patients with superficial bladder cancer. J Natl Cancer Inst 2003; 95: 588–97.
3. May F, Treibor U, Hartung R, et al. Significance of random bladder biopsies in superficial bladder cancer. Eur Urol 2003; 44: 47–50.
4. Herr HW, Reuter VE. Evaluation of new resectoscope loop for transurethral resection of bladder tumors. J Urol 1998; 159: 2067.
5. Ukai R, Kawashita E, Ikeda H. A new technique for transurethral resection of superficial bladder tumor in 1 piece. J Urol 2000; 163: 878–9.
6. Lodde M, Lusuardi L, Palermo S, et al. En bloc transurethral resection of bladder tumors: use and limits. Urology 2003; 62: 1089–91.
7. Saito S. Transurethral en bloc resection of bladder tumors. J Urol 2001; 166: 2148–50.
8. Herr HW, Donat SM, Dalbagni G. Correlation of cystoscopy with histology of papillary bladder tumors. J Urol 2002; 168: 978–80.
9. Golijanin D, Yossepowitch O, Beck S, et al. Carcinoma in a bladder diverticulum: presentation and treatment outcome. J Urol 2003; 170: 1761–4.
10. Kolozsy Z. Histopathological 'self-control' in TUR of bladder tumors. Br J Urol 1991; 67: 162–4.
11. Collado A, Chechile GE, Salvador J, et al. Early complications of endoscopic treatment for bladder tumors. J Urol 2000; 164: 1529–32.
12. Desgrandchamps F, Teren M, Dal Cortivo L, et al. The effects of transurethral resection on dissemination of epithelial cells in the circulation of patients with bladder cancer. Br J Cancer 1999; 81: 832–4.
13. Wolf H. Transurethral surgery in the treatment of invasive bladder cancer (stage T1 and T2). Scand J Urol Nephrol 1982; 104: 127–32.
14. Herr HW, Badalament RA. Superficial bladder cancer treated with BCG: a multivariate analysis of factors affecting tumor progression. J Urol 1989; 141: 22–9.
15. Dutta SC, Smith JA, Cookson MS, et al. Clinical understaging of high risk nonmuscle invasive urothelial carcinoma treated with radical cystectomy. J Urol 2001; 166: 490–3.
16. Dalbagni G, Genega E, Herr HW. Cystectomy for bladder cancer: a contemporary series. J Urol 2001; 165: 1111–15.
17. Herr HW. Uncertainty and outcome of invasive bladder tumors. Urol Oncol 1996; 2: 92–4.
18. Herr HW. The value of a second transurethral resection in evaluating patients with bladder tumors. J Urol 1999; 162: 74–6.
19. Maruniak NA, Takezawa K, Murphy WM. Accurate pathological staging of urothelial neoplasms requires better cystoscopic sampling. J Urol 2002; 167: 2404–7.
20. Klan R, Lou V, Huland H. Residual tumor discovered in routine second transurethral resection in patients with stage T1 transitional cell carcinoma of the bladder. J Urol 1991; 146: 316–18.
21. Schwaibold H, Treibor U, Kubler H, et al. Significance of second TUR for T1 bladder cancer. Eur Urol 2000; 37: 101–4.
22. Brauers A, Buettner R, Jakse G. Second resection and prognosis of high risk superficial bladder cancer: is cystectomy often too early? J Urol 2001; 165: 808–10.
23. Ozen H, Ekici S, Uygur MC, et al. Repeated transurethral resection and intravesical BCG for extensive superficial bladder tumors. J Endourol 2001; 15: 863–7.
24. Schips L, Augustin H, Zigeuner RE, et al. Is repeated transurethral resection justified in patients with newly diagnosed superficial bladder cancer. Urology 2002; 59: 220–23.
25. Rigaud J, Karam G, Braud G, et al. Value of second endoscopic resection in stage T1 bladder tumor. Prog Urol 2002; 12: 27–30.
26. Grimm M-C, Ackermann R, Vogeli TA. Effect of routine repeat transurethral resection for superficial bladder cancer: a long-term observational study. J Urol 2003; 170: 433–7.
27. Dalbagni G, Herr HW, Reuter VE. Impact of a second transurethral resection on staging of T1 bladder cancer. Urology 2002; 60: 822–5.
28. Herr HW. Tumor recurrence and progression after one versus two transurethral resections and BCG therapy (unpublished data).
29. Lee SE, Jeong IG, Ku H, et al. Impact of transurethral resection of bladder tumor: analysis of cystectomy specimens to evaluate for residual tumor. Urology 2004; 63: 873–7.
30. Holmang S, Johansson SL. Stage TA–T1 bladder cancer: the relationship between findings at first followup cystoscopy and subsequent recurrence and progression. J Urol 2002; 167: 1634–7.
31. Herr HW. High-risk superficial bladder cancer: transurethral resection alone in selected patients with T1 tumor. Semin Urol Oncol 1997; 15: 142–7.
32. Lopez-Betran A, Cheng L. Stage pT1 bladder carcinoma: diagnostic criteria, pitfalls and prognostic significance. Pathology 2003; 35: 484–91.
33. Cheng L, Weaver AL, Neumann RM, et al. Substaging of T1 bladder carcinoma based on depth of invasion as measured by micrometer: a new proposal. Cancer 1999; 86: 1035–43.
34. Kondylis FI, Demirci S, Schellhammer PF. Outcomes after intravesical BCG are affected by substaging high grade T1 transitional cell carcinoma. J Urol 2000; 163: 1120–23.

35. Flocks RH. Treatment of patients with carcinoma of the bladder. JAMA 1951; 145: 295–9.

36. Milner WA. The role of conservative surgery in the treatment of bladder tumors. Br J Urol 1954; 26: 375–7.

37. O'Flynn JD, Smith JD, Hanson JS. Transurethral resection for the assessment and treatment of vesical neoplasms. A review of 800 consecutive cases. Eur Urol 1975; 1: 38–41.

38. Barnes RW, Dick AL, Hadley HL. Survival following transurethral resection of bladder carcinoma. Cancer Res 1977; 37: 2895–98.

39. Herr HW. Transurethral resection of muscle-invasive bladder cancer: 10-year outcome. J Clin Oncol 2001; 19: 89–93.

40. Solsona E, Iborra I, Ricos JV, et al. Feasibility of transurethral resection for muscle infiltrating carcinoma of the bladder: long-term followup of a prospective study. J Urol 1998; 159: 95–8.

41. Shipley WU, Prout GR, Kaufman D, et al. Invasive bladder carcinoma: the importance of initial transurethral surgery for improved survival with irradiation. Cancer 1987; 60: 514–19.

42. Kaufman DS, Shipley WU, Griffin PP, et al. Selective bladder preservation by combination treatment of invasive bladder cancer. N Engl J Med 1993; 329: 1377–81.

43. Kachnic LA, Kaufman DS, Griffin PP, et al. Bladder preservation by combined modality therapy for invasive bladder cancer. J Clin Oncol 1997; 15: 1022–5.

44. Zietman AL, Shipley WU, Kaufman DS, et al. A phase I/II trial of transurethral surgery combined with concurrent cisplatin, 5-fluorouracil and twice daily radiation followed by selective bladder preservation in operable patients with muscle invading bladder cancer. J Urol 1998; 160: 1673–7.

45. Michaelson MD, Shipley WU, Heney NM, et al. Selective bladder preservation for muscle-invasive transitional cell carcinoma of the urinary bladder. Br J Cancer 2004; 90: 578–81.

46. Rodel C, Grabenbauer GG, Kuhn R, et al. Combined-modality treatment and selective organ preservation in invasive bladder cancer: long-term results. J Clin Oncol 2002; 20: 3061–71.

47. Grossman HB, Natale RB, Tangen CM, et al. Neoadjuvant chemotherapy plus cystectomy compared with cystectomy alone for locally advanced bladder cancer. N Engl J Med 2003; 349: 859–66.

48. Kuczk M, Machtens S, Jonas U. Surgical bladder preserving strategies in the treatment of muscle-invasive bladder cancer. World J Urol 2002; 20: 183–9.

49. Herr HW, Bajorin DF, Scher HI. Neoadjuvant chemotherapy and bladder-sparing surgery for invasive bladder cancer: ten-year outcome. J Clin Oncol 1998; 16: 1298–301.

50. Sternberg CN, Pansadoro V, Calabro F, et al. Neo-adjuvant chemotherapy and bladder preservation in locally advanced transitional cell carcinoma of the bladder. Ann Oncol 1999; 10: 1269–70.

2

Perioperative instillation of chemotherapeutic drugs

Willem Oosterlinck, Richard J Sylvester

Introduction

History

The instillation of a chemotherapeutic drug immediately after transurethral resection (TUR) is an old idea that was tested in the 1970s,[1,2] when thiotepa was used. Later, adriamycin and epodyl were also evaluated.[3,4] These first nonrandomized clinical trials suggested a reduction in the rate of tumor recurrence when a perioperative instillation was given. After these preliminary results, the need for properly conducted, large scale, randomized controlled studies became evident. The first important study of this kind came from the British Medical Research Council. Four hundred and seventeen patients with newly diagnosed superficial bladder tumors were treated with a complete TUR and then randomized into one of three groups.[5] Groups 1 and 2 received an instillation of 30 mg thiotepa at the time of TUR; thereafter patients in group 2 also received instillations of thiotepa every 3 months for a year, and group 3 was a control group that received no instillations at all. Neither the first publication of the MRC in 1985,[5] nor the second publication of the results in 1994[6] with a longer follow-up was able to show any differences in the recurrence rate in the three groups. However, subsequent randomized studies[7–14] have shown impressive improvements in the recurrence-free rate.

Despite the scientific evidence provided by these trials, a single immediate postoperative instillation has not become routine procedure in the urological world. The European Association of Urology guidelines were the first guidelines that advocated one single immediate instillation after TUR in all patients with superficial bladder tumors.[15] As one single instillation has been tested mainly in low-risk tumors, there was still doubt regarding the value of one immediate instillation in patients with multiple tumors at a higher risk for recurrence. There was also no consensus that all patients with a single, low-risk tumor should receive intravesical chemotherapy after the initial TUR. This was the reason for performing a meta-analysis of the published results of randomized clinical trials with one single immediate postoperative instillation of chemotherapy in patients with stage Ta–T1 bladder cancer.

Meta-Analysis of efficacy

In their meta-analysis, Sylvester et al[16] included seven randomized trials (Table 2.1) with recurrence information on 1476 patients.

After a median follow-up of 3.4 years and a maximum of 14.5 years, 267 of 728 patients (36.7%) receiving one postoperative instillation of epirubicin, mitomycin C, thiotepa, or pirarubicin had recurrences as compared with 362 of 748 patients (48.4%) with TUR alone (odds ratio [OR] = 0.61, p<0.0001). This meta-analysis has thus shown that one immediate instillation of chemotherapy after TUR decreases the relative risk of recurrence by 39% in patients with Ta–T1 bladder cancer (Figure 2.1).

Although the majority of the patients included in these randomized trials had a single tumor, both patients with a single tumor (OR = 0.61) and those with multiple tumors (OR = 0.44) benefited from a single instillation. However, after one instillation, 65.2% of the patients with multiple tumors had a recurrence compared with 35.8% of the patients with a single tumor, showing that one instillation alone is suboptimal treatment in patients with multiple tumors. In a trial excluded from the meta-analysis because some patients received additional instillations before recurrence, Zincke et al also found that patients with multiple tumors benefited from an immediate instillation of thiotepa or adriamycin.[17] Defining risk groups according to whether the tumor was single or multiple, and incorporating the result of the first follow-up cystoscopy, Tolley et al found that the benefit of mitomycin C, in both treatment groups combined, was similar in low-, medium-, and high-risk cases.[8] Other subgroup analyses could not be done in the meta-analysis because of the absence of individual patient data, but the two other studies[9,13] in which they were performed suggest that the treatment is beneficial across all categories of patients.

Working mechanism

The effect of one instillation may be explained either by the chemoresection of tumor left behind after an incomplete TUR or by destruction of circulating tumor cells that could implant at the site of the resection. Incomplete TUR may be an issue even in patients with solitary tumors as shown by the great variability between institutions in the recurrence rates at the first follow-up cystoscopy after TUR.[18] Oosterlinck et al[9] found that only one of the 10 patients that had residual tumors 1 month after TUR was in the group that received one instillation. Masters et al[19] found a 44% complete response rate in a marker lesion 3 months after one instillation of epirubicin. Thus one instillation can in fact eradicate tumor left behind during TUR.

Supporting the hypothesis of implantation of circulating tumor cells,[20] Whelan et al[21] found that postoperative irrigation with saline

Table 2.1 Meta-analysis of randomized trials

First author	Year	Drug	Dosage	Duration (min)	Timing	Study arms	Eligible patients
Oosterlinck[9]	1993	Epirubicin	80 mg/50 ml	60	Within 6 hours	2 arms TUR + water	402
Ali-el-Dein[10]	1997	Epirubicin	50 mg/50 ml	120	Immediately	3 arms TUR alone, + 8 weekly epirubicin + monthly 1 year	181
Rajala[13]	2002	Epirubicin	100 mg/100 ml	120	Immediately	3 arms TUR alone, TUR + interferon-α2b	200
Tolley[8]	1996	Mitomycin C	40 mg/40 ml	60	Within 24 hours	3 arms TUR alone + mitomycin every 3 months, 1 year	452
Solsona[11]	1999	Mitomycin C	30 mg/50 ml	60	Within 6 hours	2 arms TUR alone	131
MRC[5]	1995	Thiotepa	30 mg/50 ml	Unknown	Immediately	3 arms TUR alone + 4 additional instillations	379
Okamura[14]	2002	Pirarubicin	30 mg/30 ml	60	Within 6 hours	2 arms TUR alone	160

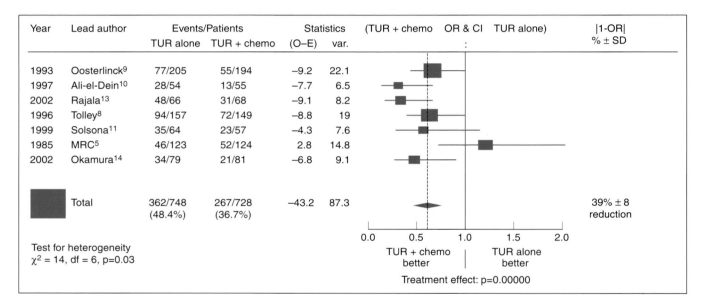

Figure 2.1
Forest plot of the different studies used in the meta-analysis of Sylvester et al[16] on one single postoperative instillation of chemotherapy. (Chemo, chemotherapy; CI, confidence interval; O–E, observed minus expected number of recurrences; OR, odds ratio; SD, standard deviation; TUR, transurethral resection; Var, variation.) Reproduced from Sylvester R, Oosterlinck W, van der Meijden A. A single immediate postoperative instillation of chemotherapy decreases the risk of recurrence in patients with stage Ta T1 bladder cancer: a meta-analysis of published results of randomized clinical trials. Journal of Urology 2004;171:2181–2186, with permission from Lippincott Williams & Wilkins.

or glycine during 18 hours significantly prolonged the time to first recurrence, with a reduction of 17% in the relative risk of recurrence. Several animal experiments also support the hypothesis of tumor implantation at traumatized places in the bladder.[22,23]

Duration of the effect

When reported, Kaplan–Meier time to first recurrence curves showed that the time point at which the treatment benefit starts varied somewhat between the studies: in three studies[9,11,13] there was a reduction in the percentage of patients with residual tumors at 1 month or with recurrence already at 3 months. In one study, the benefit appeared to start at 6 months[14]; however, in the remaining study,[8] the treatment effect appeared to start at 1 year. As suggested

by Solsona et al,[11] the effect of one instillation appears to occur early on, mainly during the first 2 years, with a possible dilution of the treatment effect with longer-term follow-up. Use of the percentage of patients with recurrence, rather than considering the time to first recurrence, may, in fact, underestimate the size of the treatment effect. However, with long-term follow-up, it is clear that the use of one immediate instillation can prevent rather than simply delay recurrences.

Timing of the instillation

In all studies the instillation was given within 24 hours, generally either immediately after TUR or within 6 hours. Kaasinen et al[24] found a doubling in the risk of recurrence if the first of 5-weekly mitomycin C instillations was not given on the same day as the TUR in frequently recurring patients. In two European Organisation for Research and Treatment of Cancer (EORTC) trials,[25] in which patients received nine instillations of epirubicin or mitomycin C over 6 months, starting treatment on the day of TUR was more effective than starting 7–15 days later in patients who did not receive further maintenance after 6 months. In another study,[26] in which patients received 15 instillations of adriamycin or mitomycin C over 1 year, fewer patients randomized to start treatment within 6 hours had recurrence as compared with patients randomized to start treatment after 7–14 days, especially those on the mitomycin C arm. There is thus some evidence that the instillation should be given on the same day as the TUR and not later.

Intravesical drugs

With the possible exception of the one study with thiotepa in which no difference was found,[5,6] the meta-analysis[16] suggests that no large differences in efficacy between the different chemotherapies exist. However, the study by Burnand et al,[1] which used 90 mg thiotepa in 100 ml rather than 30 mg in 50 ml as in the MRC study, found that one instillation of thiotepa significantly reduced the percentage of patients that had recurrence, as did Zincke et al[17] who used 60 mg thiotepa in 60 ml. This suggests that a lower concentration of thiotepa may be responsible for the lack of efficacy. However, the results from these two studies should be interpreted with caution.

The ideal drug or dosage of the other tested drugs cannot be derived from these studies. Epirubicin in concentrations from 1 to 2 mg/ml has been used with no obvious differences in the results. The same is observed for mitomycin C where concentrations between 0.6 and 1.0 mg/ml have been tested. Experts advise 40 mg over lower dosages because the concentration of the product is less influenced at a higher dose by the urine production which continues during bladder instillation. For epirubicin, 50 mg is considered to be sufficient, as higher doses have failed to show a better outcome in the perioperative setting as well as in other clinical trial designs with this drug.

Cost effectiveness

One can expect that this early instillation gives protection against recurrence, especially in the first year, with a diminishing effect thereafter. Evaluating the first recurrence, 11.7 TURs were saved for every 100 patients treated. Thus the number needed to treat (NNT) to prevent one recurrence is 1/0.117 = 8.5. Since the cost of a TUR, anesthesia, and hospitalization is probably more than 8.5 times that of one instillation in most countries, one instillation should be cost effective.

Toxicity

Despite the fact that no serious adverse effects have been mentioned in the reports published on immediate, adjuvant chemotherapy instillations, several reports have appeared on severe and prolonged complications due to leakage of the drug after an early intravesical instillation. Doherty at al[27] reported the local effects of an immediate instillation of chemotherapy (mainly epirubicin) in cystectomy specimens. It was associated with a more extensive necrosis of the bladder wall and fat necrosis of extravesical tissue than the usual muscle necrosis seen after TUR alone. An area of thin muscularis propria may undergo necrosis and result in secondary perforation. None of the 12 patients described by Doherty, however, reported local symptoms. In contrast, the effect of extravasation after intravenously administered chemotherapeutic drugs is well documented. It induces long-lasting necrosis, provoking pain and slowing the healing process. In 2003, a case of severe and long-lasting pain in the pelvic region due to extravasation of mitomycin C was reported.[28] A distal ureteral stenosis that was probably due to intravesical mitomycin C has also been described.[29,30] Undoubtedly, there is certainly an under-reporting of these complications as not every urologist that has seen such a complication is eager to report it. In any event, urologists should be aware of the potential risk of extravasation of chemotherapeutic drugs and its consequences.

Bacillus Calmette–Guérin (BCG) must *never* be used in the perioperative setting as the open wounds of the mucosa can provoke BCG septicemia, and for this reason it has never been tested in these circumstances.

Precautions

If there is a possibility of perforation or after an extended TUR, an immediate instillation should not be given. In cases where there is the possibility of intraperitoneal leakage or important resorption from the extravesical space, it seems advisable not to use a dose greater than the dose that is acceptable as one single intravenous injection. Indeed, one case of myelosuppression has been described when 80 mg of mitomycin C was retained for 2 hours after TUR of a large tumor.[31] It seems prudent to advise a 1-hour retention time and to rinse the bladder actively to ascertain a good free flow of the urine afterwards, and to avoid any overdistension during or immediately after the chemotherapy instillation. Nevertheless, it is clear from the review of the literature that one immediate instillation after TUR is an adjuvant treatment that adds hardly any morbidity to the operation itself. Nearly all patients already have a catheter after TUR and, if local regional anesthesia is used, patients will not suffer from any additional discomfort. The reluctance to use this treatment strategy should be reconsidered since the potential benefits clearly outweigh the possible risks and costs.

Conclusive recommendations on perioperative instillations

- One instillation with mitomycin C or epirubicin can reduce the recurrence rate by about 40% in single as well as in multiple Ta–T1 bladder tumors, and is thus recommended for all types of papillary superficial bladder cancer. It is *not* indicated in invasive tumors.
- Doses of 40 mg mitomycin C and 50 mg epirubicin are advocated. Higher doses increase the risk of side effects and cost without increasing efficacy.
- After an extensive resection, and in cases of obvious or suspected perforation of the bladder, it is prudent not to instill the bladder as extravasation can provoke annoying and even dangerous complications (expert opinion, a few case reports).

- It is advocated to give the instillation the same day as the TUR as it is probably insufficient the day afterwards.
- Further adjuvant intravesical therapy is indicated in multiple tumors, as one single instillation is insufficient treatment in these patients.

References

1. Burnand K, Boyd P, Mayo M, Shuttleworth K, Lloyd-Davies R. Single dose intravesical thiotepa as an adjuvant to cystodiathermy in the treatment of transitional cell bladder carcinoma. Br J Urol 1976; 48: 55–59.
2. Garrett J, Lewis R, Meehan W, Leblanc G. Intravesical thiotepa in the immediate post-operative period in patients with recurrent transitional cell carcinoma of the bladder. J Urol 1978; 120: 410–11.
3. Abrams P, Choa R, Gaches C, Ashken M, Green N. A controlled trial of single dose intravesical adriamycin in superficial bladder tumours. Br J Urol 1981; 53: 585–87.
4. Kurth K, Maksimovic P, Hop W, Schroder F, Bakker N. Single dose intravesical epodyl after TUR of Ta TCC bladder carcinoma. World J Urol 1983; 1: 89.
5. MRC Working Party on Urological Cancer. The effect of intravesical thiotepa on the recurrence rate of newly diagnosed superficial bladder cancer. An MRC Study. Br J Urol 1985; 57: 680–85.
6. Medical Research Council Working Party on Urological Cancer, Subgroup on Superficial Bladder Cancer. The effect of intravesical thiotepa on tumor recurrence after endoscopic treatment of newly diagnosed superficial bladder cancer. A further report with long-term follow-up of a Medical Research Council randomized trial. Br J Urol 1994; 73: 632–38.
7. Tolley D, Hargreave T, Smith P, et al. Effect of intravesical mitomycin C on recurrence of newly diagnosed superficial bladder cancer: interim report from the Medical Research Council Subgroup on Superficial Bladder Cancer (Urological Cancer Working Party). Br Med J 1988; 296: 1759–61.
8. Tolley D, Parmar M, Grigor K, Lallemand G, and the Medical Research Council Superficial Bladder Cancer Working Party. The effect of intravesical mitomycin C on recurrence of newly diagnosed superficial bladder cancer: a further report with 7 years of follow-up, J Urol 1996; 155: 1233–38.
9. Oosterlinck W, Kurth K, Schröder F, Bultinck J, Hammond B, Sylvester R. A prospective European Organisation for Research and Treatment of Cancer Genitourinary Group randomized trial comparing transurethral resection followed by a single intravesical instillation of epirubicin or water in single stage Ta, T1 papillary carcinoma of the bladder. J Urol 1993; 149: 749–52.
10. Ali-el-Dein B, Nabeeh A, el-Baz M, Shamaa S, Ashamallah A. Single dose versus multiple instillations of epirubicin as prophylaxis for recurrence after transurethral resection of pTa and pT1 transitional cell bladder tumors: a prospective randomized controlled study. Br J Urol 1997; 79: 731–35.
11. Solsona E, Iborra I, Ricos J, Monros J, Casanova J, Dumont R. Effectiveness of a single immediate mitomycin C instillation in patients with low risk superficial bladder cancer: short and long-term follow-up. J Urol 1999; 161: 1120–23.
12. Rajala P, Liukkonen T, Raitanen M, et al. Transurethral resection with perioperative instillation of interferon-alpha or epirubicin for the prophylaxis of recurrent primary superficial bladder cancer: a prospective randomized multicenter study—FinnBladder III. J Urol 1999; 161: 1133–35; discussion 1135–36.
13. Rajala P, Kaasinen E, Raitanen M, Liukkonen T, Rintala E, the FinnBladder Group. Perioperative single dose instillation of epirubicin or interferon-alpha after transurethral resection for the prophylaxis of primary superficial bladder cancer recurrence: a prospective randomized multicenter study—FinnBladder III long-term results. J Urol 2002; 168: 981–85.
14. Okamura K, Ono Y, Kinukawa T, et al. Randomized study of single early instillation of (2″R)-4′-O-tetrahydropyranyl-doxorubicin for a single superficial bladder carcinoma. Cancer 2002;94:2363–2368.
15. Oosterlinck W, Lobel B, Jakse G, Malmstrom P, Stockle M, Sternberg C. The EAU Working Group on Oncological Urology. Guidelines on bladder cancer. Eur Urol 2002; 41: 105–12.
16. Sylvester R, Oosterlinck W, van der Meijden A. A single immediate postoperative instillation of chemotherapy decreases the risk of recurrence in patients with stage Ta T1 bladder cancer: a meta-analysis of published results of randomized clinical trials. J Urol 2004; 171: 2181–186.
17. Zincke H, Utz D, Taylor W, Myers R, Leary F. Influence of thiotepa and doxorubicin instillation at time of transurethral surgical treatment of bladder cancer on tumor recurrence: a prospective, randomized, double-blind, controlled trial. J Urol 1983; 129: 505–09.
18. Brausi M, Collette L, Kurth K, et al. Variability in the recurrence rate at first follow-up cystoscopy after TUR in stage Ta T1 transitional cell carcinoma of the bladder: a combined analysis of seven EORTC studies. Eur Urol 2002; 41: 523–31.
19. Masters J, Popert M, Thompson P, Gibson D, Coptcoat M, Parmar M. Intravesical chemotherapy with epirubicin: a dose–response study. J Urol 1999; 161: 1490–93.
20. Soloway M, Masters S. Urothelial susceptibility to tumor cell implantation: influence of cauterization. Cancer 1980; 46: 1158–63.
21. Whelan P, Griffiths G, Stower M, et al. Preliminary results of a MRC randomised controlled trial of post-operative irrigation of superficial bladder cancer. Proceedings of the American Society of Clinical Oncology 2001; 20: Abstract 708.
22. Weldon T, Soloway M. Susceptibility of urothelium to neoplastic cellular implantation. Urology 1975; 5: 824–26.
23. Pan J, Slocum H, Rustum Y, Greco W, Gaeta J, Huben R. Inhibition of implantation of murine bladder tumor by thiotepa in cauterized bladder. J Urol 1989; 142: 1589–93.
24. Kaasinen E, Rintala E, Hellstrom P, et al. Factors explaining recurrence in patients undergoing chemoimmunotherapy regimens for frequently recurring superficial bladder carcinoma. Eur Urol 2002; 42: 167–74.
25. Bouffioux C, Kurth K, Bono A, et al. Intravesical adjuvant chemotherapy for superficial transitional cell bladder carcinoma: results of 2 European Organisation for Research and Treatment of Cancer randomized trials with mitomycin C and doxorubicin comparing early versus delayed instillations and short-term versus long-term treatment. J Urol 1995; 153: 934–41.
26. Iborra J, Ricos J, Monros J, et al. Resultados de un estudio de quimio-profilaxis intravesical, prospectivo, doble aleatorio, entre dos drogas: la adriamicina y el mitomycin; y dos modos de iniciar las instilaciones: precoz y tardio. Efecto sobre la recidiva y la progression, Arch Esp de Urol 1992; 45: 1001.
27. Doherty A, Trendell Smith N, Stirling R, Rogers H, Bellringer J. Perivesical fat necrosis after adjuvant intravesical chemotherapy. BJU Int 1999; 83: 420–23.
28. Nieuwenhuijzen J, Bex A, Horenblas S. Unusual complication after immediate postoperative intravesical mitomycin C instillation. Eur Urol 2003; 43: 711–12.
29. Oehlschlager S, Loessnitzer A, Froehner M, et al. Distal urethral stenosis after early adjuvant intravesical mitomycin C application for superficial bladder cancer. J Urol Int 2003; 70: 74–76.
30. Oddens J, van der Meyden A, Sylvester R. One immediate postoperative instillation of chemotherapy in low risk Ta, T1 bladder cancer patients. Is it always safe? Eur Urol 2004; 46: 336–38.
31. Tawkif A, Neal F, Hong K. Bone marrow suppression after intravesical mitomycin C treatment. J Urol 1986; 13: 459–60.

3

The role of intravesical chemotherapy in the treatment of bladder cancer

S Bruce Malkowicz

Introduction

Intravesical chemotherapy has been a classic approach to the treatment of nonmuscle-invasive superficial bladder cancer for several decades. Early investigations confirmed the impression that recurrence rates were decreased by this method of therapy, yet aggregate data from many trials were necessary in order to better quantitate this effect and evaluate the potential of such treatment to affect tumor progression. Although multiple agents have been employed over time, there has been a general collapse of the treatment menu over the past several years with the introduction of bacillus Calmette–Guérin (BCG) therapy. During this time, efforts to decrease tumor recurrence in an optimal fashion using immediate postoperative instillation of these agents have been validated, and further techniques to optimize administration and drug delivery have been under development. As our understanding of the appropriate role for intravesical chemotherapy has emerged, newer agents, which have demonstrated activity in advanced disease, are being tested for their applicability in this area.

Principles of practice

The theoretical goals of intravesical chemotherapy are threefold: 1) the eradication of residual disease; 2) prophylaxis against tumor recurrence; and 3) the delay or abrogation of tumor progression. The eradication of residual disease is a desirable attribute of an intravesical agent. Recent studies evaluating small marker tumors demonstrate this attribute in principle, yet larger volume and higher stage disease is less susceptible to drug mechanisms of action. Intravesical chemotherapy is not particularly suitable to the treatment of unresected disease.[1]

The goal of reducing tumor recurrence with intravesical chemotherapy has been documented by multiple, well-conducted clinical trials and several meta-analyses. Short-term impact is demonstrated as a 14% to 17% decrease in tumor recurrence, yet over 3–5 years this reduced to approximately 7%.[2,3] The instillation of chemotherapeutic agents shortly after transurethral resection may be the most effective method of capitalizing on the prophylactic effect. Several studies and a recent meta-analysis suggest an up to 37% decrease in tumor recurrence with this practice.[4] This topic is discussed in the previous chapter.

The value of maintenance therapy with chemotherapeutic agents is negligible. Although some impact on early recurrence may be suggested in some studies, a long-term impact is not demonstrated, especially in carcinoma in situ or larger lesions.[5,6]

The impact of intravesical chemotherapy on tumor progression can unfortunately be stated rather tersely—the current available data demonstrate no advantage with regard to tumor progression survival with the use of this modality.[3] In an evaluation of six large European trials, involving a total of 2535 patients with a median survival follow-up of 7.8 years, no long-term effect of prophylactic therapy was noted.

Pharmacologic considerations

The principal aspect of intravesical chemotherapy is the physical diffusion of the agent into the layers of the bladder. The efficiency of this process is affected by many attributes of the bladder wall, the urine environment, and the nature of the agent. Chemotherapeutic agents must first cross the glycosaminoglycan layer of bladder mucosa and then diffuse through the urothelial cells. Once the amina propria is reached and then the muscularis propria, there is rich vascularity which results in a decline in drug concentration in a semilogarithmic fashion.[7]

Urine volume affects drug concentration, which has an influence on the diffusion factors mentioned above. Drug concentration can be manipulated by controlling the state of dehydration. Additionally, the chemical nature of these agents can affect their ability to attain maximal contact with a lesion such as the lipophilic properties or overall molecular weight of the agent.

General agents

Mitomycin C

Mitomycin C (MMC) is an alkylating agent which, through crosslinking, inhibits DNA synthesis. It is felt to be cell cycle non-specific, although it is most sensitive in the late G1 phase. It has a molecular weight of 334 kD and has negligible systemic absorption. The average benefit in decreasing tumor recurrence in the prophylactic setting is approximately 15%.[2] There are no data to indicate that it has any impact on tumor progression over a 5-year period.[3] It has been used over a wide range of doses, and an attempt at optimization of therapy is described below.

The most frequent side effects of MMC include palmar rash or other cutaneous symptoms in up to 10% of patients, and chemical cystitis in up to 40% of patients. Myelosuppression occurs in less than 0.5% of patients and bladder contracture is rare. Most symptoms abate with the cessation of drug use.

Mitomycin therapy has emerged as a standard agent in intravesical therapy because of its equivalent effect in tumor prophylaxis and its slightly increased activity in patients treated with BCG. Efforts to increase its clinical effectiveness have been evaluated by an attempt to optimize conditions of drug stability and drug concentration.[8] An optimization protocol by the international mitomycin C consortium restricted patients from fluid intake for 8 hours prior to and during treatment. They also received 1.3 g sodium bicarbonate the evening before, morning of, and 30 minutes prior to drug administration. The bladder was drained before drug administration and then evaluated with transabdominal ultrasound in order to reduce residual urine to ≤10 cc. It was demonstrated that bladder emptying by catheter was not uniformly efficient for all patients. The dwell time was 2 hours.

Optimized patients (119) were treated with 40 mg mitomycin diluted in 20 cc, while standard therapy patients (111) received 20 mg mitomycin diluted in 20 cc, thereby doubling the concentration in the optimized arm (Figure 3.1). Dysuria occurred more frequently in the optimization group but did not lead to a greater number of treatment discontinuations. There was an increased median time to recurrence of 29.1 months (95% CI: 14–44 months) versus 11.8 months (95% CI: 7.2–16 months), p=0.005, as well as a greater percentage of recurrence-free patients: 41% (95% CI: 30.9−51.1%) versus 24.6% (95% CI: 14.9−34.3%), p=0.002 in the optimization arm. While it is not possible to say if the optimization of a single variable (drug dose) might be sufficient to lead to overall optimization of outcomes, such a protocol demonstrates an attempt to achieve the best results possible with intravesical chemotherapeutic agents. More elaborate methods to increase drug effectiveness will be discussed later.

Doxorubicin

Doxorubicin is an anthracycline antibiotic that binds DNA base pairs and inhibits topoisomerase II as well as protein synthesis. It has a high molecular weight (580 kD) and virtually no systemic

absorption. Chemical cystitis can occur in 25% to 50% of patients, and less common side effects include gastrointestinal reactions, allergic reactions, and reduced bladder capacity.[9] Multiple studies demonstrate prophylaxis in reducing the recurrence probability by 15% but no impact on progression.[2,10] The usual dosage is 30–100 mg given weekly for several weeks.

Epirubicin

Epirubicin is an anthracycline derivative of doxorubicin with a similar mechanism of action. It has a molecular weight of 579.8 kD, and has been administered in different treatment schedules at a dosage of 30–80 mg. The advantage over transurethral resection (TUR) alone for tumor prophylaxis is in the expected range of 12% to 15%.[11] It is effective as a single dose agent immediately after TUR and may be more effective with a higher cumulative dose.[12,13] It can be effective in intermediate risk patients.[14] There are few systemic side effects (<5% in most series), and chemical cystitis, which is dose dependent, occurs in approximately 15% of patients.

Valrubicin

Valrubicin is a semisynthetic analog of doxorubicin. It has a rapid uptake in cancer cells due to its lipophilic structure. This agent inhibits topoisomerase II and causes cell-cycle arrest in G2. The general dosage is 800 mg, and, in a mixed population of superficial lesions, a 40% initial response rate was noted.[15] In a population of BCG-refractory patients, a 21% response rate was noted with a median time to recurrence greater than 18 months.[16] This agent is currently approved for those patients that are BCG refractory and cannot tolerate a cystectomy.

Thiotepa (triethylene thiophosphoramide)

Thiotepa is the classic intravesical agent, which acts as an alkylating agent and is not cell cycle specific. In multiple trials it has

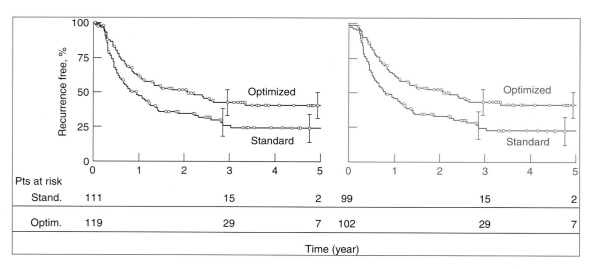

Figure 3.1
Kaplan–Meier curves of (*left*) intent-to-treat and (*right*) evaluable groups for those patients treated with an optimized or standard course of mitomycin C. At 5 years, approximately 43% of optimized patients and 24% of standard patients were recurrence free in either analysis. Reproduced with permission from Au et al.[8]

demonstrated its effectiveness for tumor prophylaxis (mean decrease over TUR, 16%) and no capacity to affect progression. It has a molecular weight of 189 kD. Because of its low molecular weight it clearly demonstrates a significant level of systemic absorption, which can result in hematologic side effects. Therefore, weekly monitoring of the complete blood count and platelet count is necessary during a treatment course. Local irritation can occur in 12% to 69% of patients. Thrombocytopenia is seen in 3% to 13% of patients and leukopenia in 8% to 55% of patients. The usual dose is 30 mg in 15 ml of sterile water.

Gemcitabine

Gemcitabine is a novel deoxycytidine analog (2′,2′-difluoro-2′deoxycytidine), which has demonstrated significant activity in advanced bladder cancer as a single agent and in combination.[17] It has a molecular weight of 299.66 kD, and its active metabolite is incorporated into DNA, thus inhibiting synthesis. It may also inhibit cytidine deaminase and ribonucleotide reductase as a component of its anticancer mechanism. Preclinical studies have suggested its value for intravesical therapy, and several phase I and phase II studies suggest its safety and general efficacy.[18–21]

Preclinical studies demonstrated no systemic absorption, immunosuppression, or histologic damage to normal urothelium.[22] In a phase I study of patients with low-grade, low-stage disease, a dose range of 1000–2000 mg gemcitabine demonstrated low or absent systemic absorption and the presence of the inactive metabolite difluorodeoxyuridine in very low levels as well, suggesting minimal accumulation of drug in the systemic circulation. Dysuria, headache, and fatigue were reported, but there was no dose-limiting toxicity (DLT).[22] Fifty percent of patients experienced no recurrences over a short period of follow-up (12 months). A similar lack of DLT at 2000 mg was noted in another phase I trial.

In a cohort of BCG-refractory patients, gemcitabine was administered twice weekly from 500 to 2000 mg. Of 18 patients, 7 had a complete response, 4 patients had a mixed response (persistent positive cytology), 3 patients demonstrated a skin reaction, and 1 patient had grade 3 thrombocytopenia and neutropenia without infection or DLT at 2000 mg.[20] In another phase I trial of 15 patients treated with between 500 and 2000 mg, gemcitabine was undetectable in the plasma of patients until the 2000 mg dose level, and then it was present (≤1 mcg/ml) only transiently.

Plasma difluorodeoxyuridine (dFdU) levels implied absorption of 0.5% to 5.5% of the instilled dose. At 12 weeks, 9 of 13 evaluable patients were recurrence-free.[21] These studies have suggested that gemcitabine at 40 mg/ml (2000 mg in 50 ml saline solution) weekly for 6 weeks is a reasonable dose for further phase II testing.

In one phase II study of 39 superficial disease patients (30 previously treated with intravesical therapy), 56% of patients demonstrated a complete response to a marker tumor, and no progression was noted among the nonresponders.[23] The majority of toxicity was grade I with dysuria as the most common finding (33% grade I, 5% grade II). Grade I hematologic complications were noted in 5% to 15% of patients.

The clinical evaluation of gemcitabine as an intravesical agent is ongoing in other phase II and phase III trials, and the above data suggest the validity of these endeavors. It remains to be seen if this agent provides any clinical advantage over the already available agents with respect to prophylaxis or tumor progression in general patients or in the refractory/salvage situation.

The molecular weight, dosage, mechanism of action, and side effects of these intravesical chemotherapy agents are summarized in Table 3.1.

Other agents

Additional agents studied in superficial bladder cancer include mitoxantrone, suramin, and paclitaxel.

Mitoxantrone

Mitoxantrone is an anthracycline derivative similar to doxorubicin. It has been studied in several small trials at doses of 10–20 mg where its tolerability has been demonstrated.[24–26] In comparison to doxorubicin, there was no difference in general efficacy or time to recurrence.[27] It has had limited evaluation in the United States.

Suramin

Suramin is a polysulfonated naphthylurea that inhibits DNA synthesis by various mechanisms, including growth factor inhibition. It is a very large molecule with minimal systemic absorption, and in phase I trials has been used in doses of up to 153 mg/ml with

Table 3.1 Intravesical chemotherapy agents

Agent	Molecular weight(kD)	Dosage	Mechanism of action	Side effects
Thiotepa	189	30 mg	Alkylating agent, cell cycle nonspecific	Thrombocytopenia, leukopenia, chemical cystitis
Mitomycin C	334	20–40 mg	Alkylating agent, cell cycle nonspecific	Palmar rash, contact dermatitis, chemical cystitis
Doxorubicin	580	30–100 mg	DNA base pair binding, topoisomerase II inhibition, protein synthesis inhibition	Chemical cystitis
Valrubicin	585	800 mg	Similar to doxorubicin but more lipophilic	Chemical cystitis
Epirubicin	579	30–80 mg	Doxycycline derivative	Chemical cystitis
Gemcitabine	299.6	2000 mg	Deoxycytidine analog, inhibits DNA synthesis, inhibits cytidine deaminase	Chemical cystitis

minimal side effects.[28,29] Recent in vivo studies suggest that this agent in low doses may act as a chemosensitizer for mitomycin C.[30]

Paclitaxel

At present, taxanes are in early study for their potential use in superficial bladder cancer based on their activity in combination chemotherapy for advanced disease.[31]

Improved drug delivery

Just as attempts to improve drug activity by avoiding dilution and increasing dwell time may have positive effects on overall outcomes, other techniques to augment drug delivery may allow for optimal outcomes with intravesical therapy for bladder cancer. Significant efforts are underway at this time to evaluate combined hyperthermia and chemotherapy, as well as studies to increase drug penetration with electromotive administration (EMDA).

The ability to enhance drug delivery to bladder tissue by the means of electric current has been demonstrated in vitro,[32,33] and tested clinically by several investigators.[32–35] Electromotive administration employs iontophoresis and electrophoresis to improve transportation of the principal agent to the tissue. In this case the sodium chloride solute provides positive sodium ions, which are iontophoresed toward the tissue. Additionally, hydration shells containing the neutral MMC molecules are electrophorized, leading to a net accumulation of drug in the tissue. Phase II data (n=27) employing MMC demonstrated a similar marker tumor response rate (40%), and a longer disease-free interval (14.5 months versus 10 months) in those patients treated with EMDA.[34] The recurrence rate in those treated with EMDA was also lower (33% versus 66% without EMDA). In a recent study of 108 patients, those with multifocal carcinoma in situ, including 98 with T1 lesions, were randomized into groups receiving passive MMC, electromotive MMC, or BCG weekly for 6 weeks with a maintenance schedule.[33] The complete response rate at 3 months was 56% for BCG, 53% for electromotive MMC, and 28% for passive MMC. At 6 months the complete response rate for these three groups was 64%, 58%, and 31%, respectively. The median time to recurrence was 26 months for BCG, 35 months for electromotive MMC, and 19.5 months for passive MMC. With regard to kinetics, the peak plasma level was higher in the electromotive MMC (43 versus 8 ng/ml), and modeling demonstrated that approximately 50% of the dose was absorbed passively at 60 minutes, whereas with EMDA, more than 80% was absorbed by 30 minutes. No statistical difference was noted in toxicity between the MMC arms, yet there was a trend toward increased numbers and severity in the EMDA arm.

Another approach to enhance intravesical chemotherapy administration is the use of thermochemotherapy in which an endocavitary microwave applicator with thermocouples delivers hyperthermia (42.5°C) to the bladder wall, as the intravesical agent is in the bladder. The feasibility of such a system has been demonstrated, and early studies confirmed a significantly improved immediate response rate with this technology.[35] Pharmacokinetic studies demonstrate an increased yet safe plasma concentration of MMC with this technology.[36]

Clinical studies have shown that prophylaxis with MMC and microwave thermotherapy in Ta and T1 patients was superior to MMC alone at 24 months of follow-up.[37] All patients underwent a complete TUR, and approximately 40% of the patients in each group had received prior intravesical therapy. Eight weekly treatments and four monthly maintenance treatments were scheduled. Six (17.1%) versus 23 (57.5%) recurrences were noted among 75 of 83 patients divided into each treatment group (p= 0.002), hazard ratio 4.82 (95% CI: 1.95–11.9). In this study, 20 mg MMC was administered in 50 cc saline. In the passive arm, dwell time was 1 hour, whereas in the thermotherapy arm the instillation was for at least 40 minutes with the solution changed at 3 minutes.

Side effects were more common in the thermotherapy arm, with pelvic pain and posterior wall thermal reaction as the major differences. No patients terminated treatment because of pain. Additionally, one case of reduced bladder capacity with urge incontinence was noted in the thermotherapy group. While this study did not compare optimal MMC therapy to thermo-intravesical therapy, a clear improvement in prophylactic parameters was noted in the thermotherapy arm compared to the intravesical arm treated under similar parameters.

In another study of 52 patients with predominantly higher stage (40 T1) lesions, in an ablative protocol 21 of 28 patients had a complete response (CR). Four of these CR patients (19%) recurred during follow-up. At 15 months no stage progression to T2 was encountered in the entire cohort.[38] In a further study of higher risk superficial patients (n=90), no progression in stage or grade was noted at 24 months, and at 1 and 2 years the recurrence rate was 14.3% and 24.6%, respectively.[39] Smaller studies demonstrate similar results.[40]

Other methods investigated for improving drug delivery include the use of agents to increase bladder wall permeability such as hyaluronidase and dimethylsulfoxide (DMSO).[41,42] More recently, magnetically targeted carriers have been studied for their ability to effect local targeting of chemotherapy to specific bladder locations.[43]

Combination chemotherapy

Although combination chemotherapy is regularly employed in the treatment of advanced transitional cell carcinoma, there is relatively scant literature regarding its use in the treatment of nonmuscle-invasive cancer. The rationale for novel combinations such as gemcitabine and doxorubicin are being studied in vitro.[44] In one study looking at a successive schedule of mitomycin (day 1) and doxorubicin (day 2) given weekly for 6 weeks, the initial complete response rate was 50%, and those patients on maintenance therapy had fewer recurrences in the short term.[45] Other studies demonstrate similar good initial responses but with an increase in local side effects.[46,47]

References

1. Bono AV, Hall RR, Denis JA, et al. Chemoresection in Ta–T1 bladder cancer. Members of the EORTC Genito-urinary group. Euro Urol 1996; 29: 35–9.
2. Lamm DL, Riggs DR, Traynelis CL, et al. Apparent failure of current intravesical chemotherapy prophylaxis to influence the long-term course of superficial transitional cell carcinoma of the bladder. J Urol 1995; 153: 1444–50.
3. Pawinski A, Sylvester R, Kurth KH, et al. A combined analysis of European Organization for Research and Treatment of Cancer and Medical Research Council randomized clinical trials for the prophylactic treatment of stage TaT1 bladder cancer. J Urol 1996; 156: 1934–41.

4. Sylvester RJ, Oosterlinck W, van der Meljden APM. A single immediate postoperative instillation of chemotherapy decreases the risk of recurrence in patients with stage Ta T1 bladder cancer: a meta-analysis of published results of randomized clinical trials. J Urol 2004; 171: 2186–90.

5. Bouffioux C, Kurth KH, Bono A, et al. Intravesical adjuvant chemotherapy for superficial transitional cell bladder carcinoma: results of 2 EORTC randomized trials with MMC and doxorubicin comparing early versus delayed instillations and short-term versus long-term treatment. J Urol 1995; 153: 934–41.

6. Hamdy FC, Hastie KJ, Kerry R, Williams JL. Mitomycin-C in superficial bladder cancer. Is long-term maintenance therapy worthwhile after initial treatment? Br J Urol 1993; 71: 183–6.

7. Dedrick RL, Flessier MF, Collin JM, Schultz D. Is the peritoneum a membrane? ASAIO J 1982; 5: 1–8.

8. Au L-S J, Badalament RA, Wientjes MG, Young DC, Warner JA. Methods to improve efficacy of intravesical Mitomycin C: results of a randomized phase III trial. J Natl Cancer Inst 2001; 93(8): 597–604.

9. Thrasher JV, Crawford ED. Complications of intravesical chemotherapy. Urol Clin North Am 1992; 9: 529–36.

10. Lamm DL, Blumenstein BA, Crawford ED, et al. A randomized trial of intravesical doxorubicin and immunotherapy with bacille Calmette–Guérin for transitional cell carcinoma of the bladder. N Engl J Med 1991; 325: 1205–9.

11. Onrust SV, Wiseman LR, Goa KL. Epirubicin: a review of its intravesical use in superficial bladder cancer. Drugs Aging 1999; 15(4): 307–33.

12. Rajala P, Kaasinen E, Raitanen M, et al. Perioperative single dose instillation of epirubicin or interferon-alpha after transurethral resection for the prophylaxis of primary superficial bladder cancer recurrence: a prospective randomized multicenter study—FinnBladder III long-term results. J Urol 2002; 168(3): 981–5.

13. Mitsumori K, Tsuchiya N, Habuchi T, et al. Early and large-dose intravesical instillation of epirubicin to prevent superficial bladder carcinoma recurrence after transurethral resection. BJU Int 2004; 94(3): 317–21.

14. Bassi P, Soinadin R, Longo F, et al. Delayed high-dose intravesical epirubicin therapy of superficial bladder cancer. A way to reduce the side effects and increase the efficacy—a phase 2 trial. Urol Int 2002; 68(4): 216–19.

15. Greenberg RE, Bahnson RR, Wood D, et al. Initial report on intravesical administration of N-triflouracetyladriamycin-14-valerate (AD-32) to patients with refractory superficial transitional cell carcinoma of the urinary bladder. Urology 1997; 49: 471–5.

16. Steinberg G, Bahnson R, Brosman S, et al. Efficacy and safety of valrubicin for the treatment of BCG refractory CIS of the bladder. J Urol 2000; 163: 761–7.

17. Von der Masse H, Hansen SE, Roberts JT, et al. Gemcitabine and cisplatin versus methotrexate, vinblastine, doxorubicin, and cisplatin in advanced or metastatic bladder cancer: results of a large randomized, multinational, multicenter, phase III study. J Clin Oncol 2000; 19: 2638–46.

18. Nativ O, Dalal E, Laufer M, Sabo E, Aronson M. Antineoplastic effect of gemcitabine in an animal model of superficial bladder cancer. Urology 2004; 64(4): 845–8.

19. Cozzi PJ, Bajorin DF, Tong W, et al. Toxicology and pharmacokinetics of intravesical gemcitabine: a preclinical study in dogs. Clin Cancer Res 1999; (9): 2629–37.

20. Dalbagni G, Russo P, Sheinfeld J, et al. Phase I trial of intravesical gemcitabine in bacillus Calmette–Guérin-refractory transitional-cell carcinoma of the bladder. J Clin Oncol 2002; 20(15): 3193–8.

21. Laufer M, Ramalingam S, Schoenberg MP, et al. Intravesical gemcitabine therapy for superficial transitional cell carcinoma of the bladder: a phase I and pharmacokinetic study. J Clin Oncol 2003; 21(4): 697–703.

22. Witjes JA, van der Heijen AG, Vriesema JL, et al. Intravesical gemcitabine: a phase I and pharmacokinetic study. Eur Urol 2004; 45(2): 182–6.

23. Gontero P, Casetta G, Maso G, et al. Phase II study to investigate the ablative efficacy of intravesical administration of gemcitabine in intermediate-risk superficial bladder cancer (SBC). Eur Urol 2004; 46(3): 339–43.

24. Flamm J, Donner G, Oberltleitner S, Hausmann R, Havelec L. Adjuvant intravesical mitoxantrone after transurethral resection of primary superficial transitional cell carcinoma of the bladder. A prospective randomised study. Eur J Cancer 1995; 31A(2): 143–6.

25. Namasivayam S, Whelan P. Intravesical mitozantrone in recurrent superficial bladder cancer: a phase II study. Br J Urol 1995; 75(6): 740–3.

26. Yaman LS, Yardakul T, Zissis NP, Arikan N, Yasar B. Intravesical mitoxantrone for superficial bladder tumors. Anticancer Drugs 1994; 5(1): 95–8.

27. Huang JS, Chen WH, Lin CC, et al. A randomized trial comparing intravesical instillations of mitoxantrone and doxorubicin in patients with superficial bladder cancer. Chang Gung Med J 2003; 26(2): 91–7.

28. Ord JJ, Streeter E, Nones A, et al. Phase I trial of intravesical suramin in recurrent superficial transitional cell bladder carcinoma. Br J Cancer 2005; 92(12): 2140–7.

29. Uchio EM, Linehan WM, Figg WD, Walther MM. A phase I study of intravesical suramin for the treatment of superficial transitional cell carcinoma of the bladder. J Urol 2003; 169(1): 357–60.

30. Xin Y, Lyness G, Chen D, et al. Low dose suramin as a chemosensitizer of bladder cancer to mitomycin C. J Urol 2005; 174(1): 322–7.

31. Vaughn DJ, Malkowicz SB, Zoltick B, et al. Paclitaxel plus carboplatin in advanced carcinoma of the urothelium: an active and tolerable outpatient regimen. J Clin Oncol 1998; 16: 255–60.

32. Di Stasi SM, Vespasiani G, Giannantoni A, et al. Electromotive delivery of mitomycin C into human bladder wall. Cancer Res 1997; 57(5): 875–80.

33. Di Stasi SM, Giannantoni A, Stephen RL, et al. Intravesical electromotive mitomycin C versus passive transport mitomycin C for high risk superficial bladder cancer: a prospective randomized study. J Urol 2003; 170: 777–82.

34. Brausi M, Campo B, Pizzocaro G, et al. Intravesical electromotive administration of drugs for treatment of superficial bladder cancer: a comparative phase II study. Urology 1998; 1(3): 506–9.

35. Colombo R, Brausi M, Da Pozzo LF, et al. Thermo-chemotherapy and electromotive drug administration of mitomycin C in superficial bladder cancer eradication. Eur Urol 2001; 39: 95–100.

36. Paroni R, Salonia A, Lev A, et al. Effect of local hyperthermia of the bladder on mitomycin C pharmacokinetics during intravesical chemotherapy for the treatment of superficial transitional cell carcinoma. Br J Clin Pharmacol 2001; 52: 273–8.

37. Colombo R, Da Pozzo LF, Salania A, et al. Multicentric study comparing intravesical chemotherapy alone and with local microwave hyperthermia for prophylaxis of recurrence of superficial transitional cell carcinoma. J Clin Oncol 2003; 21(23): 4270–6.

38. Gofrit ON, Shapiro A, Pode D, et al. Combined local bladder hyperthermia and intravesical chemotherapy for the treatment of high-grade superficial bladder cancer. J Urol 2004; 3(3): 466–71.

39. Van der Heijden AG, Kiemeney LA, Gofrit ON, et al. Preliminary European results of local microwave hyperthermia and chemotherapy treatment in intermediate or high risk superficial transitional cell carcinoma of the bladder. Eur Urol 2004; 46: 65–72.

40. Moskovitz B, Meyer G, Kravtzov A, et al. Thermo-chemotherapy for intermediate or high-risk recurrent superficial bladder cancer patients. Ann Oncol 2005; 16: 585–9.

41. Hashimoto H, Tokunaka S, Sasaki M, et al. Dimethylsulfoxide enhances the absolution of chemotherapeutic drug instillation into the bladder. Urologic Res 20: 233–36, 1992.

42. Maier U, Baumgartner G. Metaphylactic effect of mitomycin C with and without hyaluronidase after transurethral resection of bladder cancer. J Urol 1989; 141: 529–30.

43. Leakakos T, Ji C, Lawson G, Peterson C, Goodwin S. Intravesical administration of doxorubicin to swine bladder using magnetically targeted carriers. Cancer Chemother Pharmacol 2003; 51: 445–50.

44. Zoli W, Ricotti L, Tesei A, et al. Schedule-dependent cytotoxic interaction between epidoxorubicin and gemcitabine in human bladder cancer cells in vitro. Clin Cancer Res 2004; 10(4): 1500–7.

45. Fukui I, Kihara K, Sekine H, et al. Intravesical combination chemotherapy with mitomycin C and doxorubicin for superficial bladder cancer: a randomized trial of maintenance versus no maintenance following a complete response. Cancer Chemother Pharmacol 1992; 30(Suppl): 37–40.

46. Sekine H, Fukui I, Yamada T, et al. Intravesical mitomycin C and doxorubicin sequential therapy for carcinoma in situ of the bladder: a longer follow-up result. J Urol 1994; 151: 27–30.

47. Isaka S, Okano T, Abe K, et al. Sequential instillation therapy with mitomycin C and adriamycin for superficial bladder cancer. Cancer Chemother Pharmacol 1992; 30(Suppl): S41–44.

4

Intravesical chemotherapy of superficial bladder cancer: optimization and novel agents

Jessie L-S Au, M Guillaume Wientjes

Introduction

In evaluating treatment of superficial bladder cancer using intravesical chemotherapy, this chapter will explore the pharmacological basis of intravesical chemotherapy, the mathematics of drug transport in bladder tissues, the optimization of intravesical therapy using a computational approach to compare drug exposure in different parts of bladder tissues, current additional investigational and novel agents, and perspectives on future research.

Pharmacologic basis of intravesical therapy

Current status of intravesical chemotherapy

The rationale for regional therapy is to expose tumors to high drug concentrations while minimizing the systemic exposure, thereby enhancing the treatment effect and reducing the host toxicity. The bladder is an ideal organ for regional chemotherapy.[1] The urethra provides easy and relatively noninvasive access for the introduction of therapeutic agents. The intact ureterovesical junction prevents reflux of these agents into the upper urinary tracts. The voluntary control of the external urinary sphincter provides the opportunity to control the dwell time, and the agents can be readily removed from the bladder during micturition.

The goals of intravesical chemo- or immunotherapy, used to treat nonmuscle-invasive bladder cancer since 1950s,[2] are to eradicate existing/residual tumor, prevent tumor recurrence, and prevent disease progression. Intravesical therapy is most effective when tumor burden is minimized by transurethral resection, and is most often used in high-risk patients (i.e. patients with large, multiple, poorly differentiated or recurrent tumors, Tis tumors, or tumors with nuclear p53 overexpression). Bacillus Calmette–Guérin (BCG) represents the agent of choice for immunotherapy (see Chapter 33). For chemotherapy, multiple agents, including thiotepa, mitomycin C (MMC),[3] doxorubicin, epodyl, tenoposide (VM-16), and cisplatin, have been evaluated. Of the 23 reported clinical trials involving more than 4000 patients, 13 showed statistically significant reduction in tumor recurrence (14% at 1–3 years benefit over transurethral resection alone), but not for disease progression.[4,5]

Patient response to intravesical chemotherapy is highly variable, ranging from 2% to more than 50%.[6] The common adverse effect of these drugs is local cystitis and reduced bladder capacity. Thiotepa also produces bone marrow suppression in 10% of patients.

The Southwest Oncology Group showed that BCG produces a higher recurrence-free rate than MMC (e.g. 49% for BCG versus 34% for MMC after a 39-month median follow-up), but does not improve the reduction of disease progression rate, and shows a five-fold higher incidence of severe toxicities (cystitis, dysuria, hematuria, low-grade pyrexia).[7] About 10% of patients cannot tolerate BCG because of immunologic reactions.[8] BCG maintenance therapy for 3 years, while more effective than the 6-week induction therapy, is also more toxic.[9] In comparison, chemotherapy with MMC or doxorubicin, usually given as weekly treatments for 6 weeks, is equally effective when given for short or long durations (<5 months versus >3 years).[10] Intravesical chemotherapy has been and remains a popular treatment option.

Determinants of efficacy of intravesical chemotherapy

In intravesical therapy, the bladder is emptied via catheterization and the drug is instilled and maintained, usually for 2 hours, after which time the patient is allowed to void. The treatment goal is to eliminate the malignant and premalignant cells located in the urine, on the luminal bladder surface, and/or in the bladder wall. As a very small fraction of the intravesical dose is absorbed from the bladder into the systemic circulation (with the exception of thiotepa),[11] systemic toxicity is usually not a concern. Hence, the delivery of drug to tumor cells and the response of tumor cells to the drug together determine the therapeutic outcome.

Processes governing the drug delivery to different parts of the bladder

Our laboratory has established the pharmacokinetic models describing the drug concentration profiles, as a function of time and/or tissue depth, in different parts of the urinary bladder. These models, developed for several drugs (MMC, doxorubicin, 5-fluorouridine), have been validated in animals and/or human patients.[1,3,12–17]

Figure 4.1 shows the cross-section of a human urinary bladder, which consists of urothelium that lines the bladder cavity, lamina

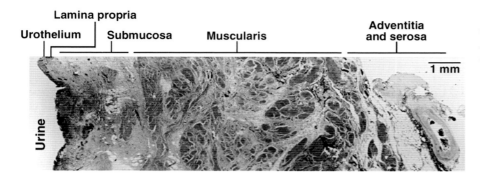

Figure 4.1
Cross-section of a human urinary bladder. Adapted with permission from Wientjes et al.[1]

propria, and superficial and deep muscle layers. In the bladder cavity, the drug concentration changes as a function of time and urine volume (Equation 1).

$$\text{Urine pharmacokinetics: } C_u = \frac{\text{Dose}}{V_u} \cdot e^{-(k_a + k_d) \cdot t}$$

where $V_u = V_0 + k_0 \cdot t + V_{res}$ Equation (1)

C_u depends on V_u or the urine volume at time t, which in turn is determined by the volume of the dosing solution (V_0), residual urine volume V_{res} at the time of drug instillation, and urine production during therapy (k_0 is production rate constant). C_u also depends on drug absorption and degradation (k_a and k_d are the respective apparent rate constants). In patients, V_{res} and k_0 are the major determinants of the drug exposure responsible for >90% of the intra- and interpatient variability, whereas drug absorption from the bladder and drug degradation are relatively minor determinants.[13]

The parameters in the urine pharmacokinetic model are determined by the treatment conditions such as patient dehydration status and urinary pH. For example, MMC is unstable at pH >8 and pH <5,[18,19] with a 10-times faster degradation in human urine at pH 5 than at pH 7.[13] Both thiotepa and its active metabolite tepa are stable in alkaline medium (pH 8.4), but are completely degraded in 30 minutes at acidic pH of 4.2.[20,21] Urinary pH also affects the ionization status and thereby affects the passive diffusion of acidic and basic drugs across the urothelium.[22] Additionally, abnormalities of the mucosal surface that occur with widespread tumor formation, inflammation, or mucosal denudation may increase drug absorption.[23] Damage to the bladder by acute cystitis or experimental procedures such as electrocoagulation enhance the absorption of doxorubicin and cisplatin in rats,[24,25] and increased extent of tumor involvement enhances the absorption of thiotepa in patients.[11] Administration of MMC within 6 days after transurethral resection also enhances the systemic absorption compared to later administration.[26] An increased urine volume unfolds the bladder, increases the surface area and reduces the thickness of the distendable bladder wall, resulting in increases of drug partition across the urothelium and systemic absorption of doxorubicin in rats.[25] In patients, the instillation volume may affect the drug contact to the lower half of the posterior wall of the bladder adjoining the trigone, which is usually folded by abdominal pressure.[27]

Drug penetration from urine into bladder tissues consists of two processes. The first process is partitioning from urine, presumably by diffusion, across the bladder urothelium, which is not perfused by blood and is the absorption barrier.[28,29] Fick's first law describes the effect of physicochemical and physiologic variables on drug absorption across a single homogeneous diffusion barrier (Equation 2).

Across the urothelium: Diffusion rate =

$$\frac{DKA(C_u - C_{uro})}{h} = k_a V_u C_u$$ Equation (2)

C_{uro} is the concentration at the interface between the urothelium and the deep tissues; D is the drug diffusion coefficient (dependent on the ionization and lipophilicity of the drug); K is the drug partition coefficient; and h and A are the thickness and surface area of the urothelium. The decline in drug concentration across the urothelium is linear with depth. The C_{uro}:C_u ratio indicates the extent of partitioning.

After crossing the urothelium, the drug is transported through the deeper tissues that are perfused by capillaries, a process described by the distributed model.[1,14,15,17] The concentration in tissue declines from C_{uro} to the averaged free drug concentration in blood (C_b). C_{depth} is the concentration at a particular tissue depth. A fraction of the drug proportional to ($C_{depth} - C_b$) is removed via absorption into the blood each time the drug encounters a capillary. As the number of capillaries increases with the distance traveled, C_{depth} declines exponentially with respect to tissue depth at a rate equal to half-width ($w_{1/2}$), which is the tissue thickness over which the concentration declines by 50% (Equation 3). Note that a smaller w_2 indicates a steeper concentration decline across the tissue and that C_u determines C_{uro} and, therefore, C_{depth}.

Beyond the urothelium: $C_{depth} = (C_{uro} - C_b) \cdot$
$e^{-(0.693/w_{1/2})\,(depth - urothelial\ thickness)} + C_b$ Equation (3)

Equations 2 and 3 provide the basis to identify the drugs that will show favorable bladder tissue delivery. This is illustrated by computer simulations that compare the tissue concentration–depth profiles of drugs with different parameters. Thiotepa was used as an example of a lipophilic compound that is rapidly and extensively absorbed into the systemic circulation.[11] Lipophilic compounds partition readily across cell membranes (hence a C_{uro}:C_u ratio of 1), and are readily absorbed into the blood circulation (hence a q or blood flow-limited removal). Using a q of 95 ml/min/100 g for the bladder flow in the rat,[30] and D=0.3 × 10^{-6} cm²/sec (approximated on the basis of the molecular weight of thiotepa),[31] the calculated w_2 (equals 0.693 (D/q)$^{1/2}$) for thiotepa is 30 µm. For comparison, we used MMC or doxorubicin, both of which are more hydrophilic, and showed a much lower C_{uro}:C_u ratio of about 1:30 and a much longer $w^{1/2}$ of about 500 µm (experimentally determined in dogs and humans).[1,16,17] Results of the simulations indicate that, in spite of the 30-fold higher partition across the urothelium, the more lipophilic drug showed lower concentrations in most parts of the bladder tissues (Figure 4.2). This is due to the rapid drainage of the highly

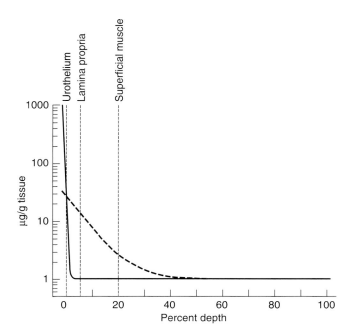

Figure 4.2
Effects of physicochemical properties of a drug on its bladder tissue penetration. Computer simulations for lipophilic (solid line) and hydrophilic (broken line) compounds, using equal initial values of C_u of 1000 μg/ml and C_b of 1 μg/ml.

lipophilic drug into the capillaries. The latter will also result in higher systemic blood concentrations and compromise the bladder targeting advantage. The ideal compound for intravesical therapy should have well-balanced lipophilic and hydrophilic properties so that it can readily partition across the urothelium, but is not rapidly absorbed into the capillaries.

Heterogeneity in chemosensitivity of human bladder tumors

The response of human tumors to chemotherapeutic agents was evaluated using three-dimensional (3D) histocultures of tumors from individual patients. The major advantage of this experimental system is the maintenance of intra- and interpatient heterogeneity of drug response.[32,33] The chemosensitivity varied significantly between tumors; the drug concentrations producing 90% inhibition of DNA synthesis showed a >40-fold variation for MMC, >100-fold for doxorubicin, 40-fold for 5-fluorouridine, and 430-fold for paclitaxel.[14,34,35] In general, these effective drug concentrations are 10–100 times higher than those in monolayer cultures of human bladder tumor cells.[36–38] This significant intertumor heterogeneity in chemosensitivity represents a potential cause of the variable and incomplete patient response.

For MMC, the tumor sensitivity was inversely correlated with tumor malignancy, with greater activity in well-differentiated superficial tumors, and lesser activity in undifferentiated, invasive, and more rapidly proliferating tumors.[39] MMC activity is also positively correlated with the expression of its two activating enzymes: DT diaphorase (also named NQO1 or NAD(P)H:quinone oxidoreductase) and cytochrome p450 reductase.[40–49]

Optimization of intravesical chemotherapy

Overview

The following example illustrates our experience using a computational approach to compare the drug exposure in different parts of bladder tissues (where tumors reside) with the exposure required for drug effects, in order to predict the treatment outcome and, more importantly, to synthesize an optimal MMC treatment regimen that was predicted to nearly double its efficacy (detailed in Wientjes et al[50]).

Drug exposure at target tumor sites

We studied the pharmacokinetics of MMC in plasma and urine of patients treated by intravesical therapy (10 patients receiving a total of 28 treatments), and the tissue pharmacokinetics in cystectomy patients and in animals (dogs and rabbits). The plasma pharmacokinetic data indicate insignificant MMC absorption into the systemic circulation. The urine and bladder tissue pharmacokinetic data were analyzed using Equations 1–3 to obtain the values of the model parameters (V_{res}, k_0 and $k_a + k_d$ for the urine pharmacokinetic model; C_u:C_{uro} ratio, C_u:C_b ratio, and $w^{1}\frac{1}{2}$ for the tissue pharmacokinetic model). Note that alterations of the urine pharmacokinetic parameters will alter the C_u and, therefore, the C_{uro} and the CxT values in different parts of the bladder.

Drug exposure required for activity

Results of the MMC pharmacodynamics in 3D histocultures of patient bladder tumors indicated a >40-fold variation in tumor sensitivity. As other investigators reported higher MMC activity at acidic pH in monolayer cultures of human tumor cells,[51–54] we investigated the effect of pH on MMC activity in 3D cultures and found that the 10-fold higher activity at acidic pH compared to neutral pH was observed in monolayer cells but not in either multilayer cultures of the same tumor cell line or histocultures of patient tumors, because of the slow equilibration between intracellular and extracellular pHs in multilayered systems (requiring at least 8 hours).[38]

Translating in vitro pharmacodynamics to in vivo treatment effect

The common denominator between in vitro and in vivo pharmacodynamics is the drug exposure under these two conditions. Equation 4 describes the relationship between drug concentration C, exposure time T, and the resulting pharmacologic effect.

$$C^n \times T = \text{effect} \qquad \text{Equation (4)}$$

When n equals 1, the concentration and the exposure time are equally important in determining the effect. Concentration is more important when n is larger than 1, and time is more important when n is smaller than 1. The n value can be determined from the in vitro pharmacodynamics attained at various exposure times.

To accommodate the differences in the drug concentration—time profiles under in vitro conditions (where drug concentrations remain relatively constant) and in vivo conditions (where concentrations change with time), C^nxT can be calculated as the time integral of C^n over time (Equation 5). For MMC, the average n value was 1.24, and statistical analysis indicated that the pharmacodynamics of one-half of the 30 patient tumors were better described by an n value of 1.24, while the other half was better described by an n of 1.

$$C^n \times T = \int_0^T C^n \times dT \qquad \text{Equation (5)}$$

Integration of pharmacokinetics and pharmacodynamics to establish the pharmacologic basis of variable and incomplete response to intravesical MMC

Figure 4.3 shows the three $C \times T$-tissue depth profiles of MMC simulated using the highest, average, and lowest C_u values obtained from patients. Also shown are the drug exposures producing 90% inhibition of DNA synthesis in 30 human bladder tumors (C^nxT_{90}), placed according to the anatomical location of the tumors (e.g. Ta and T1 tumors are located on the urothelium and lamina propria, or a tissue depth of 200 and 700 μm, respectively). The probability of tumors receiving C^nxT_{90} was 90% for Ta and 17% for T1 at the highest $C \times T$-depth profile, 22% for Ta and 0% for T1 tumors at the average profile, and 0% for Ta and T1 tumors at the lowest profile. Note that none of the T2, T3 and T4 tumors would receive C^nxT_{90}.

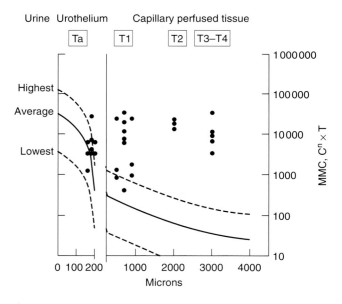

Figure 4.3
Treatment efficacy simulations based on bladder wall concentrations and tumor chemosensitivity. Simulated bladder-wall tissue $C^n \times T$ versus depth profiles based on the highest, average, and lowest urine concentration profiles obtained from patients. $C^n \times T_{90}$ (•) values were calculated from the IC_{90} using equation 5 and an n value of 1.24. Adapted with permission from Wientjes et al.[50]

These data suggest that the large intra- and intersubject variability in urine/tissue pharmacokinetics and tumor chemosensitivity contribute to the varying and incomplete patient response to intravesical MMC treatment.

Computer simulations to select optimal treatment conditions

We next evaluated whether increasing the drug exposure in tumors by reducing the sources of pharmacokinetic variability would produce therapeutic benefits. The goal was to identify an optimized MMC regimen that can be demonstrated, in a phase III trial with reasonable financial and patient resources, to be more efficacious than the usual community practice. The resource consideration was motivated in part by the fact that multiple previous clinical trials failed to show conclusive results on the dose-effect or treatment time-effect relationships of intravesical MMC therapy,[55–59] presumably because of the inadequate sample size (see below). We elected to use computer simulations to predict the $C^n \times T$ values in bladder tissues and, consequently, the drug effects and the clinical outcomes under various treatment conditions. This computational approach also enabled us to identify the sample size with appropriate statistical power.

In a typical intravesical treatment, the bladder is emptied by catheterization without checking for the completeness of bladder emptying, patients are not asked to refrain from fluid and caffeine intake, and the urine pH and urine production rate are not controlled. These conditions, on average, yielded a residual urine volume of 32.4 ml, urine production rate of 1.48 ml/min, and acidic urinary pH. By controlling the catheter position and patient positioning, and by sonographically checking the residual volume, a minimal residual urine volume of 0–10 ml can be achieved. Results obtained from healthy volunteers showed that restricting fluid and caffeine intake overnight reduced the urine output to 0.63 ml/min, and administration of bicarbonate on the night before and again in the morning was sufficient to control the urine pH at about 7, which would minimize the MMC degradation. The historical intravesical MMC dose ranges from 20 to 60 mg, dissolved in 20 or 40 ml water.[2,6,55,60,61] The simulations compared the target site drug exposure at three doses, two dosing volumes, two residual urine volumes, two urine production rates, two urine pH values, and used n (pharmacodynamic parameter in Equation 4) values of 1.24; in the simulations, each parameters was altered, independently and simultaneously, to project the improvement in the target-site exposure ($C^n \times T$) for different treatment conditions (Table 4.1). As single parameters, the rank order for enhancing the C^nxT was dose > residual volume > urine production > dosing volume > urine pH > dwell time. Table 4.1 also shows the fraction of tumors exposed to the C^nxT_{90}.

With the assumption that several logs of cytoreduction are required for eradicating tumor cells (i.e. 90% reduction in a regimen of weekly treatments for 6 weeks), the fraction of tumors receiving $C^n \times T_{90}$ was used to calculate the benefit offered by adjuvant MMC therapy. The results indicated marginal improvement achieved by changing individual parameters. For example, an increase of the dose from 20 to 40 mg increased the fraction of patients with Ta tumors receiving $C^n \times T_{90}$ from 22% to 56% but had no effect on patients with T1 tumors. Assuming a patient population with an equal distribution of Ta and T1 tumors, this increase in drug exposure was calculated to produce an 8% improvement in the recurrence-free rate. Interestingly, increasing the dwell time from 2 to 4 hours did not produce an improvement. This is because the

Table 4.1 Simulations of bladder wall exposure and treatment effect*

Variable changed	$C^n \times T$ urine	$C^n \times T$ at 200 mm	Improvement factor	Percent of tumors exposed to $C^n \times T90$	
				Ta	T1
	n=1.24				
Standard (Dose=20, V_0=20, k_0=1.48, V_{res}=32.4, pH=5, T_{inst}=120)	32,179	374	1.00	22.2	0.0
Instillation volume, from 20 to 40 ml	24,779	288	0.77	55.6	0.0
Dose, from 20 to 40 mg	76,005	882	2.36	44.4	0.0
Urine production, from 1.48 to 0.626 ml/min	44,702	519	1.39	55.6	0.0
Residual volume, from 32.4 to 0 ml	62,092	721	1.93	22.2	0.0
pH, from 5 to 7	32,237	432	1.16	22.2	0.0
Instillation time, from 120 to 240 min	32,962	383	1.02	22.2	0.0
Optimized (Dose=40, V_0=20, k_0=0.63, V_{res}=0, pH=7, T_{inst}=120)	274,919	3191	8.53	77.8	25.0
High dose combination (Dose=60, V_0=30, k_0=0.63, V_{res}=0, pH=7, T_{inst}=120)	332,968	3865	10.33	77.8	25.0
	n=1				
Standard (Dose=20, V_0=20, k_0=1.48, V_{res}=32.4, pH=5, T_{inst}=120)	9928	273	1.00	22.2	0.0
Optimized (Dose=40, V_0=20, k_0=0.63, V_{res}=0, pH=7, T_{inst}=120)	56,871	1564	5.73	77.8	16.7

* The variables were altered and the resulting C_u and $C^n \times T$ were calculated using equations 1–4. Simulations were done using two n values, 1.24 and 1.

drug concentration in urine at 2 hours was <10% of the initial concentration, thus resulting in a minimal increase in cumulative drug exposure. Likewise, increasing the dose from 40 mg/20 ml to 60 mg/30 ml (2 mg/ml is the maximum MMC solubility) did not show improvement because the tumor chemosensitivity was such that the 20% increase in drug exposure did not result in a greater fraction of responding tumors. Simultaneous optimization of five parameters (dose, 40 mg; dosing solution volume, 20 ml; urine-production rate constant, 0.63 ml/min; postcatheterization urine volume, 0; pH, 7) resulted in an increase in drug exposure by 5.7 (n=1) or 8.5-fold (n=1.24).

The conventional paradigm in clinical oncology is to test the effect of individual parameters. However, as shown above, doubling the dose would increase the response rate by only 8%, which would require >900 patients (>450 per arm) to detect a statistically significant difference at 80% power. Similarly, testing the effect of the remaining parameters, one at a time, would require at a minimum several thousand patients. As there are insufficient resources to support multiple trials of this magnitude, a more rational and realistic approach was to optimize the five parameters that, based on the simulation results using an n value of 1.24, would deliver $C^n \times T_{90}$ to 78% and 25% of T_a and T1 tumors, respectively, and would result in a 20% improvement over the standard treatment. For an n value of 1, the calculated improvement was 18%. Improvements of 18% to 20% are significant and can be detected with a modest sample size of 232 patients (116 per arm) or a total of 116 recurrences, at a 5% significance level with 80% power. These considerations led to a prospective two-arm randomized multi-institutional phase III trial.

Phase III trial results demonstrating therapeutic benefits of the optimized MMC therapy

Fourteen academic and research centers participated in the trial. The study population consisted of patients with histologically proven transitional cell carcinoma of the bladder at high risk for recurrence due to:

- two or more episodes of histologically proven Ta, Tis, or T1 transitional cell carcinoma
- multifocal bladder tumors (defined as three or more papillary tumors present simultaneously or Tis involving at least 25% of the bladder surface area and/or in two or more biopsy sites), and/or
- primary or solitary tumors that were >5 cm in size, of grade 3, or exhibited DNA aneuploidy.

Patients with adequate bone marrow reserve, adequate renal function, and a Karnofsky performance score of 50–100 were randomized within 34 days of transurethral bladder tumor resection, by four prognostic criteria: 1) presence versus absence of Tis tumor; 2) grade 3 versus grades 1 and 2 tumors; 3) multifocal versus unifocal tumors; and 4) recurrent versus primary tumors. Patients with MMC treatments within the previous 56 weeks, prior muscle-invasive (T2–4) tumors, concurrent malignancy within the last 5 years, or pregnancy were excluded.

Patients in the optimized arm were instructed to refrain from drinking fluids for 8 hours prior to and during MMC treatment, were given oral doses of 1.3 g sodium bicarbonate the night prior to, the morning of, and 30 minutes prior to drug treatment. These patients were catheterized; their post-void residual urine volumes were measured using a bladder ultrasound instrument and reduced by repositioning the catheter and/or by changing the position of the patient, until the residual urine volume was less than 10 ml. MMC (40 mg in 20 ml sterile water) was then instilled intravesically through the Foley catheter by gravity, and retained in the bladder for 2 hours. Patients in the standard arm received a lower MMC dose (20 mg in 20 ml), were not instructed to exercise voluntary dehydration, and did not receive oral sodium bicarbonate or undergo additional postcatheterization bladder-emptying measures. MMC treatments were given weekly for 6 weeks. Primary endpoints were recurrence and time to recurrence. Patients in the two arms did not differ in demographics, disease characteristics, or history of intravesical therapy.

For hematologic toxicity, one patient in the standard arm showed a transient reduction in white blood cell count, whereas no patients in the optimized arm showed toxicity. For nonhematologic toxicity, only dysuria was statistically significantly higher in the optimized arm, and it did not result in higher frequency of treatment termination (one termination due to dysuria in each arm).

Kaplan–Meier analyses of recurrence in the intent-to-treat group and the evaluable group indicated that, in both groups, patients in the optimized arm had a statistically significantly longer time to recurrence and a higher recurrence-free fraction at all time points compared to patients in the standard arm (Figure 4.4). Improvements were found across all stratification risk groups (tumor stage, grade, focality, and recurrence, stratified log-rank test). The close alignment between the clinical outcome (18–19% improvement in recurrence-free rate) and the simulation predictions (18–20% improvement) is noteworthy and lends support to using the effect-based, computational approach to identify/design the optimal intravesical treatment.

Additional investigational and novel agents

Anthracyclines

Epirubicin, a standard therapy in Europe, shows a dose-dependent efficacy between 20 and 40 mg per 40 ml, with no further improvement from 50 to 100 mg per 50 ml.[62] In a study with a 6-year follow-up, perioperative epirubicin is more effective than interferon-α in preventing recurrence.[63] Mitoxantrone shows variable activity up to the level similar to that of doxorubicin.[64–66] Pirarubicin[67–69] shows slightly better activity than saline controls. Other anthracyclines, including (2′R)-4′-O-tetrahydropyranyl-doxorubicin and amrubicin have undergone limited clinical evaluation.[70–72] Valrubicin (AD-32) provides higher bladder penetration due to its greater lipophilicity than does doxorubicin, interferes with the normal DNA breaking–resealing action of DNA topoisomerase II, and causes chromosomal damage and cell cycle arrest in the G2 phase.[73] Valrubicin is approved for patients with BCG-refractory Tis tumors unsuitable for cystectomy, whereas valrubicin produces a 20% complete response rate with no evidence of disease in 8% of patients after a median follow-up of 30 months.[74] Valrubicin is not recommended in patients that can tolerate cystectomy because of the risk of progressive disease.[75]

Mitomycin C-related treatments

Several experimental approaches to promote MMC penetration into bladder have been evaluated. In patients with high-grade tumors after failing other treatments, combination of MMC with hyperthermia shows a 75% recurrence-free survival after 20 months of follow-up.[76,77] Application of electric current (20 mAmp for 30 minutes) enhances the urothelium penetration and systemic absorption of MMC, and improves the recurrence-free survival in high-risk patients with T1 and Tis tumors,[78] but does not ablate the marker lesions.[79] Our laboratory is evaluating the use of a chemosensitizer to enhance the tumor response to MMC (see below).

EO9 is an indolequinone bioreductive agent with promising preclinical activity.[80] The enzyme NQO1, important for its bioactiva-

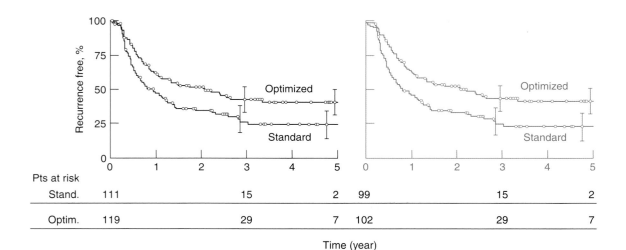

Time (year)

Figure 4.4

Kaplan–Meier analysis of treatment outcome in (*left*) intent-to-treat and (*right*) evaluable groups. Symbols indicate censored patients, error bars show 95% confidence intervals (CI). (*Left*) In the intent-to-treat group of patients (n=230), median time to recurrence was 11.8 months in the standard arm (n=111) and 29.1 in the optimized arm (n=119). For the standard arm, the recurrence-free percentages at 1-, 3- and 5-years were 48.0 (CI: 38.4–57.7), 28.4% (CI: 18.8–38%), and 24.6% (CI: 14.9–34.3%), respectively. For the optimized arm, the recurrence-free percentages at 1-, 3- and 5-years were 61.3 (CI: 52.2–70.4), 44.5% (CI: 34.7–54.3%), and 41.5% (CI: 30.9–51.1%), respectively. (*Right*) In evaluable patients (n=201), median time to recurrence was 11.3 months in the standard arm (n=99) and 29.1 in the optimized arm (n=102). For the standard arm, the recurrence-free percentages at 1-, 3- and 5-years were 47.5 (CI: 37.6–57.4), 27.1% (CI: 17.5–36.7%), and 23.5% (CI: 14–33%), respectively. For the optimized arm, the recurrence-free percentages at 1-, 3- and 5-years were 63.3 (CI: 53.9–72.7), 44.4% (CI: 34.1–54.7%), and 42.6% (CI: 32.3–52.9%), respectively. Reproduced with permission from Au et al.[3]

tion, is elevated in a subset of superficial bladder tumors.[81] A phase I study showed complete disappearance of marker lesions in six of eight patients.[82]

Antimetabolites

Gemcitabine, an active systemic agent in advanced bladder cancer, is well tolerated and shows insignificant systemic absorption when given as intravesical therapy in doses of 2 g in 50 or 100 ml saline.[83–86] 5-Fluorouracil has activity when given by long-term systemic or 6-week intravesical administration, but its activity appears to be limited to tumors with low expression of its major target enzyme, thymidylate synthase.[87,88] Oral 5-fluorouracil did not enhance the effect of perioperative intravesical doxorubicin.[89]

Antimicrotubule agents

Our MMC and doxorubicin studies suggested the following desirable properties of agents for intravesical therapy:

- higher penetration across the urothelium and longer retention in tissues
- effective against the more rapidly proliferating bladder tumors
- does not require functional p53 for apoptosis induction as 60% of bladder cancer shows high frequency of p53 mutation.[90–98]

A potential candidate is paclitaxel, which has activity against metastatic bladder cancer,[34] shows high lipophilicity and partitioning across the urothelium, tight binding to intracellular macromolecules resulting in significant drug accumulation and retention in tumor cells,[15,99] and can induce apoptosis through p53-dependent or p53-independent pathways.[100,101] An earlier phase I trial with the Food and Drug Administration (FDA)-approved paclitaxel formulation, given intravesically, did not show activity (D. Lamm, personal communication), possibly due to the sequestration of paclitaxel in Cremophor micelles.[102] Dimethyl sulfoxide (DMSO) promotes the paclitaxel release by altering the Cremophor micelle structure and promotes paclitaxel penetration into bladder tissues by disrupting the urothelium.[103] However, these beneficial effects of DMSO were compromised by the increases in urine production rate and drug permeability, and clearance by the capillaries.[104] These findings have led to the development of rapid-release, paclitaxel-loaded gelatin nanoparticles (~600 nm diameter) that release approximately 90% of the drug in 2 hours, and yield higher concentrations in the urothelium and lamina propria than the Cremophor formulation.[105] The vinca alkaloid vinorelbine showed some activity in a preliminary phase I trial.[106]

Immune stimulators

Several immune stimulators (e.g. hemocyanin, bropirimine, and interferons) have shown some efficacy (see Chapter 33).

Combination therapy

The therapeutic value of combination chemo- or immunochemotherapy in advanced cancers is well established. There have been limited attempts to develop this modality for intravesical therapy in patients; epirubicin does not improve the response to BCG,[107] whereas a combination of the bleomycin analog peplomycin and doxorubicin shows improvement over single agents.[67]

Molecular targets

Loss of tumor suppressor genes p53 and RB, overexpression of oncogenes and peptide growth factors and their ligands, and alterations in cellular adhesion molecules and tissue microenvironment all play a role in bladder tumor formation, growth, and metastasis.[108] The therapeutic targets under preclinical evaluation include: 1) epidermal growth factor receptor (EGFR), i.e. EGFR inhibitors and EGF-linked therapeutics, as superficial bladder cancer shows high EGFR expression[109,110]; and 2) p53, as its mutation is correlated with poor prognosis.[111–115] Suramin, a polysulfonated compound that broadly inhibits polypeptide growth factors, displays chemopreventive properties in a mouse superficial bladder carcinogenesis model.[116] A phase I intravesical treatment with single agent suramin showed good tolerability but limited antitumor activity.[117]

Our laboratory recently established that acidic and basic fibroblast growth factors (FGF) expressed in solid tumors are responsible for broad-spectrum resistance to anticancer drugs, and that FGF inhibitors, including monoclonal antibodies and suramin, enhance the activity of chemotherapy. The chemosensitizing effect of suramin shows an unusual dose–response relationship, occurring only at low, nontoxic doses and not at higher doses.[118–122] Results of a phase II trial in lung cancer patients indicate survival benefits of adding nontoxic doses of suramin to the standard chemotherapy (paclitaxel plus carboplatin), thus providing the clinical proof-of-concept of the suramin chemosensitization.[123,124] Separate preclinical studies have shown that nontoxic suramin treatments significantly enhanced the in vitro and/or in vivo MMC activity in xenograft and patient bladder tumors, without enhancing the host toxicity.[125] Finally, combination of chemotherapy with an FGF inhibitor is appealing as bFGF overexpression is associated with the development and chemoresistance of bladder cancer, and poor prognosis of bladder cancer patients.[126–130] Studies to identify the appropriate chemosensitizing suramin dose for intravesical therapy are ongoing in our laboratory.

Perspectives

The therapeutic value of intravesical immuno- or chemotherapy in superficial bladder cancer is well documented. However, in spite of the theoretical advantage of being able to completely eliminate the malignant cells, these treatments have not yielded 100% recurrence-free survival. Hence, further research is needed.

For MMC, optimizing the treatment conditions to maximize the drug delivery to tumors nearly doubles the recurrence-free survival in high-risk patients to about 40%. Further improvement may be possible by enhancing MMC penetration into bladder tissues using physicochemical methods such as electromotility or hyperthermia. A second approach is patient selection. We found in the phase III MMC trial that a small subset of African–American patients performed far worse than Caucasian patients, suggesting a genetic difference in patient response.[3] A potential candidate to determine patient susceptibility is the expression of quinone reductases responsible for MMC activation, which positively correlates with MMC activity in patient bladder tumors.[131,132] Further elucidation of this mechanism may provide a pharmacogenetic approach to preselect the patients likely to respond to intravesical MMC therapy. A third approach is to use chemosensitizers or other chemotherapeutic agents to enhance the activity of MMC. A fourth approach is to identify new agents that provide more favorable bladder penetration and retention characteristics and have high potency against bladder tumors with diverse pathobiologic properties.

An unanswered question in intravesical therapy is the optimal duration of therapy. The current approach of six weekly cycles is empirically based. Fewer treatments may be sufficient and should be evaluated. Finally, the Southwest Oncology Group Trial 8795, in which BCG was found to be superior to MMC, used an MMC protocol that was essentially identical to the standard arm in our phase III trial.[3] This consideration, together with the fact that MMC produces lower and more tolerable toxicity than BCG, suggests that it may be worthwhile to compare the optimized MMC regimen to use of BCG.

Acknowledgement

This work was supported in part by MERIT grant R37CA49816 from the National Cancer Institute, NIH, DHHS.

References

1. Wientjes MG, Badalament RA, Wang RC, Hassan F, Au JL. Penetration of mitomycin C in human bladder. Cancer Res 1993; 53: 3314–20.
2. Richie JP, Shipley WU, Yagoda A. Cancer of the bladder. In DeVita VT Jr, Hellman S, Rosenberg SA (eds): Cancer: Principles and Practice of Oncology. Philadelphia: JB Lippincott, 1989, pp 1008–58.
3. Au JL, Badalament RA, Wientjes MG, et al. Methods to improve efficacy of intravesical mitomycin C: results of a randomized phase III trial. J Natl Cancer Inst 2001; 93: 597–604.
4. Paulson DF. Treatment of superficial carcinoma of the bladder. Bladder Cancer, Part B: Radiation, Local and Systemic Chemotherapy, and New Treatment Modalities. New York: Liss, 1984, pp 193–209.
5. Whitmore WF Jr. Chemotherapy for bladder cancer. J Urol 1985; 134: 1181–2.
6. Herr HW. Intravesical therapy. A critical review. Urol Clin North Am 1987; 14: 399–404.
7. Lundholm C, Norlen BJ, Ekman P, et al. A randomized prospective study comparing long-term intravesical instillations of mitomycin C and bacillus Calmette–Guérin in patients with superficial bladder carcinoma. J Urol 1996; 156: 372–6.
8. Meyer JP, Persad R, Gillatt DA. Use of bacille Calmette–Guérin in superficial bladder cancer. Postgrad Med J 2002; 78: 449–54.
9. Lamm DL, Blumenstein BA, Crissman JD, BA et al. Maintenance bacillus Calmette–Guérin immunotherapy for recurrent TA, T1 and carcinoma in situ transitional cell carcinoma of the bladder: a randomized Southwest Oncology Group Study. J Urol 2000; 163: 1124–9.
10. Traynelis CL, Lamm DL. Current status of intravesical therapy for bladder cancer. In Rous S (ed): Urology Annual. New York: Norton, 1994, pp 113–43.
11. Lunglmayr G, Czech K. Absorption studies on intraluminal thio-tepa for topical cytostatic treatment of low-stage bladder tumors. J Urol 1971; 106: 72–4.
12. Chai M, Wientjes MG, Badalament RA, Burgers JK, Au JL. Pharmacokinetics of intravesical doxorubicin in superficial bladder cancer patients. J Urol 1994; 152: 374–8.
13. Dalton JT, Wientjes MG, Badalament RA, Drago JR, Au JL. Pharmacokinetics of intravesical mitomycin C in superficial bladder cancer patients. Cancer Res 1991; 51: 5144–52.
14. Song D, Wientjes MG, Gan Y, Au JL. Bladder tissue pharmacokinetics and antitumor effect of intravesical 5-fluorouridine. Clin Cancer Res 1997; 3: 901–9.
15. Song D, Wientjes MG, Au JL. Bladder tissue pharmacokinetics of intravesical taxol. Cancer Chemother Pharmacol 1997; 40: 285–92.
16. Wientjes MG, Dalton JT, Badalament RA, Drago JR, Au JL. Bladder wall penetration of intravesical mitomycin C in dogs. Cancer Res 1991; 51: 4347–54.
17. Wientjes MG, Badalament RA, Au JL. Penetration of intravesical doxorubicin in human bladders. Cancer Chemother Pharmacol 1996; 37: 539–46.
18. Underberg WJ, Lingeman H. Aspects of the chemical stability of mitomycin and porfiromycin in acidic solution. J Pharm Sci 1983; 72: 549–53.
19. Beignen JH, Lingeman H, van Munster HA. Mitomycin antitumor agents: a review of their physico-chemical and analytical properties and stability. J Pharm Biomed Anal 1986; 4: 275–95.
20. Mellett JB, Woods LA. The comparative physiological disposition of thiotepa and tepa in the dog. Cancer Res 1960; 20: 524–32.
21. Colvin M. The alkylating agents. In Chabner BA (ed): Pharmacologic Principles of Cancer Treatment. Philadelphia: WB Saunders, 1982, pp 278–80.
22. Wood JH, Leonard TW. Kinetic implications of drug resorption from the bladder. Drug Metab Rev 1983; 14: 407–23.
23. Pauli BU, Alroy J, Weinstein RS. The ultrastructure and pathobiology of urinary bladder cancer. In Bryan GT, Cohen S (eds): The Pathology of Bladder Cancer, vol II. New York: CRC Press, 1983, pp 41–140.
24. Engelmann U, Oelsner G, Burger RA, Wagner H. Permeability of the rat bladder to cisplatinum under different conditions: comparison with mitomycin C and adriamycin. Urol Res 1983; 11: 39–42.
25. Engelmann U, Burger RA, Rumpelt JH, Jacobi GH. Adriamycin permeability of the rat bladder under different conditions. J Urol 1983; 129: 862–4.
26. Kurth KH, de Wall JG, van Oosterom HP, de Jong EAJM, Tjaden UR. Plasma levels during intravesical instillation of mitomycin C. In Liss AR (ed): EORTC Genitourinary Group Monograph 2, part B: Superficial bladder tumors. Brussels: EORTC, 1985, pp 81–93.
27. Watanabe H, Nakao M, Nakagawa S, Takada H. Size and location of tumors influencing the effect of bladder instillation therapy. Cancer Chemother Pharmacol 1987; 20(Suppl): S49–S51.
28. Turnbull GJ. Ultrastructural basis of the permeability barrier in urothelium. Invest Urol 1973; 11: 198–204.
29. Hicks RM, Ketterer B, Warren RC. The ultrastructure and chemistry of the luminal plasma membrane of the mammalian urinary bladder: a structure with low permeability to water and ions. Philos Trans R Soc Lond B Biol Sci 1974; 268: 23–38.
30. Gerlowski LE, Jain RK. Physiologically based pharmacokinetic modeling: principles and applications. J Pharm Sci 1983; 72: 1103–27.
31. Flessner MF, Dedrick RL, Schultz JS. A distributed model of peritoneal-plasma transport: theoretical considerations. Am J Physiol 1984; 246: R597–R607.
32. Hoffman RM. Three-dimensional histoculture: origins and applications in cancer research. Cancer Cells 1991; 3: 86–92.
33. Weaver JR, Wientjes MG, Au JL. Regional heterogeneity and pharmacodynamics in human solid tumor histoculture. Cancer Chemother Pharmacol 1999; 44: 335–42.
34. Au JL, Kalns J, Gan Y, Wientjes MG. Pharmacologic effects of paclitaxel in human bladder tumors. Cancer Chemother Pharmacol 1997; 41: 69–74.
35. Gan Y, Wientjes MG, Badalament RA, Au JL. Pharmacodynamics of doxorubicin in human bladder tumors. Clin Cancer Res 1996; 2: 1275–83.
36. Au JL, Li D, Gan Y, et al. Pharmacodynamics of immediate and delayed effects of paclitaxel: role of slow apoptosis and intracellular drug retention. Cancer Res 1998; 58: 2141–8.

37. Walker MC, Parris CN, Masters JR. Differential sensitivities of human testicular and bladder tumor cell lines to chemotherapeutic drugs. J Natl Cancer Inst 1987; 79: 213–16.

38. Yen WC, Schmittgen T, Au JL. Different pH dependency of mitomycin C activity in monolayer and three-dimensional cultures. Pharm Res 1996; 13: 1887–91.

39. Schmittgen TD, Weaver JM, Badalament RA, et al. Correlation of human bladder tumor histoculture proliferation and sensitivity to mitomycin C with tumor pathobiology. J Urol 1994; 152: 1632–6.

40. Traver RD, Siegel D, Beall HD, et al. Characterization of a polymorphism in NAD(P)H: quinone oxidoreductase (DT-diaphorase). Br J Cancer 1997; 75: 69–75.

41. Bligh HF, Bartoszek A, Robson CN, et al. Activation of mitomycin C by NADPH:cytochrome P-450 reductase. Cancer Res 1990; 50: 7789–92.

42. Hoban PR, Walton MI, Robson CN, et al. Decreased NADPH: cytochrome P-450 reductase activity and impaired drug activation in a mammalian cell line resistant to mitomycin C under aerobic but not hypoxic conditions. Cancer Res 1990; 50: 4692–7.

43. Traver RD, Horikoshi T, Danenberg KD, et al. NAD(P)H:quinone oxidoreductase gene expression in human colon carcinoma cells: characterization of a mutation which modulates DT-diaphorase activity and mitomycin sensitivity. Cancer Res 1992; 52: 797–802.

44. Spanswick VJ, Cummings J, Smyth JF. Current issues in the enzymology of mitomycin C metabolic activation. Gen Pharmacol 1998; 31: 539–44.

45. Malkinson AM, Siegel D, Forrest GL, et al. Elevated DT-diaphorase activity and messenger RNA content in human non-small cell lung carcinoma: relationship to the response of lung tumor xenografts to mitomycin C. Cancer Res 1992; 52: 4752–7.

46. Singh SV, Scalamogna D, Xia H, et al. Biochemical characterization of a mitomycin C-resistant human bladder cancer cell line. Int J Cancer 1996; 65: 852–7.

47. Mikami K, Naito M, Tomida A, Yamada M, Sirakusa T, Tsuruo T. DT-diaphorase as a critical determinant of sensitivity to mitomycin C in human colon and gastric carcinoma cell lines. Cancer Res 1996; 56: 2823–6.

48. Siegel D, Beall H, Senekowitsch C, et al. Bioreductive activation of mitomycin C by DT-diaphorase. Biochemistry 1992; 31: 7879–85.

49. Tomasz M, Lipman R. Reductive metabolism and alkylating activity of mitomycin C induced by rat liver microsomes. Biochemistry 1981; 20: 5056–61.

50. Wientjes MG, Badalament RA, Au JL. Use of pharmacologic data and computer simulations to design an efficacy trial of intravesical mitomycin C therapy for superficial bladder cancer. Cancer Chemother Pharmacol 1993; 32: 255–62.

51. Atema A, Buurman KJ, Noteboom E, Smets LA. Potentiation of DNA-adduct formation and cytotoxicity of platinum-containing drugs by low pH. Int J Cancer 1993; 54: 166–72.

52. Pan SS, Yu F, Hipsher C. Enzymatic and pH modulation of mitomycin C-induced DNA damage in mitomycin C-resistant HCT 116 human colon cancer cells. Mol Pharmacol 1993; 43: 870–7.

53. Kennedy KA, McGurl JD, Leondaridis L, Alabaster O. pH dependence of mitomycin C-induced cross-linking activity in EMT6 tumor cells. Cancer Res 1985; 45: 3541–7.

54. Groos E, Walker L, Masters JR. Intravesical chemotherapy. Studies on the relationship between pH and cytotoxicity. Cancer 1986; 58: 1199–203.

55. Tolley DA, Parmar MK, Grigor KM, et al. The effect of intravesical mitomycin C on recurrence of newly diagnosed superficial bladder cancer: a further report with 7 years of follow up. J Urol 1996; 155: 1233–8.

56. Schwaibold H, Klingenberger HJ, Huland H. Long-term results of intravesical prevention of recurrence with mitomycin C and adriamycin in patients with superficial bladder cancer. Urologe A 1994; 33: 479–83.

57. Giesbers AA, van Helsdingen PJ, Kramer AE. Recurrence of superficial bladder carcinoma after intravesical instillation of mitomycin-C. Comparison of exposure times. Br J Urol 1989; 63: 176–9.

58. van Helsdingen PJ, Rikken CH, Sleeboom HP, de Bruyn EA, Tjaden UR. Mitomycin C resorption following repeated intravesical instillations using different instillation times. Urol Int 1988; 43: 42–6.

59. van der Meijden AP, Debruyne FM. Treatment schedule of intravesical chemotherapy with mitomycin C in superficial bladder cancer: short-term courses or maintenance therapy. Urology 1988; 31: 26–9.

60. Lum BL, Torti FM. Adjuvant intravesicular pharmacotherapy for superficial bladder cancer. J Natl Cancer Inst 1991; 83: 682–94.

61. Huland H, Otto U. Mitomycin instillation to prevent recurrence of superficial bladder carcinoma. Results of a controlled, prospective study in 58 patients. Eur Urol 1983; 9: 84–6.

62. Masters JR, Popert RJ, Thompson PM, Gibson D, Coptcoat MJ, Parmar MK. Intravesical chemotherapy with epirubicin: a dose response study. J Urol 1999; 161: 1490–3.

63. Rajala P, Kaasinen E, Raitanen M, Liukkonen T, Rintala E. Perioperative single dose instillation of epirubicin or interferon-alpha after transurethral resection for the prophylaxis of primary superficial bladder cancer recurrence: a prospective randomized multicenter study—FinnBladder III long-term results. J Urol 2002; 168: 981–5.

64. Bassi PF, Spinadin R, Carando R, et al. [Mitoxantrone chemoprophylaxis for multirecurrent multifocal superficial bladder tumours: results of a phase 2 controlled study.] Arch Ital Urol Androl 2003; 75: 202–4.

65. Huang JS, Chen WH, Lin CC, et al. A randomized trial comparing intravesical instillations of mitoxantrone and doxorubicin in patients with superficial bladder cancer. Chang Gung Med J 2003; 26: 91–7.

66. Papatsoris AG, Deliveliotis C, Giannopoulos A, Dimopoulos C. Adjuvant intravesical mitoxantrone versus recombinant interferon-alpha after transurethral resection of superficial bladder cancer: a randomized prospective study. Urol Int 2004; 72: 284–91.

67. Ikeda R, Chikazawa I, Kobayashi Y, et al. Prophylaxis of recurrence in superficial bladder carcinoma by intravesical chemotherapy—comparative study between instillation of combined double anticancer agents and single anticancer agent. Gan To Kagaku Ryoho 1999; 26: 509–14.

68. Kobayashi M, Sugaya Y, Yuzawa M, et al. [Appropriate intravesical retention time of pirarubicin concentration based on its level in tumor tissue, anti-tumor effect and side effect in intravesical instillation therapy for bladder tumor.] Gan To Kagaku Ryoho Cancer Chemother 1998; 25: 1771–4.

69. Miki T, Nonomura N, Kojima Y, et al. [A randomized study on intravesical pirarubicin (THP) chemoprophylaxis of recurrence after transurethral resection of superficial bladder cancer.] Hinyokika Kiyo Acta Urol Jpn 1997; 43: 907–12.

70. Okamura K, Ono Y, Kinukawa T, et al. Randomized study of single early instillation of (2′R)-4′-O-tetrahydropyranyl-doxorubicin for a single superficial bladder carcinoma. Cancer 2002; 94: 2363–8.

71. Tsushima T, Kobashi K, Akebi N, et al. Early phase II study of amrubicin (SM-5887) for superficial bladder cancer: a dose-finding study for intravesical chemotherapy. Gan To Kagaku Ryoho Cancer Chemother 2001; 28: 483–91.

72. Ohmori H, Yamato T, Asahi T. Phase I study of amrubicin hydrochloride (SM-5887) for superficial bladder cancer in intravesical chemotherapy. Gan To Kagaku Ryoho Cancer Chemother 2001; 28: 475–82.

73. Silber R, Liu LF, Israel M, et al. Metabolic activation of N-acylanthracyclines precedes their interaction with DNA topoisomerase II. NCI Monogr 1987; 4: 111–15.

74. Steinberg G, Bahnson R, Brosman S, Middleton R, Wajsman Z, Wehle M. Efficacy and safety of valrubicin for the treatment of Bacillus Calmette–Guérin refractory carcinoma in situ of the bladder. The Valrubicin Study Group. J Urol 2000; 163: 761–7.

75. USFDA. Valstar (Valrubicin) sterile solution for intravesical instillation: summary basis of approval equivalent. NDA 20-892. 1998. Online. Available: www.uiowa.edu/~idis/dap/valrubic.pdf.

76. Gofrit ON, Shapiro A, Pode D, et al. Combined local bladder hyperthermia and intravesical chemotherapy for the treatment of high-grade superficial bladder cancer. Urology 2004; 63: 466–71.

77. Colombo R, Da Pozzo LF, Lev A, et al. Local microwave hyperthermia and intravesical chemotherapy as bladder sparing treatment for select multifocal and unresectable superficial bladder tumors. J Urol 1998;159:783–787.

78. Di Stasi SM, Giannantoni A, Stephen RL, et al. Intravesical electromotive mitomycin C versus passive transport mitomycin C for high risk

superficial bladder cancer: a prospective randomized study. J Urol 2003; 170: 777–82.

79. Brausi M, Campo B, Pizzocaro G, et al. Intravesical electromotive administration of drugs for treatment of superficial bladder cancer: a comparative Phase II study. Urology 1998; 51: 506–9.

80. Phillips RM, Jaffar M, Maitland DJ, et al. Pharmacological and biological evaluation of a series of substituted 1,4-naphthoquinone bioreductive drugs. Biochem Pharmacol 2004; 68: 2107–16.

81. Choudry GA, Stewart PA, Double JA, et al. A novel strategy for NQO1 (NAD(P)H:quinone oxidoreductase, EC 1.6.99.2) mediated therapy of bladder cancer based on the pharmacological properties of EO9. Br J Cancer 2001; 85: 1137–46.

82. Palit V, Puri R, Shah T, Flanigan GM, Loadman PM, Phillips RM. Intravesical EUquin (EO9): a new treatment for superficial bladder cancer—results of phase I study [abstract]. Proc Br Assoc Urol Surg 2004; Poster 109.

83. Palou J, Carcas A, Segarra J, et al. Phase I pharmacokinetic study of a single intravesical instillation of gemcitabine administered immediately after transurethral resection plus multiple random biopsies in patients with superficial bladder cancer. J Urol 2004; 172: 485–8.

84. Witjes JA, van der Heijden AG, Vriesema JLJ, Peters GJ, Laan A, Schalken JA. Intravesical gemcitabine: a phase I and pharmacokinetic study. Eur Urol 2004; 45: 182–6.

85. De Berardinis E, Antonini G, Peters GJ, et al. Intravesical administration of gemcitabine in superficial bladder cancer: a phase I study with pharmacodynamic evaluation. BJU Int 2004; 93: 491–4.

86. Laufer M, Ramalingam S, Schoenberg MP, et al. Intravesical gemcitabine therapy for superficial transitional cell carcinoma of the bladder: a phase I and pharmacokinetic study. J Clin Oncol 2003; 21: 697–703.

87. Kubota Y, Noguchi S, Hosaka M. UFT in bladder cancer. Oncology 1999; 13: 112–15.

88. Hugosson J, Bergdahl S, Carlsson G, Frosing R, Norlen L, Gustavsson B. Effects of intravesical instillation of 5-fluorouracil and interferon in patients with recurrent superficial urinary bladder carcinoma. A clinical and pharmacodynamic study. Scand J Urol Nephrol 1997; 31: 343–7.

89. Naito S, Iguchi A, Sagiyama K, et al. Significance of the preoperative intravesical instillation of doxorubicin and the oral administration of 5-fluorouracil in preventing recurrence after a transurethral resection of superficial bladder cancer. Kyushu University Urological Oncology Group. Int J Urol Jpn 1997; 4: 352–7.

90. Friedrich MG, Erbersdobler A, Schwaibold H, Conrad S, Huland E, Huland H. Detection of loss of heterozygosity in the p53 tumor-suppressor gene with PCR in the urine of patients with bladder cancer. J Urol 2000; 163: 1039–42.

91. Cooke PW, James ND, Ganesan R, Burton A, Young LS, Wallace DM. Bcl-2 expression identifies patients with advanced bladder cancer treated by radiotherapy that benefit from neoadjuvant chemotherapy. BJU Int 2000; 85: 829–35.

92. Wu CS, Pollack A, Czerniak B, et al. Prognostic value of p53 in muscle-invasive bladder cancer treated with preoperative radiotherapy. Urology 1996; 47: 305–10.

93. Pfister C, Flaman JM, Dunet F, Grise P, Frebourg T. p53 mutations in bladder tumors inactivate the transactivation of the p21 and Bax genes, and have a predictive value for the clinical outcome after bacillus Calmette–Guérin therapy. J Urol 1999; 162: 69–73.

94. Bernardini S, Adessi GL, Billerey C, Chezy E, Carbillet JP, Bittard H. Immunohistochemical detection of p53 protein overexpression versus gene sequencing in urinary bladder carcinomas. J Urol 1999; 162: 1456–501.

95. Hayakawa K, Hasegawa M, Kawashima M, et al. Comparison of effects of doxorubicin and radiation on p53-dependent apoptosis in vivo. Oncol Rep 2000; 7: 267–70.

96. Sato S, Kigawa J, Minagawa Y, et al. Chemosensitivity and p53-dependent apoptosis in epithelial ovarian carcinoma. Cancer 1999; 86: 1307–13.

97. Lee TK, Lau TC, Ng IO. Doxorubicin-induced apoptosis and chemosensitivity in hepatoma cell lines. Cancer Chemother Pharmacol 2002; 49: 78–86.

98. Kawasaki T, Tomita Y, Bilim V, Takeda M, Takahashi K, Kumanishi T. Abrogation of apoptosis induced by DNA-damaging agents in human bladder-cancer cell lines with p21/WAF1/CIP1 and/or p53 gene alterations. Int J Cancer 1996; 68: 501–5.

99. Kuh HJ, Jang SH, Wientjes MG, Au JL. Computational model of intracellular pharmacokinetics of paclitaxel. J Pharmacol Exp Therap 2000; 293: 761–70.

100. Edelman MJ, Meyers FJ, Miller TR, Williams SG, Gandour-Edwards R, deVere White RW. Phase I/II study of paclitaxel, carboplatin, and methotrexate in advanced transitional cell carcinoma: a well-tolerated regimen with activity independent of p53 mutation. Urology 2000; 55: 521–5.

101. Lanni JS, Lowe SW, Licitra EJ, Liu JO, Jacks T. p53-independent apoptosis induced by paclitaxel through an indirect mechanism. Proc Natl Acad Sci USA 1997; 94: 9679–83.

102. Nemeyer I, Wientjes MG, Au JL. Cremophor reduces paclitaxel penetration into bladder wall during intravesical treatment. Cancer Chemother Pharmacol 1999; 44: 241–8.

103. Schoenfeld RH, Belville WD, Jacob WH, et al. The effect of dimethyl sulfoxide on the uptake of cisplatin from the urinary bladder of the dog: a pilot study. J Am Osteopath Assoc 1983; 82: 570–3.

104. See WA, Xia Q. Regional chemotherapy for bladder neoplasms using continuous intravesical infusion of doxorubicin: impact of concomitant administration of dimethyl sulfoxide on drug absorption and antitumor activity. J Natl Cancer Inst 1992; 84: 510–15.

105. Lu Z, Yeh TK, Tsai M, Au JL, Wientjes MG. Paclitaxel-loaded gelatin nanoparticles for intravesical bladder cancer therapy. Clin Cancer Res 2004; 10: 7677–84.

106. Bonfil RD, Gonzalez AD, Siguelboim D, et al. Immunohistochemical analysis of Ki-67, p21waf1/cip1 and apoptosis in marker lesions from patients with superficial bladder tumours treated with vinorelbine intravesical therapy in a preliminary phase I trial. BJU Int 2001; 88: 425–31.

107. Bilen CY, Ozen H, Aki FT, Aygun C, Ekici S, Kendi S. Clinical experience with BCG alone versus BCG plus epirubicin. Int J Urol Jpn 2000; 7: 206–9.

108. Jones P, Vogelzang N, Gomez J. Priorities of the kidney/bladder cancers progress review group, NCI. 2002. Online. Available: http://prg.nci.nih.gov/kidney/finalreport.html.

109. Bellmunt J, Hussain M, Dinney CP. Novel approaches with targeted therapies in bladder cancer. Therapy of bladder cancer by blockade of the epidermal growth factor receptor family. Crit Rev Oncol Hematol 2003; 46(Suppl): S85–104.

110. Bue P, Holmberg AR, Marquez M, Westlin JE, Nilsson S, Malmstrom PU. Intravesical administration of EGF-dextran conjugates in patients with superficial bladder cancer. Eur Urol 2000; 38: 584–9.

111. Garcia del Muro X, Condom E, Vigues F, et al. p53 and p21 expression levels predict organ preservation and survival in invasive bladder carcinoma treated with a combined-modality approach. Cancer 2004; 100: 1859–67.

112. Cordon-Cardo C. p53 and RB: simple interesting correlates or tumor markers of critical predictive nature? J Clin Oncol 2004; 22: 975–7.

113. Chatterjee SJ, Datar R, Youssefzadeh D, et al. Combined effects of p53, p21, and pRb expression in the progression of bladder transitional cell carcinoma. J Clin Oncol 2004; 22: 1007–13.

114. Shariat SF, Tokunaga H, Zhou J, et al. p53, p21, pRB, and p16 expression predict clinical outcome in cystectomy with bladder cancer. J Clin Oncol 2004; 22: 1014–24.

115. Pan CX, Koeneman KS. A novel tumor-specific gene therapy for bladder cancer. Med Hypotheses 1999; 53: 130–5.

116. Graham SD Jr, Napalkov P, Oladele A, et al. Intravesical suramin in the prevention of transitional cell carcinoma. Urology 1995; 45: 59–63.

117. Uchio EM, Linehan WM, Figg WD, Walther MM. A phase I study of intravesical suramin for the treatment of superficial transitional cell carcinoma of the bladder. J Urol 2003; 169: 357–60.

118. Song S, Wientjes MG, Gan Y, Au JL. Fibroblast growth factors: an epigenetic mechanism of broad spectrum resistance to anticancer drugs. Proc Natl Acad Sci USA 2000; 97: 8658–63.

119. Song S, Wientjes MG, Walsh C, Au JL. Nontoxic doses of suramin enhance activity of paclitaxel against lung metastases. Cancer Res 2001; 61: 6145–50.

120. Song S, Yu B, Wei Y, Wientjes MG, Au JL. Low-dose suramin enhanced paclitaxel activity in chemotherapy-naive and paclitaxel-pretreated human breast xenograft tumors. Clin Cancer Res 2004; 10: 6058–65.

121. Zhang Y, Song S, Yang F, Au JL, Wientjes MG. Nontoxic doses of suramin enhance activity of doxorubicin in prostate tumors. J Pharmacol Exp Therap 2001; 299: 426–33.

122. Zhao L, Wientjes MG, Au JLS. Enhancement of antitumor activity of paclitaxel by suramin: unconventional dose–response relationship [abstract]. Proc Am Assoc Cancer Res 2002; 43: 953.

123. Villalona-Calero MA, Otterson GA, Wientjes MG, et al. Phase II evaluation of low dose suramin as a modulator of paclitaxel/carboplatin (P/C) in non-small cell lung cancer (NSCLC) patients [abstract]. Lung Cancer 2003; 41(Suppl 2): 149.

124. Villalona-Calero MA, Wientjes MG, Otterson GA, et al. Phase I study of low-dose suramin as a chemosensitizer in patients with advanced non-small lung cancer. Clin Cancer Res 2003; 9: 3303–11.

125. Xin Y, Chen D, Song S-H, Lyness G, Wientjes MG, Au JL. Low-dose suramin enhances antitumor activity of mitomycin C in bladder tumors [abstract]. Proc Am Assoc Cancer Res 2004; 45: 461.

126. O'Brien TS, Smith K, Cranston D, Fuggle S, Bicknell R, Harris AL. Urinary basic fibroblast growth factor in patients with bladder cancer and benign prostatic hypertrophy. Br J Urol 1995;76: 311–14.

127. Izawa JI, Slaton JW, Kedar D, et al. Differential expression of progression-related genes in the evolution of superficial to invasive transitional cell carcinoma of the bladder. Oncol Rep 2001; 8: 9–15.

128. Munro NP, Knowles MA. Fibroblast growth factors and their receptors in transitional cell carcinoma. J Urol 2003; 169: 675–82.

129. Allen LE, Maher PA. Expression of basic fibroblast growth factor and its receptor in an invasive bladder carcinoma cell line. J Cell Physiol 1993; 155: 368–75.

130. Miyake H, Hara I, Gohji K, Yoshimura K, Arakawa S, Kamidono S. Expression of basic fibroblast growth factor is associated with resistance to cisplatin in a human bladder cancer cell line. Cancer Letters 1998; 123: 121–6.

131. Gan Y, Mo Y, Kalns JE, et al. Expression of DT-diaphorase and cytochrome P450 reductase correlates with mitomycin C activity in human bladder tumors. Clin Cancer Res 2001; 7: 1313–19.

132. Li D, Gan Y, Wientjes MG, Badalament RA, Au JL. Distribution of DT-diaphorase and reduced nicotinamide adenine dinucleotide phosphate: cytochrome p450 oxidoreductase in bladder tissues and tumors. J Urol 2001; 166: 2500–5.

5

Intravesical immunotherapy: BCG

Lori A Pinke, Donald L Lamm

Introduction

Bacille Calmette–Guérin (BCG), a live attenuated vaccine developed against tuberculosis in 1921, is currently the most effective intravesical therapy for bladder cancer. Pearl observed that those patients with tuberculosis had significantly fewer malignancies compared with a control group. He proposed an antineoplastic effect of tuberculosis infection in 1929.[1] The use of BCG in the treatment of bladder tumors was first reported by Morales in 1976. Administration of both intradermal and intravesical Armand Frappier BCG for 6 weeks decreased the rate of tumor recurrence. As previously demonstrated in animal models, he found that limited tumor load was a crucial factor in determining the effectiveness of BCG therapy because patients with limited metastatic disease did not demonstrate remission.[2]

The first controlled trial confirming the efficacy of intravesical BCG for prophylaxis was reported by Lamm and colleagues in 1980. Thirty-seven patients were randomized to either surgical resection or resection plus intravesical and percutaneous BCG therapy. The recurrence rate after 1 year was 22% in patients receiving BCG after tumor resection, significantly lower than the 42% recurrence rate in those receiving resection alone ($p=0.01$).[3] Early trials also showed a role for BCG in the treatment of residual disease after surgical resection. Tumor regression was seen in 59% of patients that were incompletely resected and then received weekly doses of intravesical and intradermal BCG for 6 weeks.[4] Subsequent controlled trials comparing surgical resection alone to resection and adjuvant BCG treatment demonstrated significantly lower recurrence rates when patients received BCG. These results are summarized in Table 5.1.

These early studies established BCG as a therapeutic agent in the treatment and prevention of recurrent bladder tumors. This chapter will summarize the use of BCG in carcinoma in situ (CIS), Ta and T1 transitional cell carcinoma (TCC). Its efficacy will be compared to other standard intravesical agents. Practical issues such as dosage schedules and treatment of toxicity will be described. Finally, recent work on optimization of BCG dosing, including dose reduction and maintenance dosing, will be reviewed.

Treatment indications

Carcinoma in situ has been shown to have a high rate of progression to muscle-invasive disease, with rates ranging from 50% to 83% in long-term studies.[5–8] Intravesical immunotherapy with BCG has a major impact on this high-risk pathology with complete response rates in the range of 70% with six instillations and 84% with an additional three instillations at 3 months.[9] Brosman demonstrated a complete response rate of 94% and recurrence rate of 13% using induction and an 18-month maintenance regimen with an average of 5.25 years' follow-up.[10] Patients with a complete response have a durable response as well: 65% may remain disease-free for 5 years or more.[11,12] Due to these impressive results, BCG is regarded as the best initial therapy for treatment of residual CIS and prophylaxis for recurrence and progression.

Nonmuscle-invasive TCC (Ta, T1) is another clinical situation in which recurrence and progression rates may be modified by intravesical BCG. The risk of recurrence after initial resection is 80% in patients with Ta or T1 tumors that were followed for a minimum of 20 years.[13] A subset of patients within this group are at highest risk, namely those with large, multiple, poorly differentiated tumors or concurrent CIS.

Management of T1 grade 3 tumors is particularly challenging since as much as 30% of patients may be understaged.[14] If treated with transurethral resection (TUR) alone, 50% to 80% may develop recurrences. Several nonrandomized BCG studies have shown efficacy in recurrence and progression prevention, and in disease-specific death rates. Pansadoro et al found a recurrence rate of 28% and a progression rate of 12% with a disease-specific death rate of 2% at 5 years.[15] These patients received 6 weeks of induction BCG with 3 months of maintenance. Hurle et al also demonstrated success in this patient group. Patients received induction and then monthly maintenance for 1 year. The recurrence rate was 23.5%, progression rate 13.7%, and disease-specific death rate 11.8%.[16] The management of patients with T1 grade 3 tumors is discussed in detail in Chapter 6.

Special Circumstances

Prostatic urethral involvement with CIS or TCC needs to be differentiated from stromal invasion as the latter situation holds no

Table 5.1 Controlled BCG trials: percent tumor recurrence

Lead author	No. pts	No BCG (%)	BCG (%)	p Value
Lamm[42]	57	52	20	<0.001
Herr[43]	86	95	42	<0.001
Herr[44]	49	100	35	<0.001
Yamamoto[45]	44	67	17	<0.05
Pagano[27]	133	83	26	<0.001
Melekos[46]	94	59	32	<0.02
Krege[47]	224	48	29	<0.05

role for BCG. Limited non-invasive urethral involvement may, however, be managed with BCG, with or without TUR. Orihuela and colleagues demonstrated that 86% of patients with mucosal involvement of the prostatic urethra had a sustained complete response in both the prostate and the bladder. They suggest that transurethral resection of the prostate (TURP) plays a crucial role by facilitating the immune response to BCG in the prostate.[17] Other authors demonstrated a local response rate of 56% to 83% in small series with limited follow-up.[18–20] BCG is a reasonable option for patients with non-invasive disease in the prostatic urethra, but care must be taken to exclude stromal involvement using staging TURP.

BCG has applications in the treatment of upper tract TCC. While the standard of care in this situation is nephroureterectomy, situations such as a solitary kidney or significant renal impairment raise the desire for preservation of the renal unit. Many different techniques have been reported. Percutaneous resection coupled with antegrade BCG administration can be accomplished after the nephrostomy tract is well established and shows no evidence of extravasation.[21] BCG can be delivered in a retrograde manner after endoscopic resection of the ureteral orifice and placement of a ureteral stent, with subsequent intravesical BCG instillation.[22] A cystogram should be done to confirm that reflux reaches the tumor site and to determine the volume in which BCG must be delivered. (*Editor's note*: Alternatively, a single J stent can be passed suprapubically, providing convenient access to the upper tract [P. Schulam, personal communication].) A limited series of patients with solitary renal units was treated with percutaneous and ureteroscopic tumor resection and subsequent BCG; 5 of 10 were alive at 24 months with no evidence of disease.[23] Patients following this course of treatment for upper tract disease should be counseled that the price paid for preserved renal function is the risk of progressive disease.

Patient Selection

As the previous examples demonstrate, BCG is a therapeutic option in a number of clinical scenarios. Proper patient selection serves to identify those that will benefit most from intravesical therapy. Primary low-grade Ta disease does not necessarily require additional intravesical therapy, though controlled trials and meta-analysis show that recurrence can be reduced with a single postoperative chemotherapy instillation.[24] However, if other risk factors for progression—such as multifocality, prior recurrence, large tumors, high tumor grade or lamina propria invasion—are present, immunotherapy is indicated. Stage T1 TCC carries a high recurrence rate, which may be minimized with prophylactic BCG after resection. It is well recognized that the presence of CIS poses high risk, and BCG is effective for both treatment and prophylaxis.

The success of BCG immunotherapy depends on several factors:

1. Bladder tumor burden should be minimized through transurethral resection. Murine model studies have shown improved response with cell volumes less than 10^3 cells.
2. BCG and the remaining tumor cells must be in juxtaposition. Tumor sites away from the area of instillation may not respond.[25]
3. Success requires an immunocompetent host. Patients must be able to mount a local or systemic inflammatory response.

Dose Optimization

Murine bladder tumor models have been used to evaluate immunotherapeutic agents and optimize dosing. Lamm et al reported on a series of experiments in which varying doses of BCG strains, including Tice, Pasteur, and Glaxo, were administered to mice with previously excised bladder tumors. The dose–response curve with survival as the endpoint was bell shaped. The antitumor effect peaked at a dose of 10^7 colony-forming units, with higher doses actually decreasing the antitumor response. The presumed mechanism for this is diversion of the immune response from the tumor to BCG or impairment of the immune response due to antigenic excess.[26]

These early mouse studies set the stage for subsequent human trials to investigate the effect of dose reduction. A low dose regimen utilizing BCG Pasteur strain, 75 mg, was compared to the higher dose of 150 mg. A 6-week induction course was given, followed by a 2-year maintenance course for all responders. The time-to-failure curves showed a disease-free interval significantly higher in the low dose group compared to the high dose group (p = 0.0009). Progression rates were similar. An additional benefit of low dose therapy is a reduction in side effects such as cystitis. The low dose regimen had a significantly lower (p < 0.05) level of side effects compared to high dose.[27] Other researchers have confirmed the benefits of reduced doses, in doses ranging from 30 to 75 mg.[28,29]

There is an increasing body of work to suggest that maintenance therapy is another way to maximize the effectiveness of BCG. Southwest Oncology Group (SWOG) Trial 8795 randomized patients to either 50 mg Tice BCG or 20 mg mitomycin C (MMC) weekly for 6 weeks and then monthly for 1 year. The recurrence-free survival was significantly prolonged (p = 0.017 proportional hazard regression) in patients receiving BCG compared to MMC.[30]

SWOG 8507 evaluated toxicity, recurrence, progression, and survival when patients with CIS or high risk TCC received either induction BCG or induction and maintenance BCG. Induction consisted of 120 mg Connaught BCG intravesically and 10^7 colony-forming units percutaneously weekly for 6 weeks. Maintenance arm patients were treated with sets of three successive weekly intravesical and percutaneous administrations of BCG at 3 months, 6 months, and every 6 months thereafter for a total of 3 years. Median recurrence-free survival was 35.7 months in the induction group versus 76.8 months in the maintenance group (log rank, p < 0.0001). The median progression-free survival was 111.5 months without maintenance, and had not been reached with over 10-years' follow-up in the maintenance arm (log rank, p = 0.04). The overall 5-year survival was 78% in the induction group compared to 83% in the maintenance group, which was not statistically significant.[9]

This treatment regimen has been described as the '6 + 3' plan. The three weekly maintenance doses are crucial, because a number greater than that has a depressant effect on the immune response. During the maintenance instillations, the immune stimulation peaks at 3 weeks and may be suppressed with subsequent instillations.[31]

The suppression seen with subsequent doses may account for the lack of success seen in Palou et al's trial. This study randomized patients to a control group receiving 6-week induction alone or a maintenance group receiving an additional six instillations every 6 months (6×6) for a 2-year period. There was no significant difference in recurrence or progression compared to controls.[32]

Maintenance therapy is certainly one of the important recent topics in BCG. It seems to offer a number of advantages over traditional induction-only therapy. Immunostimulation wanes with time, and maintenance therapy serves to 'boost' the immune response. Furthermore, since TCC is a field change disease, the patient's entire urothelium remains at risk for the course of their life. Maintenance therapy maximizes the immune surveillance over the long term.

BCG dosing

Early BCG protocols consisted of weekly instillations of 120 mg BCG for 6 weeks. This was accompanied by an intradermal injection using the Tine or multiple puncture technique. Percutaneous injection was initiated after preliminary studies failed to demonstrate skin test conversion after only intravesical instillation. In a randomized trial, maintenance BCG had an equivalent efficacy for recurrence prevention compared to percutaneous and intravesical BCG.[33] Additional early studies for treatment of CIS showed complete response rates of 68% to 100% with intravesical BCG alone.[10,34,35]

There are currently a number of BCG strains commercially available. All of these are derived from the initial strain developed at the Pasteur Institute. Commonly used strains include Connaught, Pasteur, Tice, Armand Frappier, and Tokyo. While the individual doses for each strain may vary, their efficacy is comparable. Complete response rates in the treatment of CIS range from 60% to 79%.[12]

Efficacy

Intravesical chemotherapy is effective in the prevention of tumor recurrences. Comparative studies with BCG established its superiority to thiotepa, epirubicin, and doxorubicin in the prevention of recurrence (Table 5.2).

Bohle and Bock's recent meta-analysis of BCG and mitomycin demonstrated a 34% risk reduction of progression with maintenance BCG compared to mitomycin.[36] This benefit was not seen with induction-only dosing.

Recently, several large meta-analyses have demonstrated the advantages of maintenance BCG. Bohle et al compared BCG to MMC on recurrence of stages Ta and T1 TCC. BCG versus MMC had a 44% reduction in recurrence (p=0.005). This superiority was even more profound when maintenance BCG was used. There was a 57% reduction in recurrence with maintenance compared to MMC

(p < 0.001). Toxicity did not differ significantly between the BCG maintenance and nonmaintenance groups.[37]

A meta-analysis has also been applied to the effect of BCG and MMC on progression of TCC. There was no significant difference for the odd ratios for recurrence when BCG was compared to MMC. However, when maintenance BCG was used, there was a 34% reduction in progression compared to MMC (p=0.02).[36] Sylvester et al's meta-analysis also supports the finding that progression of TCC can be reduced with maintenance BCG. Patients receiving maintenance BCG had a 37% decrease in the odds of progression compared to controls (p = 0.001).[38]

Toxicity

Many patients receiving BCG immunotherapy will experience some level of toxicity, either local or systemic. Preventive measures, early diagnosis, and appropriate treatment will limit adverse outcomes.

Irritative bladder symptoms such as cystitis may occur in 90% of patients.[39] Incidence of other local symptoms includes hematuria (43%), low-grade fever (29%), malaise (24%), and nausea (5%). These often occur after the third treatment as the patient's immune response peaks. Patients experiencing irritative symptoms are more likely to have them after subsequent treatments.[40] It is advisable to delay subsequent BCG treatments until symptoms resolve. If the symptoms persist for more than 48 hours or are accompanied by fever or malaise, treatment with 300 mg isoniazid daily is recommended, and consideration should be given to adding a fluoroquinolone to reduce the risk of developing isoniazid resistance. This should be continued while symptoms persist and may be reinstituted 1 day before subsequent treatments and continued for 3 days afterward.[41]

In contrast to local toxicity, systemic toxicity is far less frequent. High fever (>103°F/39.4°C) occurs in 3% of patients.[39] Because of the possibility of BCG sepsis, it is recommended that these patients be hospitalized and treated with isoniazid 300 mg and rifampin 600 mg daily. BCG is also sensitive to fluoroquinolones. These drugs, which act more quickly and also treat common gram-negative urinary infections, are most useful.

The most serious side effect of BCG therapy is sepsis. It occurs in 0.4% of patients and is commonly associated with intravascular absorption of the organism.[39] This could happen with administration following a traumatic urethral catheterization, during severe cystitis, or immediately after bladder biopsy. BCG instillation should be initiated at least 1 week after bladder tumor resection.

In a patient suspected of having BCG sepsis, attention should also be directed to the possibility of gram-negative sepsis. Treatment should cover both possibilities until final culture results are available, remembering that mycobacterial cultures are frequently negative, even in the presence of BCG infection. Initial treatment includes isoniazid 300 mg, rifampin 600 mg, and ethambutol 1200 mg daily, plus a fluoroquinolone or an aminoglycoside. If symptoms fail to respond or progress, prednisone 40 mg daily may be required to reduce the hypersensitivity response. Prednisone in this setting may be life saving and higher doses may be needed depending on the patient's symptoms. The steroid is slowly tapered when the patient improves, but may be reinstituted if symptoms recur after the taper. Patients with documented BCG sepsis should receive the triple-antibiotic treatment for 3–6 months. Additional BCG treatment is contraindicated.

Table 5.2 BCG versus chemotherapy: percent tumor recurrence

Lead author	BCG	Chemotherapy	p Value
Thiotepa			
Brosman[48]	0	47	<0.01
Rodrigues Netto[49]	7	43	<0.01
Martinez-Pineiro[50]	13	36	<0.01
Doxorubicin			
Lamm[11]	53	78	<0.02
Martinez-Pineiro[50]	13	43	<0.01
Sekine[51]	24	42	<0.05
Epirubicin			
Van der Meijden[52]	33	47	<0.0001

Preventive measures can help to limit some of the toxicity. BCG instillation is deferred if symptoms from the previous treatment persist or if catheterization is bloody or traumatic. Log dose reduction (1/3, 1/10, 1/30, 1/100th) prevents increasing side effects. These side effects are not required to receive the benefits of maintenance BCG.

Conclusion

BCG has been shown to have excellent success in the prophylaxis and treatment of CIS. Its use is expanding as high-risk groups are identified and stratified by prognostic factors. These highest risk categories are the ones that will benefit most from further refinements in BCG dosing. An already efficacious treatment can be improved as its mechanism is further elucidated and the principles of immunity followed. Maintenance therapy is the culmination of this knowledge to date.

References

1. Pearl R. Cancer and tuberculosis. Proc Natl Acad Sci 1929; 9: 97.
2. Morales A. Intracavitary bacillus Calmette–Guérin in the treatment of superficial bladder tumors. J Urol 1976; 116(2): 180–183.
3. Lamm DL, Thor DE, Harris SC, Reyna JA, Stogdill VD, Radwin HM. Bacillus Calmette–Guérin immunotherapy of superficial bladder cancer. J Urol 1980; 124(1): 38–40.
4. Morales A, Ottenhof P, Emerson L. Treatment of residual, non-infiltrating bladder cancer with bacillus Calmette–Guérin. J Urol 1981; 125(5): 649–51.
5. Utz DC, Hanash KA, Farrow GM. The plight of the patient with carcinoma in situ of the bladder. J Urol 1970; 103(2): 160–64.
6. Skinner DG, Richie JP, Cooper PH, Waisman J, Kaufman JJ. The clinical significance of carcinoma in situ of the bladder and its association with overt carcinoma. J Urol 1974; 112(1): 68–71.
7. Starklint H, Jensen NK, Thyro E. The extent of carcinoma in situ in urinary bladders with primary carcinomas. Acta Pathol Microbiol Scand: Section A, Pathology 1976; 84(2): 130–36.
8. Herr HW. Carcinoma in situ of the bladder. Semin Urol 1983; 1(1): 15–22.
9. Lamm DL, Blumenstein BA, Crissman JD, et al. Maintenance bacillus Calmette–Guérin immunotherapy for recurrent TA, T1 and carcinoma in situ transitional cell carcinoma of the bladder: a randomized Southwest Oncology Group Study. J Urol 2000; 163(4): 1124–9.
10. Brosman SA. The use of bacillus Calmette–Guérin in the therapy of bladder carcinoma in situ. J Urol 1985; 134(1): 36–9.
11. Lamm DL, Blumenstein BA, Crawford ED, et al. A randomized trial of intravesical doxorubicin and immunotherapy with bacille Calmette–Guérin for transitional-cell carcinoma of the bladder. N Engl J Med 1991; 325(17): 1205–9.
12. Lamm DL. BCG immunotherapy for transitional-cell carcinoma in situ of the bladder. Oncology 1995; 9(10): 947–52.
13. Holmang S, Hedelin H, Anderstrom C. The relationship among multiple recurrences and prognosis of patients with stages Ta and T1 TCC of the bladder followed for at least 20 years. J Urol 1995; 153(6): 1923–6.
14. Pagano F, Bassi P, Galetti TP, et al. Results of contemporary radical cystectomy for invasive bladder cancer: a clinicopathologic study with an emphasis on the inadequacy of the tumor, nodes and metastases classification. J Urol 1991; 145(1): 45–50.
15. Pansadoro V, Emiliozzi P, Defidio L, et al. Bacillus Calmette–Guérin in the treatment of stage T1 grade 3 transitional cell carcinoma of the bladder: long-term results. J Urol 1995; 154(6): 2054–8.
16. Hurle R, Losa A, Ranieri A, Graziotti P, Lembo A. Low dose Pasteur bacillus Calmette–Guérin regimen in stage T1, grade 3 bladder cancer therapy. J Urol 1996; 156(5): 1602–5.
17. Orihuela E, Herr HW, Whitmore WF Jr. Conservative treatment of superficial transitional cell carcinoma of prostatic urethra with intravesical BCG. Urology 1989; 34(5): 231–7.
18. Bretton PR, Herr HW, Whitmore WF Jr, et al. Intravesical bacillus Calmette–Guérin therapy for in situ transitional cell carcinoma involving the prostatic urethra. J Urol 1989; 141(4): 853–6.
19. Schellhammer PF, Ladaga LE, Moriarty RP. Intravesical bacillus Calmette–Guérin for the treatment of superficial transitional cell carcinoma of the prostatic urethra in association with carcinoma of the bladder. J Urol 1995; 153(1): 53–6.
20. Palou J, Xavier B, Laguna P, Montello M, Vicente J. In situ transitional cell carcinoma involvement of prostatic urethra: bacillus Calmette–Guérin therapy without previous transurethral resection of the prostate. Urology 1996; 47(4): 482–4.
21. Streem SB. Percutaneous management of upper-tract transitional cell carcinoma. Urol Clin North Am 1995; 22(1): 221–9.
22. Bohle A, Schuller J, Knipper A, Hofstetter A. Bacillus Calmette–Guérin treatment and vesicorenal reflux. Eur Urol 1990; 17(2): 125–8.
23. Schoenberg MP, Van Arsdalen KN, Wein AJ. The management of transitional cell carcinoma in solitary renal units. J Urol 1991; 146: 700–703.
24. Sylvester R, Oosterlinck W, van der Meijden AP. A single immediate postoperative instillation of chemotherapy decreases the risk of recurrence in patients with stage TaT1 bladder cancer: a meta-analysis of published results of randomized clinical trials. J Urol 2004; 171(6 Pt 1): 2786–90.
25. Lamm DL, DeHaven JI, Shriver J, Crispen R, Grau D, Sarosdy MF. A randomized prospective comparison of oral versus intravesical and percutaneous bacillus Calmette–Guérin for superficial bladder cancer. J Urol 1990; 144(1): 65–7.
26. Lamm DL, Reichert DF, Harris SC, Lucio RM. Immunotherapy of murine transitional cell carcinoma. J Urol 1982; 128(5): 1104–8.
27. Pagano F, Bassi P, Milani C, Meneghini A, Maruzzi D, Garbeglio A. A low dose bacillus Calmette–Guérin regimen in superficial bladder cancer therapy: is it effective? J Urol 1991; 146(1): 32–5.
28. Lebret T, Gaudez F, Herve JM, Barre P, Lugagne PM, Botto H. Low-dose BCG instillations in the treatment of stage T1 grade 3 bladder tumours: recurrence, progression and success. Eur Urol 1998; 34(1): 67–72.
29. Mack D, Holtl W, Bassi P, et al. The ablative effect of quarter dose bacillus Calmette–Guérin on a papillary marker lesion of the bladder. J Urol 2001; 165(2): 401–3.
30. Lamm D, Blumenstein B, Crawford ED, et al. Randomized intergroup comparison of Bacillus Calmette–Guérin immunotherapy and mitomycin C chemotherapy prophylaxis in superficial transitional cell carcinoma of the bladder. Urol Oncol 1995; 1: 119–26.
31. de Boer EC, De Jong WH, Steerenberg PA, Aarder LA. Induction of urinary interleukin-1 (IL-1), IL-2, IL-6, and tumor necrosis factor during immunotherapy with bacillus Calmette–Guérin in superficial bladder cancer. Cancer Immunol Immunother 1992; 34(5): 306–12.
32. Palou J, Laguna P, Millan-Rodriguez F, Hall RR, Salvador-Bayarri J, Vicente-Rodriguez J. Control group and maintenance treatment with bacillus Calmette–Guérin for carcinoma in situ and/or high grade bladder tumors. J Urol 2001; 165(5): 1488–91.
33. Lamm DL, DeHaven JI, Shriver J, Sarosdy MF. Prospective randomized comparison of intravesical with percutaneous bacillus Calmette–Guérin versus intravesical bacillus Calmette–Guérin in superficial bladder cancer. J Urol 1991; 145(4): 738–40.
34. deKernion JB, Huang MY, Lindner A, Smith RB, Kaufman JJ. The management of superficial bladder tumors and carcinoma in situ with intravesical bacillus Calmette–Guérin. J Urol 1985; 133(4): 598–601.
35. Schellhammer PF, Ladaga LE, Fillion MB. Bacillus Calmette–Guérin for superficial transitional cell carcinoma of the bladder. J Urol 1986; 135(2): 261–4.

36. Bohle A, Bock PR. Intravesical bacille Calmette–Guérin versus mitomycin C in superficial bladder cancer: formal meta-analysis of comparative studies on tumor progression. Urology 2004; 63(4): 682–7.

37. Bohle A, Jocham D, Bock PR. Intravesical bacillus Calmette–Guérin versus mitomycin C for superficial bladder cancer: a formal meta-analysis of comparative studies on recurrence and toxicity. J Urol 2003; 169(1): 90–95.

38. Sylvester RJ, van der MA, Lamm DL. Intravesical bacillus Calmette–Guérin reduces the risk of progression in patients with superficial bladder cancer: a meta-analysis of the published results of randomized clinical trials. J Urol 2002; 168(5): 1964–70.

39. Lamm DL, van der Meijden PM, Morales A, et al. Incidence and treatment of complications of bacillus Calmette–Guérin intravesical therapy in superficial bladder cancer. J Urol 1992; 147(3): 596–600.

40. Berry DL, Blumenstein BA, Magyary DL, Lamm DL, Crawford ED. Local toxicity patterns associated with intravesical bacillus Calmette–Guérin: a Southwest Oncology Group Study. Int J Urol 1996; 3(2): 98–100.

41. Lamm DL. Complications of bacillus Calmette–Guérin immunotherapy. Urol Clin North Am 1992; 19(3): 565–72.

42. Lamm DL. Bacillus Calmette–Guérin immunotherapy for bladder cancer. J Urol 1985; 134(1): 40–47.

43. Herr HW, Pinsky CM, Whitmore WF Jr, Sogani PG, Oettgen HF, Melamed MR. Experience with intravesical bacillus Calmette–Guérin therapy of superficial bladder tumors. Urology 1985; 25(2): 119–23.

44. Herr HW, Pinsky CM, Whitmore WF Jr, Sogani PC, Oettgen HF, Melamed MR. Long-term effect of intravesical bacillus Calmette–Guérin on flat carcinoma in situ of the bladder. J Urol 1986; 135(2): 265–7.

45. Yamamoto T, Hagiwara M, Nakazono M, Yamamoto H. [Intravesical bacillus Calmette–Guérin (BCG) in the treatment of superficial bladder cancer. Prospective randomized study for prophylactic effect.] Nippon Hinyokika Gakkai Zasshi—Jpn J Urol 1990; 81(7): 997–1001.

46. Melekos MD, Chionis H, Pantazakos A, Fokaefs E, Paranychianakis G, Dauaher H. Intravesical bacillus Calmette–Guérin immunoprophylaxis of superficial bladder cancer: results of a controlled prospective trial with modified treatment schedule. J Urol 1993; 149(4): 744–8.

47. Krege S, Giani G, Meyer R, Otto T, Rubben H. A randomized multicenter trial of adjuvant therapy in superficial bladder cancer: transurethral resection only versus transurethral resection plus mitomycin C versus transurethral resection plus bacillus Calmette–Guérin. J Urol 1996; 156(3): 962–6.

48. Brosman SA. Experience with bacillus Calmette–Guérin in patients with superficial bladder carcinoma. J Urol 1982; 128(1): 27–30.

49. Rodrigues Netto Junior N, Lemos GC. A comparison of treatment methods for the prophylaxis of recurrent superficial bladder tumors. J Urol 1983; 129(1): 33–4.

50. Martinez-Pineiro JA, Jimenez Leon J, Martinez-Pineiro L Jr, et al. Bacillus Calmette–Guérin versus doxorubicin versus thiotepa: a randomized prospective study in 202 patients with superficial bladder cancer. J Urol 1990; 143(3): 502–6.

51. Sekine H, Fukui I, Yamada T, Ohwada F, Yokokawa M, Ohshima H. Intravesical mitomycin C and doxorubicin sequential therapy for carcinoma in situ of the bladder: a longer followup result. J Urol 1994; 151(1): 27–30.

52. van der Meijden AP, Brausi M, Zambon V, et al. Intravesical instillation of epirubicin, bacillus Calmette–Guérin and bacillus Calmette–Guérin plus isoniazid for intermediate and high risk Ta, T1 papillary carcinoma of the bladder: a European Organisation for Research and Treatment of Cancer genito-urinary group randomized phase III trial. J Urol 2001; 166(2): 476–89.

6

G3T1 bladder carcinoma

Vito Pansadoro, Paolo Emiliozzi

Introduction

High-grade superficial bladder cancer infiltrating the lamina propria (G3T1) is an extremely malignant disease. Although it is superficial, it is very aggressive, with a high incidence of recurrence and progression to muscle-invasive disease. Though the optimal treatment is still controversial, a first line conservative approach is advocated today by most authors.[1]

Incidence

High-grade superficial bladder cancer accounts for 5% to 23% of all superficial transitional cell carcinomas of the bladder at first diagnosis, in several different series (Table 6.1).

Staging

Transurethral resection (TUR) is the most reliable procedure for clinical local staging of bladder cancer, and any treatment modality is based upon the pathology specimen obtained at TUR. However, up to 44% to 46% of patients with T1 transitional cell carcinoma of the bladder at TUR are understaged when subsequent cystectomy is performed.[15,16]

Substaging of T1 bladder cancer refers to invasion above and below the muscularis mucosae (T1A and T1B) or, alternatively, invasion above, at the level of, and below the muscularis mucosae (T1A, T1B and T1C).[17] However, a literature review showed that most series do not reveal a significant difference in terms of recurrence and progression on follow-up of substaged groups.[18] Whether or not to maintain this subclassification remains a controversial topic. No clear prognostic value can be attributed to substaging of T1 bladder cancer (Table 6.2).

Staging may also show large discrepancies due to different interpretations of the pathologic specimen. In a pathology review of 1400 TUR specimens, only 46% of 88 G3T1 tumors were confirmed, and 10% of cases were reclassified as muscle-infiltrating tumors.[22] In yet another multicenter study, the review pathologist found that 16/54 (29%) bladder cancers initially classified as G3T1 tumors were of lower grade, while 25 bladder cancers (previously classified as lower stage) were reclassified as G3T1.[23]

To reduce the risk of staging inaccuracies, interpretation of the TUR specimen should be done by an experienced pathologist with extensive experience with urothelial cancer.

Transurethral resection

Adequate TUR is essential for the treatment of superficial bladder cancer. The technique and findings of TUR can affect proper cure and local staging of bladder cancer. When no muscle is found in the specimen after TUR for T1 bladder cancer, up to 49% of cases may be found to have muscle-infiltrating tumors at the time of the second TUR.[24] To avoid the risk of understaging and/or leaving residual tumor behind, several authors have proposed a second TUR for stage T1 bladder cancers, especially when the tumor is high grade. Infiltrating tumor is present in 4% to 28% of patients at second TUR for G3T1 bladder cancer. A literature review of second TUR for T1 bladder cancer is shown in Table 6.3.

Careful and adequate TUR must be performed, particularly when the endoscopic appearance of the tumor suggests a high-grade lesion. A second TUR after 2–6 weeks is strongly recommended for G3T1 cancers, especially when no muscle is present in the specimen: up to half of the patients may have infiltrating tumor (>T1) at second resection.

Treatment

Transurethral resection alone

TUR generally is the first diagnostic and therapeutic approach to bladder carcinoma. When treated with transurethral resection only,

Table 6.1 Incidence of G3T1 bladder cancer in superficial bladder tumors

Lead author (year)	Superficial cancer	G3T1 (%)
England (1981)[2]	332	8
Heney (1983)[3]	249	11
Smith (1986)[4]	299	18
Jakse (1987)[5]	172	23
Algaba (1987)[6]	95	13
Malmstrom (1987)[7]	147	20
Pauwels (1988)[8]	122	6
Abel (1988)[9]	107	5
Witjes (1994)[10]	450	12
Otto (1994)[11]	2715	16
Pansadoro (1995)[12]	593	11
Alken (1996)[13]	631	12
Millan-Rodriguez (2000)[14]	1529	22

Table 6.2 Progression for G3T1 bladder cancer according to substaging

Lead author (year)	Follow-up (months)	Progression rate according to infiltration depth		
		Above MM (%)	At the level of MM (%)	Below MM (%)
Younes (1990)[19]	56	25	25	89
Angulo (1995)[20]	60	25		59
Holmang (1997)[21]	84	36		58
Kondylis (2000)[22]	71	22		29

MM, muscularis mucosae.

Table 6.3 Second transurethral resection for T1 bladder cancer

Lead author (year)	No. pts	Tumor grade	Stage at second TUR (%)				
			T0	Tis	Ta	T1	T≥2
Herr (1999)[24]	58	Any	22	→ 26 ←		24	28
Schwaibold (2000)[25]	60	NA	45	8	9	28	10
Brauers (2001)[26]	42	2–3	36	19	17	24	5
Ojea Calvo (2001)[27]	32	Any	41		→ 53 ←		6
	9	3	45			44	11
Rigaud (2002)[28]	52	Any	64	4	11	17	4
Schips (2002)[29]	76	Any	67		11	14	8
	39	3	61		10	15	13
Grimm (2003)[30]	34	Any	47		NA	NA	NA
	7	3	14				

NA, not applicable.

Table 6.4 Recurrence and progression in patients with G3T1 tumor after TUR alone

Lead author (year)	No. pts	Recurrence (%)	Progression (%)	Follow-up (months)
Pocock (1982)[31]	9		7	60
Heney (1983)[3]	33	79	48	36
Wolf (1983)[32]	14	50		24
RUTT (1985)[33]	430		31	60
Jakse (1987)[5]	31	80	33	60/106
Algaba (1987)[6]	12	67		26
Malmstrom (1987)[7]	7		43	60
Kaubisch (1991)[34]	18		50	36
Takashi (1991)[35]	23		35	60
Mulders (1994)[36]	48	75	27	48
Haukaas (1999)[37]	26		38	108
Zungri (1999)[38]	34	50	24	40
Paez Borda (2001)[39]	32	85	46	79
Kolodziej (2002)[40]	52	55	23	23

G3T1 tumors have high recurrence and progression rates. The recurrence rate is 50% to 80%, and progression to muscle invasive disease occurs in 27% to 63% of patients (Table 6.4). Up to 33% of patients with G3T1 bladder tumor treated with TUR alone will die of cancer.[41] Due to such an unacceptably high risk of recurrence and progression, TUR alone is not feasible for the treatment of G3T1 bladder cancer.

Radiotherapy

Adjuvant radiotherapy after TUR of G3T1 bladder tumors has been proposed. However, in 1986 a study reported progression rates of 32% to 54% at 36–60 months' follow-up, with 55% disease-free survival at 5 years.[42] These results are disappointing and basically similar to those obtained with TUR alone. Based upon those results,

Table 6.5 Progression in G3T1 tumors after radiotherapy

	No. pts	Progression (%)	Follow-up (months)
Older series			
England (1981)[2]	28	39	36
Malmstrom (1987)[7]	11	54	60
Jenkins (1989)[45]	53	32	60
Recent series			
Mulders (1994)[36]*	17	18	48
Moonen (1994)[46]	12	0	40
Holmang (1997)[21]†	11	63	84
Bell (1999)[47]	19	11	0
Van der Steen (2002)[48]	14	20	60

*Patients treated with radiotherapy between 1983 and 1988, published in 1994.
†Patients treated with radiotherapy between 1988 and 1989, published in 1997.

the use of radiotherapy for superficial bladder cancer has been discouraged.[43]

More sophisticated radiotherapy has recently become available, and the outcome of radiation therapy may be improved by newer approaches. In one report, 120 patients with G3T1 or T2 bladder cancer were treated with brachytherapy.[44] Five-year disease-free survival for G3T1 was 100%. In several recent series, the results of radiotherapy for G3T1 bladder cancer seem superior to the results reported earlier (Table 6.5). However, these series are very small and the interpretation is difficult.

Until further data can confirm the encouraging results obtained with new radiotherapeutic modalities, radiation therapy should be reserved for patients with G3T1 bladder cancer refractory to intravesical immunotherapy with bacillus Calmette–Guérin (BCG), who either refuse or are unfit for surgery.[49]

Combination radiochemotherapy

Rodel et al[50] treated 89 high-risk T1 cancer patients with radiotherapy alone or radiotherapy plus systemic chemotherapy with cisplatin or carboplatin and 5-fluorouracil. Six weeks after the end of treatment, 86% of the patients were free of disease at restaging TUR. At 5 years, any kind of recurrence and progression rates were 44% and 15%, respectively. At 10 years any kind of recurrence and progression rates were 64% and 40%, respectively. Overall survival was 75% at 5 years and 51% at 10 years. For G3T1 tumors (17 cases) the 5-year progression rate was 15%. Only a few centers have treated high-grade superficial bladder cancer with radiochemotherapy. Due to this limited experience, no definitive evaluation of this approach can be reasonably provided.

Intravesical therapy

Bacillus Calmette–Guérin

Bacillus Calmette–Guérin (BCG) immunotherapy is widely used as intravesical therapy for superficial bladder cancer. BCG reduces both recurrence and progression rates, especially in high-risk super-

ficial tumors.[51,52] Several studies have shown that immunotherapy with BCG after TUR is superior to TUR alone for the treatment of G3T1 bladder cancer.

In a prospective study, 86 patients with high-risk superficial bladder cancer were randomized to TUR plus BCG or TUR alone.[53] At 10 years, the progression rate was 38% for patients treated with BCG and 63% for control patients. Cancer-specific survival was 75% versus 55%. Similarly, Patard and al[54] compared the results obtained in 80 patients with TUR alone or TUR plus BCG. At 61–65 months, BCG treatment was superior to TUR alone in terms of cancer-specific survival (90% versus 70%, p=0.03), recurrence rates (50% versus 90%, p<0.01), and progression rates (22% versus 47%, p=0.03).

Many authors have proposed BCG as first line treatment for primary G3T1 bladder cancer. At 22–78 months of follow-up, recurrence rates are 20% to 70% and progression rates 0% to 33% (Table 6.6). In most series, the recurrence rate is 25% to 50% and progression rate 12% to 25%.

The optimal dose and schedule of BCG has not yet been established. Similar recurrence and progression rates have been reported for patients with G3T1 bladder cancers treated with full-dose and low-dose BCG regimens (see Table 6.6). In a multicenter Spanish study, Martinez-Pineiro et al[77] randomized 500 patients to either standard dose or reduced dose of BCG. At 79 months, the overall recurrence rates were 28% and 31% for standard and low-dose groups, respectively. Progression rates for high-grade superficial bladder cancer were similar for both groups: 11% and 13%. Side effects were significantly lower with the reduced dose. However, there was a significantly longer disease free-survival for patients with G3T1 tumors treated with full-dose BCG. For high-risk superficial bladder cancer, time to progression was longer and the risk of death was lower with full-dose than with low-dose BCG. Based upon these data, reduced dose BCG protocols should be avoided in G3T1 bladder cancer and a standard regimen should be used, unless a reduction of toxicity is strictly required.

In another randomized study, Gruenwald et al[78] compared results in a 12-week course of BCG with those of a standard 6-week course in 70 patients with high-risk superficial carcinoma of the bladder. At a mean follow-up of 28 months, the disease-free rate was 70% for the 12-week course compared to 55% for the 6-week course. A 12-week first course of intravesical BCG may be advisable in patients with G3T1 bladder cancer.

Several papers[57,79] have shown that early recurrence of high-grade T1 bladder cancer after BCG treatment is an ominous prognostic factor: in these patients cystectomy should be performed without delay. Herr and Sogani[80] have shown that delayed cystectomy is related to a decreased survival rate.

Dinney et al[81] reported that a deferred cystectomy in patients with T1 cancer progressing to T2 stage was associated with a higher cancer-related death rate.

Maintenance

In a multicenter study, 550 patients were randomized to maintenance or no maintenance after the first course of intravesical BCG.[49] The maintenance schedule included intravesical and percutaneous BCG each week for 3 weeks at months 3, 6, 12, 18, 24, 30, and 36 after the initial treatment. Median recurrence-free survival was 36 months in the no-maintenance arm and 77 months in the maintenance arm (p<0.0001). After reviewing the literature, Lamm[82]

Table 6.6 Results of BCG treatment for G3T1 tumors

Lead author (year)	No. pts	Recurrence (%)	Progression (%)	Follow-up (months)
Results of full-dose BCG				
Dal Bo (1990)[55]	24	25	25	22
Samodai (1991)[56]	62	20	0	46
Cookson (1992)[57]	16	44	19	59
Thanos (1994)[58]	17	37	12	36
Pfister (1995)[59]	26	50	27	54
Meng (1995)[60]	49		16	60
Baniel (1998)[61]	78	28	8	56
Klan (1998)[62]	109	39	3	78
Gohji (1999)[63]	25	40	4	63
Brake (2000)[64]	44	27	16	43
Kondylis (2000)[22]	49	65	24	71
Bogdanovic (2002)[65]	43	28	16	53
Iori (2002)[66]	41	24	2	40
Kulkarni (2002)[67]	69	35	12	45
Patard (2002)[68]*	50	50	22	61
Kim (2002)[69]	37	43	16	27
Shahin (2003)[70]	90	70	33	64
Pansadoro (2003)[71]	82	34	15	73
Peyromaure (2004)[72]	57	42	23	53
Results of low-dose BCG				
Mack (1995)[73]	21	29	NA	60
Vicente (1996)[74]	95	40	11	46
Lebret (1998)[75]	35	24	12	45
Hurle (1999)[76]	51	25	18	85

*37% of patients treated with low dose.
NA, not applicable.

concluded that there was an advantage of BCG over chemotherapy in improving long-term survival only if maintenance was given.

In a meta-analysis of 2410 patients comparing intravesical BCG to mitomycin, BCG was found to be superior to mitomycin in preventing tumor progression only if maintenance protocols were used.[83] In another meta-analysis of 4863 patients, BCG was compared to TUR alone or TUR and intravesical chemotherapy.[84] At 30 months, BCG reduced the progression rate from 13.8% to 9.8% (27%). The improvement was more evident for high-grade tumors.

Intravesical BCG schedules including maintenance therapy should be administered in patients with G3T1 bladder cancer.

The long-term results of BCG treatment for G3T1 bladder cancer have been evaluated. Herr followed 48 patients with G3T1 bladder cancer for 15 years. These patients had been initially randomized to TUR alone or TUR plus intravesical BCG. In this series, 81% of the patients eventually received BCG therapy.[85] Progression and cancer-related death rates were 25/48 (52%) and 15/48 (31%), respectively. Overall survival was 69%, with 24 (50%) patients with an intact bladder. Tumor progression was 35% at 1–5 years, 16% at 5–10 years, and 12% at 10–15 years. Cancer-specific deaths occurred in 25% of the patients in the first 5 years and in 10% after 5–15 years.

Long-term progression rates after BCG treatment have demonstrated that patients treated with BCG for G3T1 bladder cancer must undergo close surveillance for at least 15 years.

Intravesical chemotherapy

Intravesical immunotherapy with BCG seems superior to intravesical chemotherapy in reducing the recurrence rates of T1 bladder cancer.

In 334 patients (303 were T1) with superficial bladder cancer treated intravesically with BCG, epirubicin or adriamycin, the risk of recurrence was significantly higher with intravesical chemotherapy than with these drugs as single agents, though the lowest recurrence rates were obtained with a combination of BCG and epirubicin.[86] In a Spanish report, 191 patients with high-risk superficial bladder cancer were treated with BCG, mitomycin or doxorubicin. At 73 months, multivariate analysis showed that BCG treatment was associated with reduced risk of disease progression.[87]

Similarly, in a Scandinavian study, Malmstrom et al[88] found that BCG, when compared with mitomycin, prolonged recurrence-free survival in high-risk superficial bladder cancer patients, but was not more effective than mitomycin in decreasing progression rates.

In two meta-analyses, BCG with a maintenance schedule was superior to mitomycin and other intravesical chemotherapeutic agents in reducing tumor recurrence and progression rates.[52,84] In yet another meta-analysis of 1901 high-risk patients with superficial bladder cancer, BCG was more effective than mitomycin in reducing recurrence rates; however, there was no advantage in terms of tumor progression.[83]

Although intravesical chemotherapy for superficial bladder cancer has not clearly demonstrated benefits in terms of progression and cancer-specific deaths, thiotepa, mitomycin, doxorubicin, and epirubicin all seem equally effective in reducing superficial bladder cancer recurrence.[89]

Several authors have reported a clinical advantage in decreasing recurrence rates with a single dose of preoperative cytotoxic intravesical chemotherapy, 30–60 minutes after completion of TUR for superficial bladder cancer.[90] However, in a study of 168 patients, with mainly G2–3T1 bladder cancers, a single dose of postoperative intravesical epirubicin did not show any advantage for patents with

Table 6.7 Results of intravesical chemotherapy for G3T1 bladder cancer

Lead author (year)	Agent	No. pts	Recurrence (%)	Progression (%)	Follow-up (months)
Bono (1994)[92]	Doxorubicin	123	56	23	73
Serretta (2004)[93]	Doxorubicin ± epirubicin	137	51	9	24–240

high-grade tumors.[91] Therefore, the role of a single dose of intravesical chemotherapy immediately following transurethral resection of bladder tumor has not been established for G3T1 cancers. Results of long-term follow-up of patients undergoing TUR and adjuvant intravesical chemotherapy for G3T1 bladder cancer are shown in Table 6.7.

Comparison between intravesical chemotherapy and BCG for the treatment of G3T1 bladder cancer is not possible. Randomized trials are not available for high-grade superficial bladder cancer. Intravesical chemotherapy may be feasible for the treatment of G3T1 bladder cancer, but it is not the primary treatment of choice.

Alternative and second line treatments

Soloway et al[89] treated 61 patients with G3T1 bladder cancer with BCG. While six patients experienced progression to muscle invasive disease, 43 patients had recurrent superficial bladder cancer (38 high-grade T1) and were retreated with TUR and a second course of BCG. At 46 months' follow-up, only nine (21%) required cystectomy (five for local progression, four for persistent high-grade T1/carcinoma in situ).

In a similar study, 34 patients with high-risk superficial bladder cancer with recurrence at 28 months (range 7–50 months) were treated with TUR and additional BCG. At 36 months, recurrence and progression (requiring cystectomy) rates were 41% and 6%, respectively.[94] In carefully selected and strictly followed patients there may be a therapeutic role for a second course of BCG treatment.

Interferon (IFN) has been used in combination with BCG. In one study, 39 patients with G3T1 bladder cancer not responding to BCG were treated with low dose BCG plus IFNα2b.[95] At 24 months, the recurrence rate was 47%, and cystectomy was required in 10 patients (26%). Similarly, Luciani et al[96] treated 24 patients with Tis and/or T1 transitional cell carcinoma, recurrent after BCG therapy, with intravesical BCG plus IFNα2b or valrubicin. At 28.5 months, no cancer-related deaths occurred. Fourteen patients had preserved their bladders and nine patients required cystectomy.

Combination or alternative intravesical treatments may be considered a viable, though investigational, option after BCG failure in patients at high risk for surgery.

Cystectomy

Up to 81% of patients with high-grade superficial bladder cancer refractory to BCG may progress to muscle invasion,[97]

Table 6.8 Results for radical cystectomy in G3T1 tumors

Lead author (year)	No. pts	5-year survival (%)	10-year survival (%)
Siref (1988)[99]	32	67	57
Malkowicz (1993)[100]*	14	80	
Amling (1994)[101]†	91	76	62
Gschwend (1998)[102]	45	92	
Stein (2001)[103]‡	208	74	51
Madersbacher (2003)[104]	77	76	58

*G3 in 58, G2 in 17.
†Mainly G3.
‡72% high grade.

and radical cystectomy is the standard approach for patients with muscle-infiltrating bladder cancer. It is also considered to be a suitable option for the treatment of high-grade superficial bladder cancer.[98] The procedure has better acceptance than in the past due to the advent of orthotopic bladder substitutions.

Herr and Sogani[80] treated 90 patients with high-risk superficial bladder cancer with cystectomy. At 96 months, survival was 49%. Siref and Zincke treated another 32 patients with T1 (72% were high grade tumors) with cystectomy. Systemic progression occurred in 17 (53%) at 5 or more years of follow-up.[99]

Good results are obtained with cystectomy for high-grade superficial bladder cancer, with 5- and 10-year survivals of 67% to 95% and 51% to 62%, respectively (Table 6.8).

Since long-term survival after cystectomy for G3T1 bladder cancer is similar to that obtained with intravesical BCG, open surgery as first line treatment may lead to a large number of unnecessary cystectomies. However, up to 33% of patients treated with BCG may experience disease progression. Careful follow-up is needed for identification of early (3–6 months) recurrences of high-grade tumors, or progression after BCG therapy, either of which requires immediate cystectomy.

Prognostic factors

Given that a significant number of G3T1 tumors progress and require aggressive treatment, it is useful to identify patients that will not respond to intravesical immunotherapy. Clinical characteristics of the tumor and biologic markers have been studied for predictive factors.

Clinical characteristics

Eighty patients with G3T1 bladder cancer were treated with intravesical BCG or chemotherapy by Solsona et al.[87] The lack of complete response to treatment at the 3-month cystoscopy (no visible tumor, negative random biopsies) was a strong predictor of invasive progression in 29 nonresponding patients. Palou et al[105] also treated 159 patients with G3T1 bladder cancer with BCG. Progression rates were 42%, 29%, and 4% according to relapse at 3 months, at 6 months, or later recurrence, respectively. In yet another report of 102 patients with high-risk superficial bladder cancer treated with BCG,[106] the risk of progression was significantly higher in patients with superficial recurrence within 6 months.

Further papers[57,79] have shown that early recurrence of high-grade T1 bladder cancer after BCG treatment is a bad prognostic factor: in these patients cystectomy should not be deferred. Sanchez-Ortiz et al[107] found a higher progression rate in patients undergoing cystectomy with a delay of more than 12 weeks.

We have reported previously on 82 patients with G3T1 bladder cancer treated with BCG.[1] At a median follow-up of 73 months, the number of lesions, history of prior superficial bladder cancer, and associated carcinoma in situ (CIS) did not significantly correlate with recurrence or progression.

In a multivariate analysis of 51 patients with G3T1 bladder tumor treated with low dose BCG, Hurle et al[76] found that only tumor size (p=0.027) and coexisting CIS (p=0.024) significantly influenced results; however, in another study in 44 patients with G3T1 cancer, Brake et al[64] found no correlation between BCG failure and CIS.

Lebret at al[108] reported that tumor size, but not the number of lesions, predicted recurrence and progression in 35 patients with G3T1 bladder cancer treated with BCG. Saint et al[106] found that tumor size and multifocality were not significantly related to BCG outcome in 102 patients with high-risk superficial bladder cancer, while previous superficial tumors and the association with CIS had a significant impact on treatment outcome.

Biologic markers

The p53 gene regulates the cell cycle and p53 mutations are found in many different tumors, including transitional cell carcinoma. The role of p53 in predicting results of BCG treatment for high-risk superficial bladder cancer has been particularly controversial. In 1998, Sarosdy[109] reviewed the literature on the subject, and established that p53 tumor suppressor gene expression did not seem to correlate with the outcome of intravesical BCG in high-grade superficial bladder cancer.

P53 overexpression by immunohistochemistry has been reported to be an independent predictive factor of recurrence for high-risk superficial bladder cancer.[106] However, since p53 immunostaining is higher in grade 3 and T1 bladder cancers, it is not clear whether the prognostic significance, if found, could be due just to the strict association with G3T1 bladder carcinoma.[110]

Llopis et al[111] studied 207 patients with T1 bladder cancer. Nearly half the patients underwent intravesical therapy with chemotherapeutic agents or BCG. In 59 patients treated with BCG, 5-year progression was 45%; p53 was significantly correlated with progression (p=0.0031).

Shariat et al[112] found that p53 did not significantly affect disease progression or survival in 43 patients with T1 bladder cancer. They found that there was a trend toward a worse prognosis for association with CIS, though it did not reach statistical value.

Grossman et al[113] evaluated 45 patients with pT1 bladder cancer retrospectively with regard to the expression of two tumor suppressor genes, p53 and RB. Patients with normal expression of both proteins (i.e. p53 negative and RB heterogeneously positive) had an excellent outcome, with no patient showing disease progression, whereas patients with abnormal expression of either or both proteins had a significant increase in progression (p=0.04 and p=0.005, respectively).

In a paper from Memorial Sloan-Kettering,[114] 19 patients with T1 bladder cancer treated with intravesical BCG were studied. p53 nuclear overexpression was related to increased progression rate before BCG therapy and in those patients with BCG refractory tumors.

Only a few investigators have studied the prognostic value of p53 in a selected population with high-grade T1 bladder cancers treated with intravesical BCG. They have not been able to confirm a correlation with treatment outcome.

Conflicting data have been reported on the prognostic value of clinical and biologic features of G3T1 bladder cancer. Although p53 may have some role in predicting the risk of progression in patients treated with TUR alone or with intravesical chemotherapy, its value in the prognosis of high-grade superficial bladder cancers treated with BCG still needs to be confirmed in large series. The association with CIS might be related to a more aggressive disease. New markers are still investigational. Future studies might clarify if additional predictive prognostic factors can help with identifying those tumors which are more likely to progress with conservative treatment. To date, no evidence of predictive value has been clearly shown for any parameter, except for early (within 3–6 months) tumor recurrence after BCG therapy, which requires aggressive therapy with cystectomy.

Conclusion

G3T1 bladder cancer is an aggressive disease. When TUR alone is performed, recurrence and progression rates are extremely high. Intravesical therapy with full-dose BCG and maintenance protocols is the best conservative approach to primary G3T1 bladder cancers and should be considered as first line treatment. However, recurrence and progression have been described even up to 15–20 years after intravesical immunotherapy for G3T1 bladder cancer. These patients require strict surveillance for life. After BCG failure, second line treatments (second BCG course, intravesical chemotherapy, low-dose BCG plus IFNα2b) may be considered in carefully selected patients, or in patients that cannot or do not want to undergo surgery. Except for early recurrence after BCG, no definite prognostic factors are available to identify those patients that will experience disease progression. Patients with recurrence within 6 months should undergo cystectomy.

References

1. Pansadoro V, Emiliozzi P, dePaula F, Scarpone P, Pansadoro A, Sternberg CN. Long term follow-up of G3T1 transitional cell carcinoma of the bladder treated with intravesical Bacille Calmette–Guérin: 18-year experience. Urology 2002; 59: 227–31.
2. England HR, Paris AMI, Blandy JP. The correlation of T1 bladder tumor history with prognosis and follow-up requirements. Br J Urol 1981; 53: 593–7.
3. Heney NM, Ahmed S, Flannagan MJ, et al for National Bladder Cancer Collaborative Group A. Superficial bladder cancer: progression and recurrence. J Urol 1983; 130: 1083–6.

4. Smith G, Elton RA, Chisholm GD, Newsam JE, Hargreave TB. Superficial bladder cancer: intravesical chemotherapy and tumor progression to muscle invasion or metastases. Br J Urol 1986; 58: 659–63.

5. Jakse G, Loidl W, Seeber G, Hofstadter F. Stage T1, grade 3 transitional cell carcinoma of the bladder: an unfavourable tumor? J Urol 1987; 137: 39–43.

6. Algaba F. Origin of high grade superficial bladder cancer. Eur Urol 1987; 13: 153–5.

7. Malmstrom PU, Busch C, Norlen BJ. Recurrence, progression and survival in bladder cancer. Scand J Urol Nephrol 1987; 21: 185–95.

8. Pauwels RPE, Schapers RFM, Smeets AWGB. Grading in superficial bladder cancer. (1) Morphological criteria. Br J Urol 1988; 61: 129–34.

9. Abel PD, Hall RR, Williams G. Should pT1 transitional cell cancers of the bladder be classified as superficial? Br J Urol 1988; 62: 235–9.

10. Witjes JA, Kiemeney LA, Schaafsma HE, Debruyne FM. The influence of review pathology on study outcome of a randomized multicentre superficial bladder cancer trial. Members of the Dutch South East Cooperative Urological Group. Br J Urol 1994; 73(2): 172–6.

11. Otto T, Rubben H. Management of T1 G3 bladder carcinomas. EAU Update Series 1994; 2(16): 122–7.

12. Pansadoro V, Emiliozzi P, Defidio L, et al. Bacillus Calmette–Guérin in the treatment of stage T1 grade 3 transitional cell carcinoma of the bladder: long term results. J Urol 1995; 154: 2054–8.

13. Alken P. Personal communication. In Sarosdy MF (ed): Management of High Grade Superficial Bladder Cancer. Role of BCG. AUA Update Ser 1998; XVII(Lesson 12): 89–95.

14. Millan-Rodriguez F, Chechile-Toniolo G, Salvador-Bayarri J, Palou J, Algaba F, Vicente-Rodriguez J. Primary superficial bladder cancer risk groups according to progression, mortality and recurrence. J Urol 2000; 164(3 Pt 1): 680–4.

15. Dutta SC, Smith JA Jr, Shappell SB, Coffey CS, Chang SS, Cookson MS. Clinical understaging of high risk nonmuscle invasive urothelial carcinoma treated with radical cystectomy. J Urol 2001; 166(2): 490–93.

16. Lee SE, Jeong IG, Ku JH, Kwak C, Lee E, Jeong JS. Impact of transurethral resection of bladder tumor: analysis of cystectomy specimens to evaluate for residual tumor. Urology 2004; 63(5): 873–7.

17. Hasui Y, Osada Y, Kitada S, Nishi S. Significance of invasion to the muscularis mucosae on the progression of superficial bladder cancer. Urology 1994; 43(6): 782–6.

18. Cheng L, Weaver AL, Neumann RM, Scherer BG, Bostwick DG. Substaging of T1 bladder carcinoma based on the depth of invasion as measured by micrometer: a new proposal. Cancer 1999; 86(6): 1035–43.

19. Younes M, Sussman J, True LD. The usefulness of the level of the muscularis mucosae in the staging of invasive transitional cell carcinoma of the urinary bladder. Cancer 1990; 66(3): 543–8.

20. Angulo JC, Lopez JI, Grignon DJ, Sanchez-Chapado M. Muscularis mucosa differentiates two populations with different prognosis in stage T1 bladder cancer. Urology 1995; 45(1): 47–53.

21. Holmang S, Hedelin H, Anderstrom C, Holmberg E, Johansson SL. The importance of the depth of invasion in stage T1 bladder carcinoma: a prospective cohort study. J Urol 1997; 157(3): 800–3.

22. Kondylis FI, Demirci S, Ladaga L, Kolm P, Schellhammer PF. Outcomes after intravesical bacillus Calmette–Guérin are not affected by substaging of high grade T1 transitional cell carcinoma. J Urol 2000; 163(4): 1120–3.

23. Van Der Meijden A, Sylvester R, Collette L, Bono A, Ten Kate F. The role and impact of pathology review on stage and grade assessment of stages Ta and T1 bladder tumors: a combined analysis of 5 European Organisation for Research and Treatment of Cancer Trials. J Urol 2000; 164(5): 1533–7.

24. Herr HW. The value of a second transurethral resection in evaluating patients with bladder tumors. J Urol 1999; 162(1): 74–6.

25. Schwaibold H, Treiber U, Kuber H, Leyh H, Hartung R. Significance of second transurethral resection for T1 bladder cancer. Eur Urol 2000; 37(Suppl 2): abstract 441:111.

26. Brauers A, Buettner R, Jakse G. Second resection and prognosis of primary high risk superficial bladder cancer: is cystectomy often too early? J Urol 2001; 165(3): 808–10.

27. Ojea Calvo A, Nunez Lopez A, Alonso Rodrigo A, et al. Value of a second transurethral resection in the assessment and treatment of patients with bladder tumor. Actas Urol Esp 2001; 25(3): 182–86.

28. Rigaud J, Karam G, Braud G, Glemain P, Buzelin JM, Bouchot O. T1 bladder tumors: value of a second endoscopic resection. Prog Urol 2002; 12(1): 27–30.

29. Schips L, Augustin H, Zigeuner RE, et al. Is repeated transurethral resection justified in patients with newly diagnosed superficial bladder cancer? Urology 2002; 59(2): 220–23.

30. Grimm MO, Steinhoff C, Simon X, Spiegelhalder P, Ackermann R, Vogeli TA. Effect of routine repeat transurethral resection for superficial bladder cancer: a long-term observational study. J Urol 2003; 170(2 Pt 1): 433–37.

31. Pocock RD, Ponder BA, O'Sullivan JP, Ibrahim SK, Easton DF, Shearer RJ. Prognostic factors in non-infiltrating carcinoma of the bladder: a preliminary report. Br J Urol 1982; 54(6): 711–15.

32. Wolf H, Hojgaard K. Prognostic factors in local surgical treatment of invasive bladder cancer with special reference to the presence of urothelial dysplasia. Cancer 1983; 51(9): 1710–15.

33. RUTT (Registry for Urinary Tract Tumors: Harnwegstumorregister). Jahresbericht Verh Dtsch Ges Urol 1985; 37: 665–69.

34. Kaubisch S, Lum BL, Reese J, Freiha F, Torti FM. Stage T1 bladder cancer: grade is the primary determinant for risk of muscle invasion. J Urol 1991; 146: 28–31.

35. Takashi M, Sakata T, Murase T, Hamajima N, Miyake K. Grade 3 bladder cancer with lamina propria invasion (pT1): characteristics of tumor and clinical course. Nagoya J Med Sci 1991; 53(1–4): 1–8.

36. Mulders PFA, Hoekstra WJ, Heybroek RPM, et al and Members of the Dutch South Eastern Bladder Cancer Group. Prognosis and treatment of T1G3 bladder tumors. A prognostic factor analysis of 121 patients. Eur J Cancer 1994; 30A(7): 914–17.

37. Haukaas S, Daehlin L, Maartmann-Moe H, Ulvik NM. The long-term outcome in patients with superficial transitional cell carcinoma of the bladder: a single-institutional experience. BJU Int 1999; 83(9): 957–63.

38. Zungri E, Martinez L, Da Silva EA, Pesqueira D, de la Fuente Buceta A, Pereiro B .T1 GIII bladder cancer. Management with transurethral resection only. Eur Urol 1999;36(5):380–384.

39. Paez Borda A, Lujan Galan M, Gomez de Vicente JM, Moreno Santurino A, Abate F, Berenguer Sanchez A. Preliminary results of the treatment of high grade (T1G3) superficial tumors of the bladder with transurethral resection. Actas Urol Esp 2001; 25(3): 187–92.

40. Kolodziej A, Dembowski J, Zdrojowy R, Wozniak P, Lorenz J. Treatment of high-risk superficial bladder cancer with maintenance bacille Calmette–Guérin therapy: preliminary results. BJU Int 2002; 89(6): 620–2.

41. Donat SM. Evaluation and follow-up strategies for superficial bladder cancer. Urol Clin North Am 2003; 30(4): 765–76.

42. Quilty PM, Duncan W. Treatment of superficial (T1) tumours of the bladder by radical radiotherapy. Br J Urol 1986; 58: 147–52.

43. Sawczuk IS, Olsson CA, deVere White R. The limited usefulness of external beam radiotherapy in the control of superficial bladder cancer. Br J Urol 1988; 61(4): 330–2.

44. Gonzalez Gonzalez D, Haitze van der Veen J, Ypma AF, Blank LE, Hoestra CJ, Veen RE. Brachytherapy for urinary bladder cancer. Arch Esp Urol 1999; 52(6): 655–61.

45. Jenkins BJ, Nauth-Misir RR, Martin JE, Fowler CG, Hope-Stone HF, Blandy JP. The fate of G3pT1 bladder cancer. Br J Urol 1989; 64(6): 608–10.

46. Moonen LM, Horenblas S, van der Voet JC, Nuyten MJ, Bartelink H. Bladder conservation in selected T1G3 and muscle-invasive T2–T3a bladder carcinoma using combination therapy of surgery and iridium-192 implantation. Br J Urol 1994; 74(3): 322–7.

47. Bell CR, Lydon A, Kernick V, Hong A, Penn C, Pocock RD, Stott MA. Contemporary results of radical radiotherapy for bladder transitional cell carcinoma in a district general hospital with cancer-centre status. BJU Int 1999; 83(6): 613–18.

48. Van der Steen-Banasik EM, Visser AG, Reinders JG, Heijbroek RP, Idema JG, Janssen TG, Leer JW. Saving bladders with brachytherapy: implantation technique and results. Int J Radiat Oncol Biol Phys 2002; 53(3): 622–29.

49. Zietman AL, Shipley WU, Heney NM, Althausen AF. The case for radiotherapy with or without chemotherapy in high-risk superficial and muscle-invading bladder cancer. Semin Urol Oncol 1997; 15(3): 161–8.

50. Rodel C, Dunst J, Grabenbauer GG, Kuhn R, Papadopoulos T, Schrott KM, Sauer R. Radiotherapy is an effective treatment for high-risk T1-bladder cancer. Strahlenther Onkol 2001; 177(2): 82–8.

51. Lamm DL, Blumenstein BA, Crissman JD, et al. Maintenance bacillus Calmette–Guérin immunotherapy for recurrent TA, T1 and carcinoma in situ transitional cell carcinoma of the bladder: a randomized Southwest Oncology Group Study. J Urol 2000; 163(4): 1124–9.

52. Sylvester RJ, van der Meijden AP, Lamm DL. Intravesical bacillus Calmette–Guérin reduces the risk of progression in patients with superficial bladder cancer: a meta-analysis of the published results of randomized clinical trials. J Urol 2002; 168(5): 1964–70.

53. Herr HW, Schwalb DM, Zhang ZF, et al. Intravesical bacillus Calmette–Guérin therapy prevents tumor progression and death from superficial bladder cancer: ten-year follow-up of a prospective randomized trial. J Clin Oncol 1995; 113: 1404–08.

54. Patard J, Moudouni S, Saint F, et al and the Members of the Groupe Necker. Tumor progression and survival in patients with T1G3 bladder tumors: multicentric retrospective study comparing 94 patients treated during 17 years. Urology 2001; 58(4): 551–6.

55. Dal Bo V, Belmonte P, Veronesi A, et al. Intravesical BCG instillations in patients with carcinoma in situ and pT1G3 transitional cell carcinoma of the bladder. Eur Urol 1990; 18(1): 43–6.

56. Samodai L, Kiss L, Kolozsy Z, Mohacsi L. The efficacy of intravesical BCG in the treatment of patients with high risk superficial bladder cancer. Int Urol Nephrol 1991; 23(6): 559–67.

57. Cookson MS, Sarosdy MF. Management of stage T1 superficial bladder cancer with intravesical Bacillus Calmette–Guérin therapy. J Urol 1992; 148: 797–801.

58. Thanos A, Karassantes T, Davillas E, Sotiriou V, Davillas N. Bacillus Calmette–Guérin therapy for high-risk superficial bladder cancer. Scand J Urol Nephrol 1994; 28(4): 365–8.

59. Pfister C, Lande P, Herve JM, Barre P, Barbagelatta M, Camey M, Botto H. T1 G3 bladder tumors: the respective role of BCG and cystectomy. Prog Urol 1995; 5: 231–7.

60. Meng MV, Sanda MG. Comparison of intravesical BCG to radical cystectomy for high grade, T1 transitional cell carcinoma using Markov decision tree analysis. J Urol 1995; 153(Suppl): 466.

61. Baniel J, Grauss D, Engelstein D, Sella A. Intravesical bacillus Calmette–Guérin treatment for stage T1 grade 3 transitional cell carcinoma of the bladder. Urology 1998; 52(5): 785–9.

62. Klan R, Steiner U, Sauter T, et al. Zystektomie beim schlecht differenzierten T1-harnblasenkarzinom—oft zu früh? Akt Urol 1998; 29: 53–8.

63. Gohji K, Nomi M, Okamoto M, et al. Conservative therapy for stage T1b, grade 3 transitional cell carcinoma of the bladder. Urology 1999; 53(2): 308–13.

64. Brake M, Loertzer H, Horsch R, Keller K. Recurrence and progression of stage T1, grade 3 transitional cell carcinoma of the bladder following intravesical immunotherapy with Bacillus Calmette–Guérin. J Urol 2000; 163: 1697–701.

65. Bogdanovic J, Marusic G, Djozic J, Sekulic V, Budakov P, Dejanovic N, Stojkov J. The management of T1G3 bladder cancer. Urol Int 2002; 69(4): 263–5.

66. Iori F, Di Seri M, De Nunzio C, Leonardo C, Franco G, Spalletta B, Laurenti C. Long-term maintenance bacille Calmette–Guérin therapy in high-grade superficial bladder cancer. Urology 2002; 59(3): 414–18.

67. Kulkarni JN, Gupta R. Recurrence and progression in stage T1G3 bladder tumour with intravesical bacille Calmette–Guérin (Danish 1331 strain). BJU Int 2002; 90(6): 554–7.

68. Patard JJ, Rodriguez A, Leray E, Rioux-Leclercq N, Guille F, Lobel B. Intravesical Bacillus Calmette–Guérin treatment improves patient survival in T1G3 bladder tumours. Eur Urol 2002; 41(6): 635–41.

69. Kim SI, Kwon SM, Kim YS, Hong SJ. Association of cyclooxygenase-2 expression with prognosis of stage T1 grade 3 bladder cancer. Urology 2002; 60(5): 816–21.

70. Shahin O, Thalmann GN, Rentsch C, Mazzucchelli L, Studer UE. A retrospective analysis of 153 patients treated with or without intravesical bacillus Calmette–Guérin for primary stage T1 grade 3 bladder cancer: recurrence, progression and survival. J Urol 2003; 169(1): 96–100.

71. Pansadoro V, Emiliozzi P, dePaula F, et al. High grade superficial (G3T1) transitional cell carcinoma of the bladder treated with intravesical Bacillus Calmette–Guérin (BCG). J Exp Clin Cancer Res 2003; 22(Suppl 4): 223–7.

72. Peyromaure M, Zerbib M. T1G3 transitional cell carcinoma of the bladder: recurrence, progression and survival. BJU Int 2004; 93(1): 60–3.

73. Mack D, Frick J. Five-year results of a phase II study with low-dose bacille Calmette–Guérin therapy in high-risk superficial bladder cancer. Urology 1995; 45: 958–61.

74. Vicente J, Laguna MP, Palou J. The value of conservative treatment in G3T1 bladder tumours. Eur Urol Today 1996; 6: 14–18.

75. Lebret T, Becette V, Barbagelatta M, et al. Correlation between p53 overexpression and response to bacillus Calmette–Guérin therapy in a high risk select population of patients with T1G3 bladder tumours. J Urol 1998; 159(3): 788–91.

76. Hurle R, Losa A, Ranieri A, Manzetti A, Lembo A. Intravesical bacillus Calmette–Guérin in stage T1, grade 3 bladder cancer therapy: a 7-year follow-up. Urology 1999; 54(2): 258–63.

77. Martinez-Pineiro JA, Flores N, Isorna S, et al for CUETO (Club Urologico Espanol de Tratamiento Oncologico). Long-term follow-up of a randomized prospective trial comparing a standard 81 mg dose of intravesical bacille Calmette–Guérin with a reduced dose of 27 mg in superficial bladder cancer. BJU Int 2002; 89(7): 671–80.

78. Gruenwald IE, Stein A, Rashcovitsky R, Shifroni G, Lurie A. A 12- versus 6-week course of bacillus Calmette–Guérin prophylaxis for the treatment of high risk superficial bladder cancer. J Urol 1997; 157: 487–91.

79. Herr HW, Klein EA, Rogatko A. Local BCG failures in superficial bladder cancer. A multivariate analysis of risk factors influencing survival. Eur Urol 1991; 19(2): 97–100.

80. Herr HW, Sogani PC. Does early cystectomy improve the survival of patients with high risk superficial bladder tumors? J Urol 2001; 166(4): 1296–9.

81. Dinney CPN, Babkowski RC, Antelo M, et al. Relationship among cystectomy, microvessel density and prognosis in stage T1 transitional cell carcinoma of the bladder. J Urol 1998; 160: 1285–90.

82. Lamm DL. Preventing progression and improving survival with BCG maintenance. Eur Urol 2000; 37(Suppl 1): 9–15.

83. Bohle A, Bock PR. Intravesical bacille Calmette–Guérin versus mitomycin C in superficial bladder cancer: formal meta-analysis of comparative studies on tumor progression. Urology 2004; 63(4): 682–6.

84. Shelley MD, Wilt TJ, Court J, Coles B, Kynaston H, Mason MD. Intravesical bacillus Calmette–Guérin is superior to mitomycin C in reducing tumour recurrence in high-risk superficial bladder cancer: a meta-analysis of randomized trials. BJU Int 2004; 93(4): 485–90.

85. Herr HW. Tumour progression and survival in patients with T1G3 bladder tumours: 15-year outcome. Br J Urol 1997; 80(5): 762–5.

86. Ali-el-Dein B, Sarhan O, Hinev A, Ibrahiem el-HI, Nabeeh A, Ghoneim MA. Superficial bladder tumours: analysis of prognostic factors and construction of a predictive index. BJU Int 2003; 92(4): 393–9.

87. Solsona E, Iborra I, Dumont R, Rubio-Briones J, Casanova J, Almenar S. The 3-month clinical response to intravesical therapy as a predictive factor for progression in patients with high risk superficial bladder cancer. J Urol 2000; 164(3 Pt 1): 685–9.

88. Malmstrom PU, Wijkstrom H, Lundholm C, Wester K, Busch C, Norlen BJ. 5-year followup of a randomized prospective study comparing mitomycin C and bacillus Calmette–Guérin in patients with superficial bladder carcinoma. Swedish–Norwegian Bladder Cancer Study Group. J Urol 1999; 161(4): 1124–7.

89. Soloway MS, Sofer M, Vaidya A. Contemporary management of stage T1 transitional cell carcinoma of the bladder. J Urol 2002; 167(4): 1573–83.

90. O'Donnell MA. New therapeutic strategies for non-muscle-invasive (superficial) bladder cancer. AUA Update Ser 2002; XXII(Lesson 2): 9–15.

91. Ali-el-Dein B, Nabeeh A, el-Baz M, Shamaa S, Ashamallah A. Single-dose versus multiple instillations of epirubicin as prophylaxis for recurrence after transurethral resection of pTa and pT1 transitional-cell bladder tumours: a prospective, randomized controlled study. Br J Urol 1997; 79(5): 731–5.

92. Bono AV, Lovisolo JA, Saredi G. Transurethral resection and sequential chemo-immunoprophylaxis in primary T1G3 bladder cancer. Eur Urol 2000; 37(4): 478–83.

93. Serretta V, Pavone C, Ingargiola GB, Daricello G, Allegro R, Pavone-Macaluso M. TUR and adjuvant intravesical chemotherapy in T1G3 bladder tumors: recurrence, progression and survival in 137 selected patients followed up to 20 years. Eur Urol 2004; 45(6): 730–6.

94. Bassi P, Piazza N, Abatangelo G, et al. BCG immunotherapy of high-risk superficial bladder cancer. In Böhle A, Jocham D (eds): Optimal Therapy for Patients with High-Risk Superficial Bladder Cancer—Controversy and Consensus. Proceedings of the First Lübeck Symposium on Bladder Cancer. Basel: Karger, 1997.

95. O'Donnell MA, Krohn J, DeWolf WC. Salvage intravesical therapy with interferon-alpha 2b plus low dose bacillus Calmette–Guérin is effective in patients with superficial bladder cancer in whom bacillus Calmette–Guérin alone previously failed. J Urol 2001; 166(4): 1300–4.

96. Luciani LG, Neulander E, Murphy WM, Wajsman Z. Risk of continued intravesical therapy and delayed cystectomy in BCG-refractory superficial bladder cancer: an investigational approach. Urology 2001; 58(3): 376–9.

97. Marth D, Studer UE, Ackermann D, Zingg EJ. Primäre Therapieversager nach intravesikalem BCG wegen Carcinoma in situ erlauben kein expektives Verhalten. Urologe [A] 1991; (Suppl. 30): A71.

98. Esrig D, Freeman JA, Stein JP, Skinner DG. Early cystectomy for clinical stage T1 transitional cell carcinoma of the bladder. Semin Urol Oncol 1997; 15(3): 154–60.

99. Siref LE, Zincke H. Radical cystectomy for historical and pathologic T1, N0, M0 (stage A) transitional cell cancer. Need for adjuvant systemic chemotherapy? Urology 1988; 31(4): 309–11.

100. Malkowicz SB, Nichols P, Lieskovsky G, Boyd SD, Huffman J, Skinner DG. The role of radical cystectomy in the management of high grade superficial bladder cancer. J Urol 1993; 144: 641–5.

101. Amling CL, Thrasher JB, Frazier HA, Dodge RK, Robertson JE, Paulson DF. Radical cystectomy for stages Ta, Tis and T1 transitional cell carcinoma of the bladder. J Urol 1994; 151: 31–6.

102. Gschwend JE, Vieweg J, Fair WR. Contemporary results of radical cystectomy for primary bladder cancer. AUA Update Ser 1998; XVIII(Lesson 13): 98–103.

103. Stein JP, Lieskovsky G, Cote R, et al. Radical cystectomy in the treatment of invasive bladder cancer: long-term results in 1,054 patients. J Clin Oncol 2001; 19(3): 666–75.

104. Madersbacher S, Hochreiter W, Burkhard F, Thalmann GN, Danuser H, Markwalder R, Studer UE. Radical cystectomy for bladder cancer today—a homogeneous series without neoadjuvant therapy. J Clin Oncol 2003; 21(4): 690–6.

105. Palou J, Rosales A, Millan F, Zaragoza R, Salvador J, Vicente J. Clinical prognostic factors of recurrence and progression in TCC stage T1 G3 treated with BCG. BJU Int 2000; 86(Suppl. 3): 3–7.

106. Saint F, Le Frere Belda MA, Quintela R, et al. Pretreatment p53 nuclear overexpression as a prognostic marker in superficial bladder cancer treated with Bacillus Calmette–Guérin (BCG). Eur Urol 2004; 45(4): 475–82.

107. Sanchez-Ortiz RF, Huang WC, Mick R, Van Arsdalen KN, Wein AJ, Malkowicz SB. An interval longer than 12 weeks between the diagnosis of muscle invasion and cystectomy is associated with worse outcome in bladder carcinoma. J Urol 2003; 169(1): 110–15.

108. Lebret T, Becette V, Herve JM, et al. Prognostic value of MIB-1 antibody labeling index to predict response to Bacillus Calmette–Guérin therapy in a high-risk selected population of patients with stage T1 grade G3 bladder cancer. Eur Urol 2000; 37(6): 654–9.

109. Sarosdy MF. Management of high grade superficial bladder cancer. Role of BCG. AUA Update Ser 1998; XVII(Lesson 12): 90–5.

110. Pfister C, Flaman JM, Dunet F, Grise P, Frebourg T. p53 mutations in bladder tumors inactivate the transactivation of the p21 and Bax genes, and have a predictive value for the clinical outcome after bacillus Calmette–Guérin therapy. J Urol 1999; 162(1): 69–73.

111. Llopis J, Alcaraz A, Ribal MJ, et al. p53 expression predicts progression and poor survival in T1 bladder tumours. Eur Urol 2000; 37(6): 644–53.

112. Shariat SF, Weizer AZ, Green A, et al. Prognostic value of P53 nuclear accumulation and histopathologic features in T1 transitional cell carcinoma of the urinary bladder. Urology 2000; 56(5): 735–40.

113. Grossman HB, Liebert M, Antelo M, Dinney CP, Hu SX, Palmer JL, Benedict WF. p53 and RB expression predict progression in T1 bladder cancer. Clin Cancer Res 1998; 4(4): 829–34.

114. Lacombe L, Dalbagni G, Zhang ZF, Cordon-Cardo C, Fair WR, Herr HW, Reuter VE. Overexpression of p53 protein in a high-risk population of patients with superficial bladder cancer before and after bacillus Calmette–Guérin therapy: correlation to clinical outcome. J Clin Oncol 1996; 14(10): 2646–52.

7

What to do when BCG fails

Guido Dalbagni

Introduction

Although bacillus Calmette–Guérin (BCG) is a highly effective therapy for bladder cancer, the problem of BCG failure is significant. When the therapy fails, radical cystectomy is the gold standard. Patients are sometimes reluctant, however, to undergo major surgery for a condition that does not pose an immediate threat to their lives. Furthermore, radical cystectomy is not suitable for a subset of patients with severe comorbidities. A number of alternatives have been developed. After considering the definition of BCG failure, we will detail these therapies.

Definition of BCG failure

In evaluating salvage therapies for use after BCG failure, comparisons between therapies have been hampered by the lack of standard definitions for BCG failure and BCG-refractory transitional cell carcinoma (TCC). Some series have defined BCG failure after a single induction course of BCG[1,2]; others after two courses.[3] The latter is preferable, since it is known that patients do respond to a second cycle of BCG. Haaff et al reported the overall response in 61 patients treated with one or two courses. The 25 patients in whom the initial induction cycle failed were treated with a second course. Eight of 19 patients (42%) with carcinoma in situ (CIS) responded to the induction course, while 56% became free of tumor after additional BCG, for a cumulative response of 68% after a mean follow-up of 13.5 months. Six of 13 patients (46%) with residual tumors were rendered disease-free after one induction course, and three of seven (43%) became free of tumor after a second treatment. The overall response was 69% with a mean follow-up of 15.2 months. Nine of 29 patients treated for prophylaxis after complete resection had a recurrence after a mean follow-up of 11.8 months. An additional induction course was given to these patients. Overall, 90% (26/29) were free of recurrence at a mean follow-up of 12.8 months.[4] Okamura et al reported the effect of repeated courses of BCG (Tokyo strain) as a prophylactic agent to prevent recurrences in patients with Ta/T1 cancer. Seventeen of 75 patients (23%) developed recurrences after a single course, and 12 received additional courses after a transurethral resection of bladder tumor (TURBT). The overall success rate was 90.7%.[5]

Bui et al reported the clinical outcome of 11 patients who received a second course after an initial complete response (CR). All patients were followed for a minimum of 5 years, and the median interval to tumor recurrence after the initial treatment was 17 months (range 9–74 months). Nine of the 11 patients achieved a CR and five were free of disease at a median follow-up of 87 months (range 64–110 months).[6] Overall, 42% to 82% of patients who did not respond to an induction course responded to a second cycle.[6–9]

These data suggest that a second course of BCG is warranted. These results also argue against defining BCG as failure to respond to a single induction course.

Tis after two cycles portends a poor prognosis

Patients whose disease recurs after a second cycle are less likely to respond to additional BCG,[6] and are at increased risk of progression.[7] Catalona et al found that, among patients in whom two or more courses of BCG failed, the risk of developing muscle-invasive tumors or metastatic disease was 30% and 50%, respectively, while only 20% responded to additional BCG therapy.[7] Sarosdy et al reported a 28% progression and metastasis rate among patients in whom BCG and bropirimine failed and who subsequently underwent nonsurgical treatment.[3]

Patients with persistent TCC after two cycles of BCG do worse than patients with recurrence after an initial response

Harland et al reported disease progression among 10% of patients who responded to one or two courses of BCG versus 48% among those that failed to respond, with a median follow-up of 32 months.[10] The long-term outcomes of patients with Tis, treated as part of a randomized study comparing mitomycin C versus two strains of BCG, have been reported by the Dutch South East Cooperative Urological Group.[11] Of the 65% of patients who achieved a CR, 18% had progression of disease while 67% of the nonresponders had progression.[11] The cumulative response rates for the first and second 6-week courses were 56%. Ovesen et al reported a 26% progression rate among complete responders versus 77% among nonresponders with a median follow-up of 46 months.[12]

The disease-free interval is an important prognostic variable

Bretton et al reported clinical outcomes of 28 patients that received a second course of BCG. Progression occurred in 13 patients (46%), and the median duration of response to course 1 of BCG was shorter for these patients than for those with no progression. Of the 13 patients with progression, 10 (77%) had responded to course 1 for less than 21.6 months compared to only 4 of 15 (27%) without progression.[13] The conclusion of this study was that a second course of BCG was useful in patients who had a *prolonged* response to the initial treatment. Merz et al reported a high progression rate after a second course of BCG among patients whose initial response to induction BCG was followed by a recurrence within 9 months, compared to no recurrences after the second course among patients who developed recurrences after more than 12 months.[14]

These data suggest that patients with an initial CR and a late relapse are the ones most likely to benefit from a repeat course of BCG.

Patients relapsing with T1 disease after BCG therapy are at high risk of progression

Herr and colleagues reported a progression rate of 82% among 17 patients who had stage T1 TCC at the 3-month evaluation after BCG therapy. The median time to progression was 8.5 months.[15,16] The aggressive nature of T1 TCC at the 3-month evaluation was confirmed by others.[17,18]

It seems reasonable, based on the current literature, to define BCG-refractory TCC or BCG failure as any situation associated with a high progression rate. This includes:

- persistent Tis after two consecutive BCG courses (nonresponders)
- recurrent Tis within less than 6 months of achieving a complete response after one or two courses of BCG
- recurrent Tis while on maintenance therapy
- relapse with T1 disease.

The methods of reporting the results have been inconsistent. Most studies have included all patients who received one or more courses of BCG.[19–22] Investigators have often combined patients with persistent disease (nonresponders) and patients with recurrent Tis after an initial response,[1,3] and a few studies have combined patients who were nonresponders to BCG and patients that could not complete BCG therapy because of toxicity (BCG intolerant).[3,19] Furthermore, most studies have combined all patients with papillary tumors with and without Tis. Finally, most studies have not indicated the disease-free interval after the last BCG course. These inconsistencies have led to comparisons of outcome in a very heterogeneous population.

Treatment of BCG-Refractory CIS

Patients whose bladder cancer progresses after failure of intravesical therapy have been shown to fare worse than patients presenting with a de novo muscle-invasive tumor. Van der Heijden et al reported a 37% 3-year cancer-specific survival rate for the progressive group versus 65% in the de novo group.[23]

Radical cystectomy is the gold standard in patients with BCG-refractory TCC. However, those patients reluctant to undergo major surgery are usually willing to explore alternatives. Furthermore,

a subset of patients with severe comorbidities are not candidates for cystectomy. Several alternative approaches have been proposed, as follows.

Intravesical valrubicin

Valrubicin is an analog of adriamycin (N-trifluoroacetyladriamycin-14-valerate [AD32]), an anthracycline with a mechanism of action different from the parent compound. Valrubicin inhibits nucleoside incorporation into DNA and RNA, leading to chromosomal damage.[24] In a phase I study of 32 patients with nonmuscle-invasive TCC, 13 patients achieved a CR with valrubicin treatment. The drug had only minor systemic side effects, and the serum levels of unmetabolized valrubicin and its two primary metabolites were very low. However, 29 patients (91%) had mild to severe irritative symptoms, which persisted for several days after each instillation.[25]

The efficacy of valrubicin was demonstrated in a phase II study of 90 patients with Tis after failure of multiple courses of intravesical therapy, including at least one course of BCG. Patients received 800 mg valrubicin weekly for 6 weeks. Nineteen patients (21%) had a CR, defined as no evidence of recurrence for at least 6 months from the initiation of therapy; 7 of these 19 had a durable response, with a median follow-up of 30 months. Forty-four patients underwent a radical cystectomy (six of whom had stage pT3 disease at cystectomy), and four patients died of bladder cancer during the 30-month follow-up. Most patients (90%) had mild to moderate local bladder symptoms, with urinary frequency in 66%, urinary urgency in 63%, and dysuria in 60%.[22]

In 1997, valrubicin was approved by the Food and Drug Administration (FDA) for the treatment of BCG-refractory Tis in patients who refuse or are unable to undergo cystectomy.

Preavailability: intravesical gemcitabine

Gemcitabine (2′,2′-difluoro-2′-deoxycytidine; Gemzar) is a novel deoxycytidine analog with a broad spectrum of antitumor activity. It was first approved in the United States for the treatment of pancreatic cancer,[26,27] but has since been found to be effective in many other tumor types. Gemcitabine has a molecular weight of 299.66, and, after intracellular activation, the active metabolite is incorporated into DNA, resulting in inhibition of further DNA synthesis. Gemcitabine may also inhibit ribonucleotide reductase and cytidine deaminase as part of its cytotoxic activity.[17] Gemcitabine is highly effective (overall response rates ranging from 22.5% to 28%) and well tolerated as both first- and second-line, single-agent therapy for the treatment of metastatic TCC.[28–30] Studies have reported a low incidence of systemic side effects. A randomized, multicenter, phase III study demonstrated that patients with unresectable or metastatic disease treated with gemcitabine plus cisplatin (GC) had survival rates similar to those of patients treated with MVAC (methotrexate, vinblastine, doxorubicin [adriamycin], and cisplatin), and GC had a better safety profile and tolerability.[31] On the basis of its excellent clinical activity, patient tolerability, and chemical characteristics, gemcitabine is a logical candidate for intravesical therapy.

Dalbagni et al reported a phase I study of intravesical gemcitabine twice a week for 3 weeks, followed by a second cycle after a week of rest, in a heavily pretreated population with BCG-refractory TCC. This study demonstrated that intravesical gemcitabine was well tolerated with minimal bladder irritation and acceptable myelosuppression. Serum levels of gemcitabine were undetectable at concentrations of 5, 10, and 15 mg/ml. However, serum gemcitabine was detected at a concentration of 20 mg/ml. Complete response as defined by a negative post-treatment cystoscopy, including a biopsy of the urothelium and negative cytology, was achieved in 7 of 18 patients (39%).[19] This was followed by a phase II study of patients with BCG-refractory TCC to determine the efficacy of gemcitabine as an intravesical agent; 28 patients completed therapy, and 16 achieved a complete response.[32]

Laufer et al reported a phase I study of weekly intravesical gemcitabine in 15 patients that had received intravesical therapy previously. Serum gemcitabine levels were undetected at concentrations of 5, 10, 15, and 20 mg/ml, while low concentrations were present in all patients receiving 40 mg/ml. However, the metabolite dFdU (2'2'-difluorodeoxyuridine) was detectable in plasma of patients receiving gemcitabine at concentrations of 15 mg/ml or higher, implying minimal absorption of gemcitabine at lower doses. The authors concluded that intravesical gemcitabine is well tolerated, with minimal toxicity. Furthermore, no evidence of recurrence at 12 weeks was noted in 9 of 13 evaluable patients.[33]

In a recent phase I study, De Berardinis and associates reported no detection of systemic gemcitabine at a concentration of 40 mg/ml. However, the inactive metabolite was detected in plasma. They were able to demonstrate activity of deoxycytidine kinase in tissue samples, an enzyme that produces 2',2'-difluoro-deoxycytidine triphosphate, the active metabolite of gemcitabine.[34]

All reports published thus far confirm the low systemic absorption of gemcitabine, the good tolerability with minimal local and systemic toxicity, and, more importantly, the efficacy of gemcitabine as an intravesical agent, even in heavily pretreated patients. This agent warrants further investigation in a large cohort of patients.

Intravesical BCG and interferon-α

Interferons are glycoproteins that mediate host immune responses such as stimulation of phagocytes, cytokine release, enhanced natural killer cell activity, and activation of T and B lymphocytes. Intravesical interferon-α 2b (IFNα2b) has demonstrated activity in patients with nonmuscle-invasive bladder cancer.[35] Among patients with Tis enrolled in a randomized trial, two of nine that had failed earlier intravesical therapy had a CR to IFNα2b.[2]

A phase I study of low-dose BCG with different doses of IFNα2b demonstrated that this combination is well tolerated.[36] O'Donnell et al reported the efficacy of the combination in a cohort of patients who had received one or more induction courses of BCG. Of 40 patients enrolled, 63% and 53% were disease-free at 12 and 24 months, respectively.[20] The response for patients in whom a single course of BCG failed was similar to the response of those in whom multiple courses failed. There was a trend towards worse outcomes in patients with an early relapse after the induction course of BCG.[20] Punnen et al reported a durable response to low-dose BCG plus IFNα in 6 of 12 patients with nonmuscle-invasive TCC that received one or more courses of BCG.[37] Lam et al treated 32 patients with nonmuscle-invasive bladder cancer, including patients whose disease recurred after BCG. After a follow-up of 22 months, 66% were disease-free.[38]

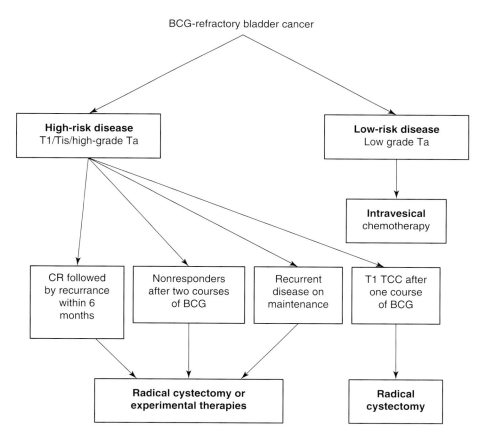

Figure 7.1
Management of BCG-refractory bladder cancer. (CR, complete response; TCC, transitional cell carcinoma.)

Photodynamic therapy

Several investigators have reported the efficacy of photodynamic therapy in managing nonmuscle-invasive tumors (also reviewed in Chapter 36). This approach has also been tested in patients with BCG-refractory tumors. Nseyo et al reported the results of a multicenter trial assessing the safety and efficacy of porfimer sodium photodynamic therapy in patients in whom earlier intravesical therapy for Tis had failed. Of the 36 patients enrolled, 34 had received more than one intravesical therapy, including thiotepa, mitomycin, and doxorubicin. At 3 months, 58% achieved a complete response, but 10 of the 21 responders had a recurrence during follow-up (mean, 12 months). Fourteen patients (39%) underwent a radical cystectomy for persistent or recurrent disease, and 22% had muscle-invasive disease. Significant urinary symptoms developed, and seven patients developed bladder contractures.[39]

Photodynamic therapy after the oral administration of 5-aminolevulinic acid was performed in 24 patients with recurrent nonmuscle-invasive TCC after BCG. At a median follow-up of 36 months, 3 of 5 patients with Tis and 4 of 19 with papillary TCC were free of disease.[40]

Other alternative therapies have been investigated, including oral bropirimine, an immunostimulant which has produced remission in patients with Tis after prior intravesical therapy.[3] CR was detected in 30% of the evaluable patients that were BCG resistant. Progression to muscle-invasive or metastatic disease was documented in 6% of the patients.[3]

Conclusion

- A management strategy for BCG-refractory nonmuscle-invasive cancer is suggested in Figure 7.1.
- Bropirimine is not FDA approved and is not being evaluated in clinical trials for bladder cancer.
- Valrubicin has been discontinued and is not currently available.
- Radical cystectomy still remains the standard of care for patients with BCG-refractory Tis.
- Salvage therapy for patients that refuse, or are unable to undergo, cystectomy is still under investigation.
- New promising strategies and agents warrant further investigation.

References

1. Klein EA, Rogatko A, Herr HW. Management of local bacillus Calmette–Guérin failures in superficial bladder cancer. J Urol 1992; 147: 601–5.
2. Glashan RW. A randomized controlled study of intravesical alpha-2b-interferon in carcinoma in situ of the bladder. J Urol 1990; 144: 658–61.
3. Sarosdy MF, Manyak MJ, Sagalowsky AI, et al. Oral bropirimine immunotherapy of bladder carcinoma in situ after prior intravesical bacille Calmette–Guérin. Urology 1998; 51: 226–31.
4. Haaff EO, Dresner SM, Ratliff TL, et al. Two courses of intravesical bacillus Calmette–Guérin for transitional cell carcinoma of the bladder. J Urol 1986; 136: 820–4.
5. Okamura T, Tozawa K, Yamada Y, et al. Clinicopathological evaluation of repeated courses of intravesical bacillus Calmette–Guérin instillation for preventing recurrence of initially resistant superficial bladder cancer [see comment]. J Urol 1996; 156: 967–71.
6. Bui TT, Schellhammer PF. Additional bacillus Calmette–Guérin therapy for recurrent transitional cell carcinoma after an initial complete response. Urology 1997; 49: 687–90; discussion 690–91.
7. Catalona WJ, Hudson MA, Gillen DP, et al. Risks and benefits of repeated courses of intravesical bacillus Calmette–Guérin therapy for superficial bladder cancer. J Urol 1987; 137: 220–4.
8. Kavoussi LR, Torrence RJ, Gillen DP, et al. Results of 6 weekly intravesical bacillus Calmette–Guérin instillations on the treatment of superficial bladder tumors. J Urol 1988; 139: 935–40.
9. Kim JC, Steinberg GD. Medical management of patients with refractory carcinoma in situ of the bladder. Drugs Aging 2001; 18: 335–44.
10. Harland SJ, Charig CR, Highman W, et al. Outcome in carcinoma in situ of bladder treated with intravesical bacille Calmette–Guérin. Br J Urol 1992; 70: 271–75.
11. van Gils-Gielen RJ, Witjes WP, Caris CT, et al. Risk factors in carcinoma in situ of the urinary bladder. Dutch South East Cooperative Urological Group. Urology 1995; 45: 581–86.
12. Ovesen H, Horn T, Steven K. Long-term efficacy of intravesical bacillus Calmette–Guérin for carcinoma in situ: relationship of progression to histological response and p53 nuclear accumulation. J Urol 1997; 157: 1655–9.
13. Bretton PR, Herr HW, Kimmel M, et al. The response of patients with superficial bladder cancer to a second course of intravesical bacillus Calmette–Guérin. J Urol 1990; 143: 710–2; discussion 712–3.
14. Merz VW, Marth D, Kraft R, et al. Analysis of early failures after intravesical instillation therapy with bacille Calmette–Guérin for carcinoma in situ of the bladder. Br J Urol 1995; 75: 180–4.
15. Herr HW, Badalament RA, Amato DA, et al. Superficial bladder cancer treated with bacillus Calmette–Guérin: a multivariate analysis of factors affecting tumor progression. J Urol 1989; 141: 22–9.
16. Herr HW. Progression of stage T1 bladder tumors after intravesical bacillus Calmette–Guérin. [Erratum appears in J Urol 1991; 145(4): 840.] J Urol 1991; 145: 40–3; discussion 43–4.
17. Hurle R, Losa A, Manzetti A, et al. Intravesical bacille Calmette–Guérin in stage T1 grade 3 bladder cancer therapy: a 7-year follow-up. Urology 1999; 54: 258–63.
18. Solsona E, Iborra I, Dumont R, et al. The 3-month clinical response to intravesical therapy as a predictive factor for progression in patients with high risk superficial bladder cancer [see comment]. J Urol 2000; 164: 685–9.
19. Dalbagni G, Russo P, Sheinfeld J, et al. Phase I trial of intravesical gemcitabine in bacillus Calmette–Guérin-refractory transitional-cell carcinoma of the bladder [see comment]. J Clin Oncol 2002; 20: 3193–8.
20. O'Donnell MA, Krohn J, DeWolf WC. Salvage intravesical therapy with interferon-alpha 2b plus low dose bacillus Calmette–Guérin is effective in patients with superficial bladder cancer in whom bacillus Calmette–Guérin alone previously failed. J Urol 2001; 166: 1300–4; discussion 1304–5.
21. Luciani LG, Neulander E, Murphy WM, et al. Risk of continued intravesical therapy and delayed cystectomy in BCG-refractory superficial bladder cancer: an investigational approach. Urology 2001; 58: 376–9.
22. Steinberg G, Bahnson R, Brosman S, et al. Efficacy and safety of valrubicin for the treatment of Bacillus Calmette–Guérin refractory carcinoma in situ of the bladder. The Valrubicin Study Group [see comment]. J Urol 2000; 163: 761–7.
23. van der Heijden AG, Witjes JA. Future strategies in the diagnosis, staging and treatment of bladder cancer. Curr Opin Urol 2003; 13: 389–95.
24. Kuznetsov DD, Alsikafi NF, O'Connor RC, et al. Intravesical valrubicin in the treatment of carcinoma in situ of the bladder. Exp Opin Pharmacother 2001; 2: 1009–13.
25. Greenberg RE, Bahnson RR, Wood D, et al. Initial report on intravesical administration of N-trifluoroacetyladriamycin-14-valerate (AD 32) to patients with refractory superficial transitional cell carcinoma of the urinary bladder. Urology 1997; 49: 471–75.
26. Hertel LW, Boder GB, Kroin JS, et al. Evaluation of the antitumor activity of gemcitabine (2',2'-difluoro-2'-deoxycytidine). Cancer Res 1990; 50: 4417–22.
27. Burris HA 3rd, Moore MJ, Andersen J, et al. Improvements in survival and clinical benefit with gemcitabine as first-line therapy for patients

with advanced pancreas cancer: a randomized trial [see comment]. J Clin Oncol 1997; 15: 2403–13.

28. Moore MJ, Tannock IF, Ernst DS, et al. Gemcitabine: a promising new agent in the treatment of advanced urothelial cancer. J Clin Oncol 1997; 15: 3441–5.

29. Stadler WM, Kuzel T, Roth B, et al. Phase II study of single-agent gemcitabine in previously untreated patients with metastatic urothelial cancer. J Clin Oncol 1997; 15: 3394–8.

30. Lorusso V, Pollera CF, Antimi M, et al. A phase II study of gemcitabine in patients with transitional cell carcinoma of the urinary tract previously treated with platinum. Italian Co-operative Group on Bladder Cancer. Eur J Cancer 1998; 34: 1208–12.

31. von der Maase H, Hansen SW, Roberts JT, et al. Gemcitabine and cisplatin versus methotrexate, vinblastine, doxorubicin, and cisplatin in advanced or metastatic bladder cancer: results of a large, randomized, multinational, multicenter, phase III study [see comment]. J Clin Oncol 2000; 18: 3068–77.

32. Dalbagni G, Mazumdar M, Russo P, et al. Phase II trial of intravesical gemcitabine in BCG-refractory transitional cell carcinoma of the bladder. J Urol 2004; 171: Abstract 274.

33. Laufer M, Ramalingam S, Schoenberg MP, et al. Intravesical gemcitabine therapy for superficial transitional cell carcinoma of the bladder: a phase I and pharmacokinetic study. J Clin Oncol 2003; 21: 697–703.

34. De Berardinis E, Antonini G, Peters GJ, et al. Intravesical administration of gemcitabine in superficial bladder cancer: a phase I study with pharmacodynamic evaluation. BJU Int 2004; 93: 491–94.

35. Torti FM, Shortliffe LD, Williams RD, et al. Alpha-interferon in superficial bladder cancer: a Northern California Oncology Group Study. J Clin Oncol 1988; 6: 476–83.

36. Stricker P, Pryor K, Nicholson T, et al. Bacillus Calmette–Guérin plus intravesical interferon alpha-2b in patients with superficial bladder cancer. Urology 1996; 48: 957–61; discussion 961–62.

37. Punnen SP, Chin JL, Jewett MA. Management of bacillus Calmette–Guérin (BCG) refractory superficial bladder cancer: results with intravesical BCG and interferon combination therapy. Can J Urol 2003; 10: 1790–5.

38. Lam JS, Benson MC, O'Donnell MA, et al. Bacillus Calmette–Guérin plus interferon-alpha2B intravesical therapy maintains an extended treatment plan for superficial bladder cancer with minimal toxicity. Urol Oncol 2003; 21: 354–60.

39. Nseyo UO. Photodynamic therapy in the management of bladder cancer. J Clin Laser Med Surg 1996; 14: 271–80.

40. Waidelich R, Stepp H, Baumgartner R, et al. Clinical experience with 5-aminolevulinic acid and photodynamic therapy for refractory superficial bladder cancer. J Urol 2001; 165: 1904–07.

Section 2

T2-4

8

Selection and perioperative management of patients undergoing radical cystectomy and urinary reconstruction

Melissa R Kaufman, Joseph A Smith Jr

Introduction

Radical cystectomy is a formidable surgical procedure. Moreover, many patients with invasive bladder cancer have significant comorbidity considering the median age at diagnosis and the strong association with a history of cigarette smoking. Optimal patient preparation and perioperative management are therefore essential in decreasing both the morbidity and mortality from this operation. This chapter defines some of the selection criteria, the preoperative evaluation, and the perioperative management of patients undergoing radical cystectomy.

Who are candidates

Radical cystectomy is the treatment of choice for muscle invasive or recurrent high-grade transitional cell carcinoma of the bladder.[1] The median survival for patients not cured by surgery is limited.[2] Patients with unresectable local disease may have significant morbidity from bleeding, pelvic pain, or voiding symptoms. Combined, these factors create strong incentives to proceed with cystectomy in patients with disease not controllable by transurethral methods. Historically, a significant number of patients were excluded from cystectomy because of advanced age and/or significant comorbidity.[3] Improvements in surgical technique and postoperative management have expanded the patient population considered eligible for surgery.[4]

There are few data which allow calculation of how many patients are excluded from radical cystectomy by being declared medically unfit for surgery. Undoubtedly, this categorization is appropriate for a distinct minority for whom alternative treatment methods must be considered.[5] However, the overwhelming majority of patients in whom cystectomy is indicated on the basis of tumor status should be considered candidates for surgery despite the attendant risks.[6]

Age

In most reported series, the typical patient undergoing cystectomy is in the sixth or seventh decade of life.[7] There are a number of reports, however, detailing the morbidity and mortality of the operation in octogenarians or even nonagenarians.[8] Chronologic age is only one consideration and must be correlated with comorbidity. Most series have shown that elderly patients tolerate cystectomy with morbidity not substantially different from that of younger patients.[9–12]

The choice of urinary diversion may be influenced in part by age. Parekh et al were unable to show any significant increase in morbidity for patients undergoing continent orthotopic neobladder reconstruction over that of patients undergoing ileal conduit cutaneous diversion.[13] Nonetheless, continent reconstruction is a more lengthy procedure, and it seems logical that morbidity may be somewhat increased, especially in the elderly. Further, the quality-of-life advantages afforded by continent reconstruction may be of less importance in older patients.[14] In properly motivated and informed patients, orthotopic neobladder can be offered even to those over 80 years of age. In general, however, most elderly patients are better served by an ileal conduit.

Comorbidity

With any operation, including radical cystectomy, the risk of postoperative complications correlates with preexisting comorbid medical conditions. The American Society of Anesthesiologists (ASA) scoring system separates anesthetic risk by comorbid factors and has been shown to stratify anesthetic risk accurately (Box 8.1).[15]

The correlation of transitional cell carcinoma of the bladder with a history of smoking compounds the problem.[16,17] Other comorbid related conditions that occur commonly in populations of patients undergoing radical cystectomy include coronary artery disease, a risk or history of cerebrovascular accident (CVA), and peripheral vascular disease. Chronic obstructive pulmonary disease is frequently observed in patients being considered for radical cystectomy.

Nevertheless, many patients with significant comorbidity tolerate cystectomy well with proper attention to perioperative management as discussed below. Even in elderly ASA Class 3 or 4 patients, cystectomy can be performed with acceptable morbidity and limited mortality.[6,18] Overall, very few patients should be considered unfit for cystectomy strictly because of age or comorbidity.

Preoperative evaluation and Management

One of the keys to limiting postoperative morbidity is proper evaluation of presurgical medical conditions (Table 8.1). Although elimination or complete correction of many comorbid conditions is not feasible, appropriate control and evaluation can help minimize or prevent postoperative complications.[19] Studies have shown that an undue delay between the diagnosis of invasive bladder cancer and radical cystectomy can adversely affect both pathologic findings and survival.[20,21] In general, time periods of greater than 90 days between diagnosis and surgery are associated with a worse prognosis. However, an expeditious and thorough evaluation of the patient's general medical condition should not be compromised.

Box 8.1 American Society of Anesthesiologists physical class classification

Class 1:	No organic, physiological, biochemical, or psychiatric disturbance
Class 2:	Mild to moderate systemic disturbance that may or may not be related to the reason for surgery, such as anemia, morbid obesity, diabetes mellitus, chronic bronchitis, or essential hypertension
Class 3:	Severe systemic disturbance, which may or may not be related to the reason for surgery, such as poorly controlled hypertension, diabetes mellitus with vascular complications, chronic obstructive pulmonary disease that limits activity, or history of myocardial infarction
Class 4:	Severe systemic disturbance that is life threatening with or without surgery, such as congestive heart failure, persistent angina, or advanced hepatic dysfunction
Class 5:	Moribund patient who has little chance of surviving, but undergoes surgery as a last resort

---

Coronary artery disease

Although an electrocardiogram is obtained routinely before anesthesia, a cardiac stress test should also be considered, even in asymptomatic patients.[22] Sometimes a correctable ischemia or arrhythmia is uncovered. Identifiable ischemia on a stress test should be evaluated with coronary angiography. When appropriate, percutaneous coronary artery stents should be placed.[23] Occasionally, findings requiring coronary artery bypass grafts are discovered. Although this surgery would obviously delay cystectomy beyond the preferred time period, and introduce a risk of tumor progression, correction of significant coronary artery occlusive disease preoperatively may be indicated to decrease the risk of perioperative myocardial infarction and death.

Preoperative correction or control of cardiac arrhythmias is essential. In general, cardiology consultation would be appropriate. An attempt to determine the etiology of new onset or previously undiagnosed atrial fibrillation or other arrhythmias should be undertaken. The ventricular response should be controlled and premature contractions suppressed to ensure optimal cardiac output.

Cerebrovascular disease

Carotid artery evaluation should be considered, especially in patients with a history of coronary artery occlusive disease or peripheral vascular disease. Auscultation of the neck could reveal a carotid bruit. Doppler ultrasound is an easy and noninvasive method for evaluation of the carotid artery. Significant stenosis may require preoperative consultation with a vascular surgeon or neurosurgeon.[24] Transient hypotension which could occur during surgery might precipitate a devastating CVA in the face of significant carotid artery occlusion.

Chronic obstructive pulmonary disease

Although the underlying lung damage from chronic obstructive pulmonary disease (COPD), especially when cigarette induced, is not

---

Table 8.1 Common cystectomy comorbidities and evaluation/treatment strategies

Comorbidity	Preoperative evaluation	Postoperative evaluation
Coronary artery disease	Electrocardiogram	Routine monitoring of vital signs
	Exercise or pharmacologic stress testing	Careful fluid management
	Cardiology consultation	Restart cardiac medications
Cerebrovascular disease	Carotid duplex analysis	Neurologic examinations
Chronic obstructive pulmonary disease	Cessation of smoking	Bronchodilators
	Chest x-ray	Aggressive pulmonary toilet
	Pulmonary consultation as indicated	Incentive spirometry
		Respiratory therapy as indicated
Diabetes mellitus	Blood glucose, HgA1c testing	Blood glucose testing
	Ensure proper management with oral agents	Sliding scale insulin
Nutritional status	Rare indication for total parenteral nutrition	Oral feeding as rapidly as feasible
		High-calorie supplements
		Total parenteral nutrition for prolonged ileus

reversible, preoperative measures to optimize lung function can be important. Even short-term cessation of smoking can improve recovery.[25] Bronchodilators and pulmonary toilet can be important preoperative adjuncts to aggressive postoperative pulmonary care. Although clinical recognition of lung disease is often sufficient to identify patients at risk for postoperative pulmonary complications, spirometry may be useful if there is uncertainty concerning the presence or extent of lung impairment.[26] Baseline arterial blood gases have not been proven to enhance risk assessment or postoperative management.

Diabetes

Type 2 diabetes is an extremely common and increasingly frequent problem. Further, many patients with type 2 diabetes have poor long-term blood glucose control reflected by elevated hemoglobin-A1c (HgA1c) levels. Elevated blood glucose and HgA1c have been correlated to increased mortality in critically ill surgical patients.[27,28] Prior to cystectomy, HgA1c levels should be obtained and optimal diabetic control attained. Diet, exercise, and weight loss often allow effective management of many individuals with type 2 diabetes. If oral agents and other measures are unsuccessful, insulin administration may be necessary to correct hyperglycemia.

Nutritional status

Some patients with bladder cancer have experienced significant weight loss or poor nutrition, perhaps as a consequence of a locally advanced tumor. The National Veterans Affairs Surgical Risk Study demonstrated that preoperative hypoalbuminemia, reflecting malnutrition, correlates with significantly increased morbidity and mortality.[29] Currently, preoperative intravenous nutrition is rarely indicated or necessary. However, use of high caloric supplements may be helpful in some situations to optimize nutritional status without unduly delaying surgery. Historically, total parenteral nutrition has been used in select patients to reverse a catabolic status, and to facilitate wound healing and recovery after cystectomy.[30] Early and aggressive use of postoperative parenteral nutrition should be considered, especially in patients with poor preoperative nutritional status.

Azotemia

Invasive bladder cancer may occlude the ureteral orifice and cause hydronephrosis. In the face of a normal contralateral kidney, renal function may not be compromised with unilateral obstruction. In this setting, relief of the obstruction is not necessary prior to cystectomy. With bilateral obstruction, or with impaired function of the contralateral kidney and unilateral obstruction, azotemia may be present. Significant azotemia should be corrected prior to surgery.[31] Cystoscopic placement of ureteral stents is usually difficult when obstruction results from invasive bladder cancer because the tumor obscures the trigone and ureteral orifice. A percutaneous nephrostomy tube may be required. Depending upon the degree and duration of obstruction, postobstructive diuresis may occur after placement of a nephrostomy tube.

Preoperative preparation

Preparation for blood transfusion

Radical cystectomy is an operation with the potential for significant intraoperative blood loss.[32–34] In addition, anemia is a common preoperative finding, either because of chronic disease or because of hematuria. Profound anemia should be corrected preoperatively with blood transfusions. Indeed, even in patients with a normal serum hematocrit preoperatively, possible need for blood transfusion should be anticipated. Although bleeding is not usually massive and sudden with cystectomy, the median intraoperative blood loss is such that a substantial number of patients require a blood transfusion.[33] A type and screen may be sufficient, depending upon how long it takes to obtain fully cross-matched blood in a given hospital. For most patients, however, blood should be typed and cross-matched preoperatively so that it can be administered in a timely fashion if required.

Bowel preparation

Thoughts about both the value and method of bowel preparation have evolved in recent years.[35] Undoubtedly, though, minimizing contamination of the operative field is desirable and is facilitated by a mechanical bowel preparation. With an ileal conduit, minimal contamination should occur with division of the bowel and anastomosis of the ureters. Isolation and cleansing of a small bowel segment used for construction of a continent reservoir can also minimize contamination. An effective mechanical bowel preparation becomes more important when the colon is used for urinary tract reconstruction. Regardless of the method used for reconstruction, there is a low but definite risk of rectal injury with cystectomy. A decision to perform primary closure of a recognized rectal injury is facilitated by minimizing fecal spillage.

Various methods are used for mechanical cleansing of the bowel.[35] Most commonly, an oral polyethylene glycol electrolyte solution (GoLYTELY) is administered. However, this requires consumption of a large amount of fluid, and can cause vomiting or abdominal cramping and pain. In particular, many elderly patients tolerate this poorly and may be unable to complete the bowel preparation. Dehydration from the induced diarrhea can also be problematic. Oral sodium phosphate solutions have been shown to have an equivalent mechanical cleansing effect and require consumption of less fluid.[36]

Antibiotic bowel preparation may also be important. The classic Nichols preparation consists of 1 g each of oral neomycin and erythromycin base at 1300, 1400, and 2300 hours the day prior to surgery.[37] The addition of intravenous antibiotics, preferably a third generation cephalosporin, used at maximum dosage and administered at the ideal time before, during, and for 24 hours after surgery, is the preferred regimen to decrease wound infection rates for bowel surgery.[38]

Preoperative medications

In general, instructions about withholding preoperative medications are delivered to the patient by the anesthesiologist. However, it is important for the surgeon to be aware of medicines that should be withheld and the time required for washout.[39,40] Warfarin should be discontinued 5 days prior to surgery. Depending upon the reason for which long-term warfarin is being used, a window wherein low molecular weight heparin is used to bridge the time of discontinuation until readministration of warfarin may be important. In particular, patients with mechanical heart valves should be maintained with such a window. Aspirin and nonsteroidal anti-inflammatory drugs should be withheld at least 7 days prior to surgery because of their antiplatelet effect. Clopidogrel and ticlopidine, inhibitors of platelet aggregation, should be stopped 7 days preoperatively. Metformin, a commonly used oral medication for glycemic control in patients with type 2 diabetes, should be withheld for at least 1 day prior to surgery.

Antihypertensives usually are continued until the day prior to surgery. Depending on blood pressure control and the medications themselves, the anesthesiologist may allow oral intake of some antihypertensives on the morning of surgery with a small sip of water. Otherwise, patients generally are kept with nothing by mouth for at least 8 hours prior to the surgery to avoid aspiration. Although currently not frequently used, psychotropic monoamine oxidase inhibitors must be discontinued 2 weeks preoperatively.

Intraoperative patient monitoring

Intraoperative monitoring is the responsibility of the anesthesiologist but requires input from the surgeon. The two should communicate about the anticipated length of surgery, the method of urinary reconstruction, and the potential for significant blood loss depending upon tumor size and stage. At a minimum, a large-bore peripheral intravenous cannula should be available for administration of blood products. Insertion of a central line is not routinely required. However, in patients with significant cardiovascular comorbidity, the presence of a central line could allow rapid insertion of a pulmonary artery catheter. An automatic, inflatable arm cuff is usually sufficient for monitoring blood pressure. A radial artery catheter, however, allows continuous blood pressure monitoring as well as evaluation of serial arterial blood gasses when oxygenation is an issue. This may be particularly applicable in patients with chronic obstructive pulmonary disease or cardiovascular comorbidity.

Postoperative care

Location

Each surgeon must make a decision about the appropriate hospital area for early postoperative recovery depending upon circumstances within the hospital. Not all hospitals provide equivalent care in different units. Fewer than 5% of our patients undergoing cystectomy require transfer to the intensive care unit postoperatively.[41] In some circumstances, we utilize an intermediate care unit when continuous cardiac monitoring is desirable, especially in patients with a history of arrhythmia or intraoperative rhythm disturbances. Most often, though, patients are transferred from the recovery room to the urology ward, where there are nurses experienced in the postoperative care of patients undergoing cystectomy.

We utilize an incision that does not extend above the level of the umbilicus for cystectomy, even with urinary reconstruction. In these circumstances, even in patients with significant COPD, extubation in the operating room or recovery room is feasible. Sometimes, however, there is delayed return of a good respiratory effort. In this situation, overnight intubation and ventilatory support are important. Efforts to wean the patient from the ventilator as soon as possible should be undertaken and usually are feasible on the first postoperative day.

Pain management

Pain is one of the most frequently expressed concerns for patients undergoing surgical procedures. Beyond the physical discomfort and mental anguish associated with pain, poor analgesic control after cystectomy can increase the rate of complications. Mobility may be limited in a patient with poor pain control, increasing the risk of postoperative pneumonia or thromboembolic complications. Inappropriate use of narcotics can occasionally lead to respiratory depression and frequently contributes to ileus. Further, mental status changes with narcotic administration can lead to confusion or even combativeness and dislodgement of drains or tubes.[25]

Fortunately, the lower midline abdominal incision used for cystectomy does not frequently cause significant pain after surgery. The pain associated with a surgical incision depends not only on the length but also on the location. Upper abdominal incisions interfere more with respiratory efforts. Further, separation of muscles along the natural plane of the linea alba avoids the need for actual incision of muscular tissue. Other than pain from the surgical incision itself, bowel distension from ileus is the most common cause of postoperative pain. A vicious cycle can ensue with administration of narcotics for pain relief which, in turn, exacerbates or prolongs ileus.

Occluded stents may also be a source of postoperative pain, usually flank pain. The pain can be severe and colicky. Irrigation of stents to maintain patency should be performed in patients complaining of flank pain. Occasionally, radiographic imaging to ensure proper stent placement can be helpful.

For all of these reasons, postoperative pain management is an important aspect of care for patients undergoing cystectomy. Epidural catheters can be an effective method for analgesia after surgery. However, there are also potential problems with epidural catheters. First, insertion and maintenance of the catheter itself require additional steps. Rather than facilitating mobility, the presence of an epidural catheter may limit ambulation. In our experience, the use of an epidural catheter has not decreased the severity or duration of postoperative ileus. The catheter may become dislodged and provide ineffective pain control.

Patient-controlled analgesia allows more effective pain control and may also result in less overall narcotic usage than periodic administration of parenteral narcotics. A basal rate of analgesic administration (usually morphine sulfate) is maintained, and the patient makes a decision about when an additional bolus is required. Patients should be encouraged to use bolus administration as necessary but to limit narcotic use as much as possible.

Ketorolac, a nonsteroidal anti-inflammatory drug, is an effective analgesic and may have particular applicability in a postoperative setting. We routinely administer ketorolac 30 mg in the postanesthesia care unit and continue a dose of 15 mg every 6 hours for 24 hours postoperatively. Most often, this provides excellent analgesia and limited narcotics are required as supplements. Because of a risk of renal dysfunction with prolonged administration, ketorolac generally should be discontinued 24–48 hours postoperatively and its use withheld altogether in patients with azotemia.[42] In addition, there is some risk of gastrointestinal toxicity or hemorrhagic complications.[43]

Deep venous thrombosis prophylaxis

In most surgical series, thromboembolic complications are the leading cause of mortality and a significant source of morbidity in patients undergoing radical cystectomy.[8] Multiple factors contribute to the risk of thromboembolic problems including comorbidity, the underlying malignancy, and the generally prolonged duration of surgery. Although many guidelines recommend routine anticoagulant prophylaxis for patients undergoing cystectomy, most clinicians are concerned about the risk of hemorrhagic complications. Although intraoperative bleeding may not be directly affected, postoperative bleeding, pelvic hematoma, and hematuria may all occur in patients on anticoagulant prophylaxis.

Numerous studies have shown that, in order to obtain the maximal effect, any form of prophylaxis used must be administered preoperatively.[44] Low-dose warfarin, mini-dose heparin, and low molecular weight heparin probably have nearly equal efficacy in preventing thromboembolic complications. Further, all have been shown to be superior to no prophylactic anticoagulants in terms of decreasing both deep venous thrombosis (DVT) and pulmonary embolus (PE). Prolonged lymphatic drainage may occur more frequently in patients on anticoagulants, leading to lymphocele formation.[45] However, with intraperitoneal procedures such as radical cystectomy and pelvic lymph node dissection, the entire peritoneum is open and there is less likelihood of loculation of lymphatic fluid.

Other measures are also important. It is generally agreed that early ambulation is important and should be encouraged. Pneumatic calf compression devices have not been proven to be of benefit for radical cystectomy but are commonly used and recommended on the basis of their value with other surgical procedures.[46,47]

In a patient with a suspected DVT, Doppler ultrasonography should be performed. While the accuracy is more limited for calf thrombosis, the test has greater than 95% sensitivity and specificity for proximal venous thrombosis, the most common source of pulmonary embolus.[48] If a Doppler study confirms the presence of DVT, anticoagulant therapy should be administered with unfractionated heparin.[49] The goal of therapy is a partial thromboplastin time 2–2.5 times the control value. Oral warfarin should be initiated immediately as a delay of 5–7 days may occur before therapeutic levels are achieved. Continuation of anticoagulant therapy is usually recommended for a minimum of 3 months after a postoperative thromboembolic event.

If DVT or PE is diagnosed within the first 48 hours after surgery, consideration should be given to placement of an inferior vena cava filter, although there may be a reluctance to administer full dose anticoagulation in the early postoperative period. Even with a filter in place, however, anticoagulant therapy should be initiated once the patient gets beyond the immediate postoperative state.

A clinical suspicion of pulmonary embolus requires prompt diagnosis and treatment. Ventilation perfusion scans frequently are indeterminate in the postoperative period because of atelectasis and/or pneumonia. The diagnosis can be confirmed by pulmonary arteriography or helical computed tomography (CT) scan. Thrombolytic therapy is playing an increasing role in treatment of an acute PE, especially in a patient with clinically significant respiratory compromise.

Gastrointestinal management

Historically, patients undergoing major abdominal surgery, especially procedures with a bowel anastomosis, were maintained on nasogastric suction until bowel function returned. In some centers, gastrostomy tube placement has been used to avoid the discomfort of prolonged nasogastric suction. Increasingly, nasogastric tubes are being omitted after abdominal surgery. Nasogastric tubes remove the naturally produced gastric juices as well as air from endogenous production and swallowing. Thus, they may help prevent postoperative distension or vomiting. Nonetheless, most patients do not require nasogastric suction after cystectomy, and placement of a gastrostomy tube seems needlessly invasive.

There is some additional information suggesting that early enteral feeding can help prevent some of the immunosuppression which occurs after surgery and may help promote peristalsis. We performed a randomized prospective study which showed no difference between patients receiving oral intake on the second postoperative day and those kept without food until bowel sounds and bowel function returned (unpublished data). There was an identical rate of abdominal distension in around 10% of patients in both groups requiring insertion of a nasogastric tube.

The pathway we use maintains the patient nil by mouth for at least 24 hours after surgery but nasogastric tubes are not used routinely.[50,51] By the second or third postoperative day, a full liquid diet may be initiated and advanced as tolerated. The stepwise progression from clear liquids to full liquids to a regular diet is not necessarily maintained. In fact, we usually avoid a clear liquid diet alone as many patients prefer full liquids and there is no evidence that a clear liquid diet is tolerated better. Bisacodyl suppositories are used beginning on the second or third postoperative day. This helps promote emptying of the colon and rectum. However, small bowel ileus is likely unaffected.

In a patient with abdominal distension beyond the fourth or fifth postoperative day, a diagnosis of partial small bowel obstruction must be considered. Anastomotic stricture or edema, internal hernia, or obstruction from fibrous tissue can all cause either partial or complete small bowel obstruction after cystectomy. A radiographic flat plate film of the abdomen can be helpful. While distended small bowel typically is visualized in either circumstance, gas in the colon or rectum is more suggestive of ileus. Clinical findings are also important. Bowel sounds are usually diminished or absent when distension is from ileus, whereas they may be hyperactive and with intermittent rushes when small bowel obstruction is present.

Unless there is evidence of an acute intraperitoneal process, the initial management in a patient with ileus versus partial small bowel obstruction is nasogastric suction. Prolonged ileus is the most common cause of delayed hospital discharge and usually resolves spontaneously.[51] Histamine receptor antagonists or proton pump inhibitors may help prevent some of the gastric discomfort. If an apparent ileus fails to resolve after a period of nasogastric suction, an abdominal CT scan should be considered. Sometimes an intraperitoneal fluid collection such as urinoma or abscess, especially in a patient with fever, can be the source of a prolonged ileus. Administration of oral contrast with small bowel follow-through occasionally is helpful. A water-soluble contrast agent should be used. Ready passage of the contrast, especially into a dilated colon, is consistent with ileus. Parenteral nutrition should be considered in patients with prolonged ileus, and surgical exploration should be deferred unless there are signs of acute obstruction. The overwhelming majority of patients eventually have resolution of the ileus and do not require exploration. Sometimes, however, partial small bowel obstruction can mimic ileus, and surgical exploration is required if there is no resolution of the small bowel distention.

Management of drainage tubes

The number and type of drainage tubes used after cystectomy is very much dependent upon the philosophy of the individual surgeon. In general, however, a closed suction drain should be placed in the pelvis. The drain evacuates lymphatic fluid, blood, and any urine which may extravasate from either the ureteral anastomosis or the suture line of the reservoir or conduit. Since the drain is intraperitoneal, some output can be expected under the best of circumstances. In general, we remove the drain when the overall output is less than 100 cc in 24 hours. If drainage is excessive or prolonged, it can be submitted for chemistry studies. A creatinine level exceeding the serum level indicates the presence of urine in the drainage. Also, indigo carmine given intravenously will stain the drainage blue if there is urine present. Most often, watchful waiting is appropriate even in the face of a urine leak as spontaneous healing can be expected. If the urine leakage is readily evacuated by the drain, the patient may tolerate this well and even begin oral feeding. If there are indwelling stents, their patency should be confirmed. If no stents are present, or if the drainage persists, an intravenous pyelogram may help detect the source of the urine leakage and allow placement of a nephrostomy tube and internal stent if appropriate.

Ureteral stents frequently are placed across the ureterointestinal anastomosis. Depending upon the method of reconstruction, these may exit through the ileal conduit stoma, through a separate skin stab wound, or alongside a urethral Foley catheter. In any event, their patency should be maintained by periodic irrigation. There is no strong evidence that stents prevent or even reduce the risk of ureterointestinal anastomotic stricture, but they can avoid temporary obstruction from edema and divert the urine to external drainage while anastomotic healing occurs.[52] The duration for which stents are left indwelling is also a matter of individual surgeon philosophy. However, we typically will remove the stents prior to patient discharge.

Some surgeons place a drainage catheter within an ileal conduit to promote urine drainage while the suture or staple line along the base of the conduit heals. This tube may be redundant if there are indwelling ureteral stents. Further, because it can interfere with secure maintenance of a stomal appliance, removal prior to discharge is usually advised.

With a continent cutaneous reservoir, pouch drainage usually occurs via a Malecot catheter which exits either above or below the abdominal stoma. Since most continent cutaneous reservoirs are constructed from right colon, a large amount of mucus is produced and periodic tube irrigation is indicated to maintain patency. These tubes typically are left indwelling for up to several weeks until the patient is facile with intermittent catheterization.

With an orthotopic reservoir, a urethral Foley catheter is placed. Simultaneous placement of a Malecot tube in the suprapubic region is used by some surgeons as a security measure. We have found this unnecessary, and a 20 Fr. urethral Foley catheter alone has provided adequate drainage. The anastomotic integrity usually is sufficient so that a catheter could be replaced if there were premature autodeflation of the catheter balloon. The patient is discharged with the catheter in place with the intent that it be removed approximately 3 weeks later.

Stomal therapy

Although many patients are motivated to avoid an abdominal stoma, an ileal conduit can provide good quality of life and be a relatively trouble-free method for urinary diversion. However, proper placement and maintenance of the stoma are essential. The stomal site should be selected preoperatively. Usually, the stoma is placed in either the right lower or the right upper quadrant of the abdomen depending upon the patient's body habitus, abdominal creases, or scars from prior surgical incisions. Use of mesh for closure of a ventral or inguinal hernia can also affect placement.

A trained stomal therapist should be available to mark the patient preoperatively. The patient is examined in a sitting, standing, and lying position. The belt line is determined. The stomal therapist may mark both a primary and a secondary site to allow the surgeon some flexibility as intraoperative findings such as adhesions or short mesentery length can dictate placement of the stoma in a specific location.

The patient and the patient's family should be engaged in changing the stomal appliance as soon as possible after surgery. Many patients have a natural aversion to a stoma initially but quickly become comfortable with it and adept at changing the appliance. Selection of proper wafer size and determination of whether use of an abdominal belt is indicated are important considerations.

Discharge planning

A patient should be afebrile, ambulatory without assistance, and tolerating an oral diet before discharge is considered. Even under these circumstances, strong family support and good education are essential. Although a patient may be able to maintain self-hygiene, assistance in food preparation and cleanup as well as aspects of daily living are necessary for a period of time. Sometimes family members are either unavailable or unable to provide the necessary care. Visiting nurses can allow a patient to return to a home environment even when some assistance is required. In other situations, an intermediate care facility can provide a bridge between inpatient hospitalization and a return home. The key to all of these measures is proper preparation and education of both the patient and immediate family members or care providers.

Clinical pathways

All aspects of perioperative care are facilitated by use of a clinical pathway.[53] The pathway document outlines the minimal care necessary for the ideal patient (Tables 8.2 and 8.3). Further, the pathway allows the patient to anticipate various aspects of care and to participate in recovery. Especially with an operation as complex as cystectomy, deviations from a pathway or use of additional procedures or testing is common. Thus, it is incumbent upon the clinician to provide careful oversight and involvement rather than simply allowing the pathway to serve as a default guide.

Table 8.2 Radical cystectomy—ileal conduit pathway: pre- and early postoperative care

	Preoperative preparation	*Day of surgery/postoperatively*	*Postoperative days 1–2*
Goals	Informed consent process Preop testing/labs completed within 30 days of surgery Patient and family verbalize understanding of preop teaching	Tolerates procedure without complication Recovers uneventfully from anesthesia Drains and stents patent and functioning Pain controlled, temperature <101°F	Tolerates ambulation with assistance Drains and stents patent and functioning Pain controlled, temperature <101°F Urine output >30 cc/hr
Care reminder	Vital signs Height and weight	Vital signs and temperature q.q.h. Assess stoma/peristomal skin q.q.h. Check pouch/dressing q.q.h. Strict intake and output	Vital signs and temperature q.q.h. Assess stoma/peristomal skin q.q.h. Check pouch q.q.h., dressing off POD 2 Strict intake and output
Treatment	History and physical Consent signed	Incentive spirometer q.h. SCD on 7 hr, off 1 hr TED hose, knee high TCDB q.h. Jackson-Pratt drain empty and record q8h	Incentive spirometer q.h. SCD on 7 hr, off 1 hr TED hose, knee high TCDB q.h. Jackson-Pratt drain empty and record q8h
Activity	Ad lib	Bedrest	Out of bed to chair POD 1, then ambulate Ambulate in hallway t.i.d. POD 1
Diet	Clear liquid diet day prior to surgery NPO after midnight	NPO	NPO
Tests	Complete blood count Chest x-ray (posteroanterior and lateral) if indicated Basic metabolic panel if indicated Type and crossmatch 2 units packed red blood cells	Potassium 0500 POD 1 Hematocrit 0500 POD 1 and POD 2	
Medication	Bowel preparation day prior to surgery GoLYTELY, neomycin, flagyl	D5 ½ NS + 20 mEq KCl @ 150 cc/hr Cefotetan 1 g IV on call to OR then 1 g IV q12h × 2 doses Ketorolac 30 mg IV in PACU then 15 mg IV q6h × 36 hr Analgesic IV/PCA Famotidine 20 mg IV q12h Individualized patient medications	D5 ½ NS + 20 mEq KCl @ 150 cc/hr Cefotetan 1 g IV on call to OR then 1 g IV q12h × 2 doses Ketorolac 30 mg IV in PACU then 15 mg IV q6h × 36 hr Analgesic IV/PCA Famotidine 20 mg IV q12h Individualized patient medications
Consults	Enterostomal RN to mark stoma Anesthesia preop evaluation clinic RN practitioner consult CM consult	Enterostomal RN teaching Social work consult	Enterostomal RN teaching
Teaching	Orientation to medical center when/where to arrive for surgery, parking, family waiting/visitation MD instructions on procedure anticipated risks/benefits Preop processes concerning cystectomy/ileal conduit	Postop routines to anticipate, IS, TCDB Use of PCA	Patient to receive written educational materials 'About Your Urostomy' booklet
Discharge planning	Initiate discharge planning, assess home/family support Anticipated length of stay Notify CM for special needs Coordinate with primary care provider, development disability services, prn Autologous blood donation prn	Home health care referral	

CM, case manager; IS, incentive spirometer; IV, intravenous; NPO, nil per os; PACU, postanesthesia care unit; PCA, patient-controlled analgesia; PO, per os (orally); POD, postoperative day; PRN, according to circumstances, RN, registered nurse; SCD, sequential compression devices; TED, thromboembolic disease; TCDB, turn/cough/deep breathe.

Table 8.3 Radical cystectomy—ileal conduit pathway: ongoing postoperative care and follow-up

	Postoperative days 3–4	Postoperative days 5–7	Postoperative follow-up
Goals	Pain controlled, temperature <101°F Wafer/pouch intact without leakage Drain output decreasing to 100 cc/day Ambulates with assistance Return of bowel function with flatus/bowel movement	Pain controlled, temperature <101°F Wafer/pouch intact without leakage Patient/family demonstrate urostomy care and verbalize understanding of procedure of pouch/wafer change Ambulates with assistance Return of bowel function, tolerates diet Patient/family understand discharge instructions and home care	Pain controlled Wound healing adequate Tolerates baseline activity
Care reminder	Vital signs and temperature q.q.h. Assess stoma/peristomal skin q.q.h. Check pouch q.q.h. Strict intake and output	Vital signs and temperature q.q.h. Assess stoma/peristomal skin q.q.h. Check pouch q.q.h. Strict intake and output	Vital signs and temperature
Treatment	Incentive spirometer q.h. SCD on 7 hr, off 1 hr TED hose, knee high TCDB q.h. Jackson-Pratt drain empty and record q8h	Incentive spirometer q.h. SCD on 7 hr, off 1 hr TED hose, knee high TCDB q.h. D/C drains on day of discharge	
Activity	Ambulate in hallway t.i.d.		Ad lib
Diet	NPO	Full liquid diet advance to regular diet as tolerated	Regular
Tests	Hematocrit 0500 POD 4 BMP 0500 POD 4		
Medication	D5 ½ NS + 20 mEq KCl/L @ 150 cc/hr Analgesic IV/PCA Famotidine 20 mg IV q12h Individualized patient medications	Decrease and D/C IV fluids when taking PO Analgesic PO D/C famotidine when taking PO Trimethoprim-sulfamethoxazole (Bactrim DS) PO b.i.d. × 17 days, alternatively nitrofurantoin (Macrodantin) 100 mg PO q.h.s. × 17 days Individualized patient medications	
Consults	–	–	

Teaching		Discharge self-care and activity:
		   May shower
		   Walking and stairs okay
		   No lifting over 5 lbs
		   No driving
		   Keep wound clean and dry
		Discharge medications:
		   Milk of Magnesia for constipation
		   Percocet for pain
		   Bactrim or Macrodantin × 17 days
		Reportable signs and symptoms:
		   How and when to contact surgeon
		   Call for temperature >101°F, wound erythema, increased tenderness, nausea, and emesis
		Pouch/wafer change	

Discharge planning		Discharge prescriptions written and received Follow-up appointment scheduled and confirmed 2–4 weeks, depending on surgeon preference Home health care arrangements completed prior to discharge	

D/C, discontinue. See Table 8.2 for explanation of other acronyms.

Conclusion

The morbidity and mortality from radical cystectomy have diminished significantly over the last few decades. Some of this is a consequence of improved surgical technique and better understanding of the anatomy. To a great extent, though, the improvements can be attributed to advances in perioperative care. Sometimes this means eliminating or withholding unnecessary procedures or treatments, especially those which are invasive in themselves. In other circumstances, it requires active intervention. In all situations, familiarity with available knowledge and experience is essential in providing optimal results.

References

1. Stein JP, Lieskovsky G, Cote R, et al. Radical cystectomy in the treatment of invasive bladder cancer: long-term results in 1,054 patients. J Clin Oncol 2001; 19: 666–75.
2. Quek ML, Stein JP, Clark PE, et al. Natural history of surgically treated bladder carcinoma with extravesical tumor extension. Cancer 2003; 98: 955–61.
3. Montie JE, Wood DP Jr. The risk of radical cystectomy. Br J Urol 1989; 63: 483–6.
4. Thrasher JB, Crawford ED. Current management of invasive and metastatic transitional cell carcinoma of the bladder. J Urol 1993; 149: 957–72.
5. Shipley WU, Kaufman DS, Zehr E, et al. Selective bladder preservation by combined modality protocol treatment: long-term outcomes of 190 patients with invasive bladder cancer. Urology 2002; 60: 62–68.
6. Farnham SB, Cookson MS, Alberts G, et al. Benefit of radical cystectomy in the elderly patient with significant co-morbidities. Urol Oncol 2004; 22: 178–81.
7. Lynch CF, Cohen MB. Urinary system. Cancer 1995;75:316–329.
8. Hendry WF. Morbidity and mortality of radical cystectomy (1971–78 and 1978–85). J R Soc Med 1986; 79: 395–400.
9. Chang SS, Alberts G, Cookson MS, et al. Radical cystectomy is safe in elderly patients at high risk. J Urol 2001; 166: 938–41.
10. Peyromaure M, Guerin F, Debre B, et al. Surgical management of infiltrating bladder cancer in elderly patients. Eur Urol 2004; 45: 147–54.
11. Game X, Soulie M, Seguin P, et al. Radical cystectomy in patients older than 75 years: assessment of morbidity and mortality. Eur Urol 2001; 39: 525–29.
12. Soulie M, Straub M, Game X, et al. A multicenter study of the morbidity of radical cystectomy in select elderly patients with bladder cancer. J Urol 2002; 167: 1325–8.
13. Parekh DJ, Gilbert WB, Koch MO, et al. Continent urinary reconstruction versus ileal conduit: a contemporary single-institution comparison of perioperative morbidity and mortality. Urology 2000; 55: 852–55.
14. Dutta SC, Chang SC, Coffey CS, et al. Health related quality of life assessment after radical cystectomy: comparison of ileal conduit with continent orthotopic neobladder. J Urol 2002; 168: 164–67.
15. American Society of Anesthesiologists. New classification of physical status. Anesthesiology 1963; 24: 111.
16. Morrison AS. Advances in the etiology of urothelial cancer. Urol Clin North Am 1984; 11: 557–66.
17. Burch JD, Rohan TE, Howe GR, et al. Risk of bladder cancer by source and type of tobacco exposure: a case-control study. Int J Cancer 1989; 44: 622–8.
18. Parekh DJ, Clark T, O'Connor J, et al. Orthotopic neobladder following radical cystectomy in patients with high perioperative risk and co-morbid medical conditions. J Urol 2002; 168: 2454–6.
19. Miller DC, Taub DA, Dunn RL, et al. The impact of co-morbid disease on cancer control and survival following radical cystectomy. J Urol 2003; 169: 105–9.
20. Chang SS, Hassan JM, Cookson MS, et al. Delaying radical cystectomy for muscle invasive bladder cancer results in worse pathological stage. J Urol 2003; 170: 1085–7.
21. Sanchez-Ortiz RF, Huang WC, Mick R, et al. An interval longer than 12 weeks between the diagnosis of muscle invasion and cystectomy is associated with worse outcome in bladder carcinoma. J Urol 2003; 169: 110–5; discussion 115.
22. Eagle KA, Berger PB, Calkins H, et al. ACC/AHA guideline update for perioperative cardiovascular evaluation for noncardiac surgery—executive summary: a report of the American College of Cardiology/American Heart Association Task Force on Practice Guidelines (Committee to Update the 1996 Guidelines on Perioperative Cardiovascular Evaluation for Noncardiac Surgery). Online. Available: www.acc.org/clinical/guidelines/perio/update/periupdate_index.htm.
23. Park KW. Preoperative cardiac evaluation. Anesthesiol Clin North America 2004; 22: 199–208.
24. Beneficial effect of carotid endarterectomy in symptomatic patients with high-grade carotid stenosis. North American Symptomatic Carotid Endarterectomy Trial Collaborators. N Engl J Med 1991; 325: 445–53.
25. Richardson JD, Cocanour CS, Kern JA, et al. Perioperative risk assessment in elderly and high-risk patients. J Am Coll Surg 2004; 199: 133–46.
26. Rock P, Passannante A. Preoperative assessment: pulmonary. Anesthesiol Clin North America 2004; 22: 77–91.
27. Connery LE, Coursin DB. Assessment and therapy of selected endocrine disorders. Anesthesiol Clin North America 2004; 22: 93–123.
28. Coursin DB, Connery LE, Ketzler JT. Perioperative diabetic and hyperglycemic management issues. Crit Care Med 2004; 32: S116–25.
29. Gibbs J, Cull W, Henderson W, et al. Preoperative serum albumin level as a predictor of operative mortality and morbidity: results from the National VA Surgical Risk Study. Arch Surg 1999; 134: 36–42.
30. Askanazi J, Hensle TW, Starker PM, et al. Effect of immediate postoperative nutritional support on length of hospitalization. Ann Surg 1986; 203: 236–9.
31. Krishnan M. Preoperative care of patients with kidney disease. Am Fam Physician 2002; 66: 1471–6.
32. Ahlering TE, Henderson JB, Skinner DG. Controlled hypotensive anesthesia to reduce blood loss in radical cystectomy for bladder cancer. J Urol 1983; 129: 953–4.
33. Chang SS, Smith JA Jr, Wells N, et al. Estimated blood loss and transfusion requirements of radical cystectomy. J Urol 2001; 166: 2151–4.
34. Park KI, Kojima O, Tomoyoshi T. Intra-operative autotransfusion in radical cystectomy. Br J Urol 1997; 79: 717–21.
35. Ferguson KH, McNeil JJ, Morey AF. Mechanical and antibiotic bowel preparation for urinary diversion surgery. J Urol 2002; 167: 2352–6.
36. Oliveira L, Wexner SD, Daniel N, et al. Mechanical bowel preparation for elective colorectal surgery. A prospective, randomized, surgeon-blinded trial comparing sodium phosphate and polyethylene glycol-based oral lavage solutions. Dis Colon Rectum 1997; 40: 585–91.
37. Nichols RL, Broido P, Condon RE, Gorbach SL, Nyhus LM. Effect of preoperative neomycin–erythromycin intestinal preparation on the incidence of infectious complications following colon surgery. Ann Surg 1973; 178: 453–9.
38. Mangram AJ, Horan TC, Pearson ML et al. Guideline for prevention of surgical site infection, 1999. Centers for Disease Control and Prevention (CDC) Hospital Infection Control Practices Advisory Committee. Am J Infect Control 1999; 27: 97–134.
39. Mercado DL, Petty BG. Perioperative medication management. Med Clin North Am 2003; 87: 41–57.
40. Pass SE, Simpson RW. Discontinuation and reinstitution of medications during the perioperative period. Am J Health Syst Pharm 2004; 61: 899–914.
41. Chang SS, Cookson MS, Hassan JM, et al. Routine postoperative intensive care monitoring is not necessary after radical cystectomy. J Urol 2002; 167: 1321–4.

42. Haragsim L, Dalal R, Bagga H, et al. Ketorolac-induced acute renal failure and hyperkalemia: report of three cases. Am J Kidney Dis 1994; 24: 578–80.

43. Strom BL, Berlin JA, Kinman JL, et al. Parenteral ketorolac and risk of gastrointestinal and operative site bleeding. A postmarketing surveillance study. JAMA 1996; 275: 376–82.

44. Heit JA. Perioperative management of the chronically anticoagulated patient. J Thromb Thrombolysis 2001; 12: 81–7.

45. Koch MO Jr, Smith JA. Low molecular weight heparin and radical prostatectomy: a prospective analysis of safety and side effects. Prostate Cancer Prostatic Dis 1997; 1: 101–4.

46. Cisek LJ, Walsh PC. Thromboembolic complications following radical retropubic prostatectomy. Influence of external sequential pneumatic compression devices. Urology 1993; 42: 406–8.

47. Chandhoke PS, Gooding GA, Narayan P. Prospective randomized trial of warfarin and intermittent pneumatic leg compression as prophylaxis for postoperative deep venous thrombosis in major urological surgery. J Urol 1992; 147: 1056–9.

48. Ramzi DW, Leeper KV. DVT and pulmonary embolism: Part I. Diagnosis. Am Fam Physician 2004; 69: 2829–36.

49. Ramzi DW, Leeper KV. DVT and pulmonary embolism: Part II. Treatment and prevention. Am Fam Physician 2004; 69: 2841–8.

50. Baumgartner RG, Wells N, Chang SS, et al. Causes of increased length of stay following radical cystectomy. Urol Nurs 2002; 22: 319–23.

51. Chang SS, Baumgartner RG, Wells N, et al. Causes of increased hospital stay after radical cystectomy in a clinical pathway setting. J Urol 2002; 167: 208–11.

52. Regan JB, Barrett, DM. Stented versus nonstented ureteroileal anastomoses: is there a difference with regard to leak and stricture? J Urol 1985; 134: 1101–3.

53. Chang SS, Cookson MS, Baumgartner RG, et al. Analysis of early complications after radical cystectomy: results of a collaborative care pathway. J Urol 2002; 167: 2012–6.

9

Radical cystectomy—technique and outcomes

John P Stein, Donald G Skinner

Introduction

In the United States, bladder cancer is the fourth most common cancer in men and the eighth most common in women, with transitional cell carcinoma (TCC) comprising nearly 90% of all primary bladder tumors.[1] Although the majority of patients present with superficial bladder tumors, 20% to 40% of patients will either present with or ultimately develop muscle-invasive disease. Invasive bladder cancer is a lethal malignancy. If left untreated, over 85% of patients die of the disease within 2 years of the diagnosis.[2] Furthermore, in a certain percent of patients with high-grade bladder tumors without involvement of the lamina propria disease will recur/progress and/or fail intravesical management. Such patients may be best treated with an earlier cystectomy when survival outcomes are optimal.[3]

The rationale for an aggressive treatment approach employing radical cystectomy for high-grade, invasive bladder cancer is based on several important observations:

1. The best long-term survival rates, coupled with the lowest local recurrences, are seen following definitive surgery removing the primary bladder tumor and regional lymph nodes.[4,5]
2. The morbidity and mortality of radical cystectomy has significantly improved over the past several decades.
3. TCC tends to be a tumor that is resistant to radiation therapy, even at high doses.
4. Chemotherapy alone, or in combination with bladder-sparing protocols, has not demonstrated long-term local control and survival rates equivalent to those with cystectomy.[6]
5. Radical cystectomy provides accurate pathologic staging of the primary bladder tumor (p stage) and regional lymph nodes, thus selectively determining the need for adjuvant therapy based on precise pathologic evaluation.

For the aforementioned reasons, radical cystectomy has become a standard and arguably is the best definitive form of therapy for high-grade, invasive bladder cancer today.

The evolution and improvement in lower urinary tract reconstruction, particularly orthotopic diversion, has been a major component in enhancing the quality of life of patients requiring cystectomy. Currently, most men and women can safely undergo orthotopic lower urinary tract reconstruction to the native, intact urethra following cystectomy.[7] Orthotopic reconstruction most closely resembles the original bladder in both location and function, provides a continent means to store urine, and allows volitional voiding via the urethra. The orthotopic neobladder eliminates the need for a cutaneous stoma, urostomy appliance, and the need for intermittent catheterization in most cases. These efforts have improved the quality of life of patients who must undergo bladder removal, and have also stimulated patients and physicians to consider radical cystectomy for high-grade, invasive bladder cancer at an earlier, more curable stage.[8]

At the University of Southern California (USC) a dedicated effort has been made to improve continually upon the surgical technique of radical cystectomy and to provide an acceptable form of urinary diversion, without compromise of a sound cancer operation.[9–11] Certain technical issues regarding radical cystectomy and an appropriate extended bilateral pelvic iliac lymphadenectomy are critical in order to minimize local recurrence and positive surgical margins, and to maximize cancer-specific survival. Attention to surgical detail is important in optimizing the successful clinical outcomes of orthotopic diversion, maintaining the rhabdosphincter mechanism and urinary continence in these patients.[11]

Herein, the detailed surgical approach and technical aspects of radical cystectomy in men and women are described. This surgical approach also includes a description of an extended lymphadenectomy. We believe this is an important component in radical cystectomy and the clinical outcomes of patients with high-grade, invasive bladder cancer. A growing body of evidence exists to suggest that a more extended lymphadenectomy may be beneficial in both lymph node-positive and lymph node-negative patients with bladder cancer.[12–16] Although the exact limits of the lymphadenectomy for patients with bladder cancer undergoing cystectomy are currently debated, we advocate a lymph node dissection with the boundaries to include initiation at the level of the inferior mesenteric artery (superior limits of dissection), extending laterally over the inferior vena cava/aorta to the genitofemoral nerve (lateral limits of dissection), and distally to the lymph node of Cloquet medially (on Cooper's ligament) and the circumflex iliac vein laterally. This dissection should also include bilaterally all obturator, hypogastric, and presciatic lymph nodes, as well as the presacral lymph nodes.

Indications for cystectomy

Invasive bladder cancer includes a spectrum of tumors ranging from infiltration of the superficial lamina propria (T1), to extension into (T2), and through (T3) the muscularis propria. Traditionally, tumor invasion of the smooth muscle bladder muscularis propria has been an absolute indication for radical cystectomy. In addition, there is sufficient evidence to suggest that certain high-grade tumors invading the lamina propria (T1) are at increased risk for muscularis propria invasion and/or tumor progression,[3,17–22] and may be best treated with an early radical cystectomy. Furthermore, superficial bladder tumors with lymphovascular invasion,[19,23] those with prostatic urethral involvement,[24] or those associated with carcinoma in situ (CIS),[25,26] in conjunction with a poor response to repeated transurethral resection and intravesical therapy,[22] may also be at high risk and could benefit from an early and aggressive therapeutic scheme such as radical cystectomy.

Preoperative Evaluation

Complete clinical staging for bladder cancer should evaluate the retroperitoneum and pelvis along with common metastatic sites, including the lungs, liver, and bones. A chest x-ray, liver function tests, and serum alkaline phosphatase should be obtained routinely. Patients with an elevated serum alkaline phosphatase and/or complaints of bone pain should undergo a bone scan. A computed tomography (CT) scan of the chest is obtained when pulmonary metastases are suspected by history, or because of an abnormal chest x-ray. A CT scan of the abdomen and pelvis is routinely performed to evaluate the pelvis and retroperitoneum for any significant lymphadenopathy or local contiguous spread. This radiographic evaluation should also be performed in patients with suspected metastases, elevated liver functions tests, or a bladder tumor associated with hydronephrosis, or in patients with an extensive primary bladder tumor that is either clinically nonmobile or fixed; the results of these studies may have an impact upon the decision for neoadjuvant therapy. However, CT scan of the primary bladder is neither sufficiently sensitive nor specific to evaluate the degree of bladder wall tumor invasion or to determine accurately the pelvic lymph node involvement with tumor.[27,28]

En bloc radical cystectomy and pelvic–Iliac lymphadenectomy: surgical technique

Preoperative preparation

Patients undergoing radical cystectomy are admitted on the morning of the day before surgery. All patients receive a mechanical and antibacterial bowel preparation the day before surgery. Intravenous hydration must be considered in these patients to prevent dehydration upon arrival at the operating room. In addition, all patients should be evaluated and counseled by the enterostomal therapy nurse prior to surgery. A clear liquid diet may be consumed until midnight, after which time the patient takes nothing per mouth. A standard modified Nichols bowel preparation[29] is initiated the morning of admission: 120 ml castor oil laxative (Neoloid) by mouth at 09:00; 1 g neomycin by mouth at 10:00, 11:00, 12:00, 13:00, 16:00, 20:00, and 24:00; and 1 g erythromycin base by mouth at 12:00, 16:00, 20:00, and 24:00. This regimen is generally well tolerated, obviates the need for enemas, and maintains nutritional and hydrational support. Intravenous crystalloid fluid hydration is begun in the evening before surgery in those patients admitted to the hospital on the day before surgery, and maintained to ensure an adequate circulating intravascular volume as the patient enters the operating room. This may be particularly important in the elderly, frail patient with associated comorbidities.

Patients over 50 years of age at our institution routinely undergo prophylactic digitalization prior to cystectomy unless a specific contraindication exists. Patients younger than 50 years of age are not routinely digitalized. Digoxin is given orally: 0.5 mg at 12:00, 0.25 mg at 16:00, and 0.125 mg at 20:00. Our experience with preoperative digitalization in patients undergoing cystectomy has been positive and there is evidence suggesting that preoperative digitalization may reduce the risk of perioperative dysrhythmias and congestive heart failure in the elderly patient undergoing an extensive operative procedure.[30,31] Attention to fluid management is important in these elderly patients, particularly on postoperative days three and four when mobilization of third-space fluid is highest, subsequently necessitating liberal use of diuretics. In addition, intravenous broad-spectrum antibiotics are administered en route to the operating room, providing adequate tissue and circulating levels at the time of incision.

Preoperative evaluation and counseling by the enterostomal therapy nurse is a critical component to the successful care of all patients undergoing cystectomy and urinary diversion. Patients determined to be appropriate candidates for orthotopic reconstruction are instructed how to catheterize per urethra should it be necessary postoperatively. All patients are site marked for a cutaneous stoma, instructed in the care of a cutaneous diversion (continent or incontinent form), and instructed in proper catheterization techniques should medical, technical or oncologic factors preclude orthotopic reconstruction. The ideal cutaneous stoma site is determined only after the patient is examined in the supine, sitting, and standing position. Proper stoma site selection is important to patient acceptance, and to the technical success of lower urinary tract reconstruction should a cutaneous form of diversion be necessary. Incontinent stoma sites are best located higher on the abdominal wall, while stoma sites for continent diversions can be positioned lower on the abdomen (hidden below the belt line) since they do not require an external collecting device. The use of the umbilicus as the site for catheterization may be employed with excellent functional and cosmetic results.

Patient positioning

The patient is placed in the hyperextended supine position with the superior iliac crest located at the fulcrum of the operating table (Figure 9.1). The legs are slightly abducted so that the heels are positioned near the corners of the foot of the table. In the female patient considering orthotopic diversion, the modified frog-leg or lithotomy position is employed, allowing access to the vagina. Care should be taken to ensure that all pressure points are well padded. Reverse Trendelenburg position levels the abdomen parallel with the floor and helps to keep the small bowel contents in the epigastrium. A nasogastric tube is placed, and the patient is prepped from nipples to mid-thighs. In the female patient the vagina is also fully prepped. After the patient is draped, a 20 Fr. Foley catheter is placed in the bladder and left to gravity drainage. A right-handed surgeon stands on the patient's left-hand side of the operating table.

Incision

A vertical midline incision is made extending from the pubic symphysis to the cephalad aspect of the epigastrium. The incision should be carried lateral to the umbilicus on the contralateral side of the marked cutaneous stoma site. When the umbilicus is considered as the site for a catheterizable stoma, the incision should be directed

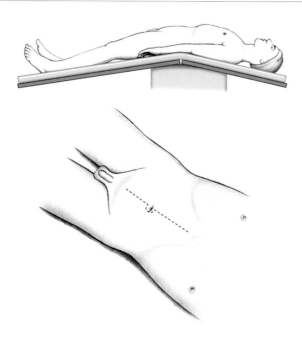

Figure 9.1
Proper patient positioning for cystectomy in the male patient. Note that the iliac crest is located at the break of the table. Reproduced with permission from Stein, JP, Skinner, DG. Surgery Illustrated: Radical Cystectomy. BJU International 2004; 94: 197–221 (Blackwell Publishing). © Stephan Spitzer.

2–3 cm lateral to the umbilicus at this location. The anterior rectus fascia is incised, the rectus muscles retracted laterally, and the posterior rectus sheath and peritoneum entered in the superior aspect of the incision. As the peritoneum and posterior fascia are incised inferiorly to the level of the umbilicus, the urachal remnant (median umbilical ligament) is identified, circumscribed, and removed en bloc with the cystectomy specimen (Figure 9.2). This maneuver prevents early entry into a high-riding bladder, and ensures complete removal of all bladder remnant tissue. Care is taken to remain medial and avoid injury to the inferior epigastric vessels (lateral umbilical ligaments), which course posterior to the rectus muscles. If the patient has previously had a cystotomy or segmental cystectomy, the cystotomy tract and cutaneous incision should be circumscribed full-thickness and excised en bloc with the bladder specimen. The medial insertion of the rectus muscles attached to the pubic symphysis can be slightly incised, maximizing pelvic exposure throughout the operation.

Abdominal exploration

A careful, systematic intra-abdominal exploration is performed to determine the extent of disease, and to evaluate for any hepatic metastases or gross retroperitoneal lymphadenopathy. The abdominal viscera are palpated to detect any concomitant unrelated disease. If no contraindication exists at this time, all adhesions should be incised and freed.

Bowel mobilization

The bowel is mobilized beginning with the ascending colon. A large right-angle Richardson retractor elevates the right abdominal wall.

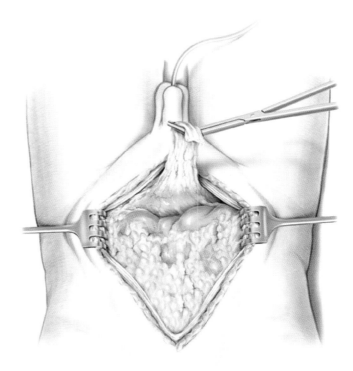

Figure 9.2
Wide excision of the urachal remnant and medial umbilical ligaments en bloc with the cystectomy specimen. Reproduced with permission from BJU International 2004; 94: 197–221; © Stephan Spitzer.

The cecum and ascending colon are reflected medially to allow incision of the lateral peritoneal reflection along the avascular/white line of Toldt. The mesentery to the small bowel is then mobilized off its retroperitoneal attachments cephalad (toward the ligament of Treitz) until the retroperitoneal portion of the duodenum is exposed. This mobilization facilitates a tension-free urethroenteric anastomosis if orthotopic diversion is performed. Combined sharp and blunt dissection facilitate mobilization of this mesentery along a characteristic avascular fibroareolar plane. Conceptually, the mobilized mesentery forms an inverted right triangle: the base formed by the third and fourth portions of the duodenum, the right edge represented by the white line of Toldt along the ascending colon, the left edge represented by the medial portion of the sigmoid and descending colonic mesentery, and the apex represented by the ileocecal region (Figure 9.3). This mobilization is critical in setting up the operative field, and facilitates proper packing of the intra-abdominal contents into the epigastrium.

The left colon and sigmoid mesentery are then mobilized to the region of the lower pole of the left kidney by incising the peritoneum lateral to the colon along the avascular/white line of Toldt. The sigmoid mesentery is then elevated off the sacrum, iliac vessels, and distal aorta in a cephalad direction up to the origin of the inferior mesenteric artery (IMA) (Figure 9.4). This maneuver provides a wide mesenteric window through which the left ureter will pass (without angulation or tension) for the ureteroenteric anastomosis at the terminal portions of the operation. This sigmoid mobilization helps identify the IMA and facilitates retraction of the sigmoid mesentery, particularly when the superior limits of the lymph node dissection are performed. Care should be taken to dissect along the

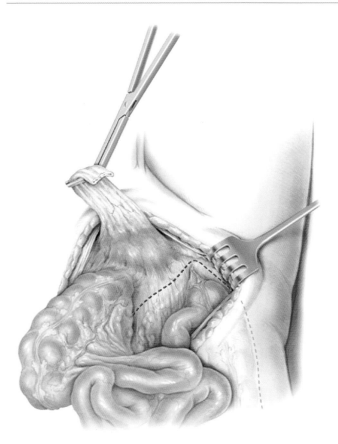

Figure 9.3
View of the pelvis from overhead after the ascending colon and peritoneal attachments of the small bowel mesentery have been mobilized up to the level of the duodenum. This mobilization allows the bowel to be properly packed in the epigastrium and exposes the area of the aortic bifurcation which is the starting point of the lymph node dissection. Reproduced with permission from BJU International 2004; 94: 197–221; © Stephan Spitzer.

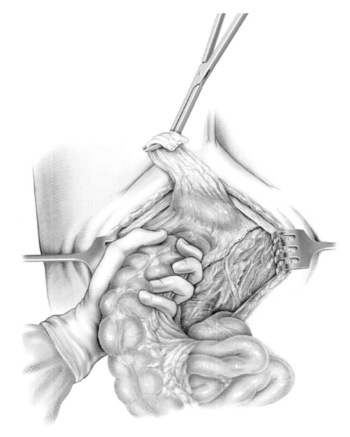

Figure 9.4
View of the pelvis from overhead, after the ascending colon and small bowel have been packed in the epigastrium. Note that the sigmoid mesentery is mobilized off the sacral promontory and distal aorta up to the origin of the inferior mesenteric artery. Reproduced with permission from BJU International 2004; 94: 197–221; © Stephan Spitzer.

base of the mesentery and to avoid injury to the inferior mesenteric artery and blood supply to the sigmoid colon.

After mobilization of the bowel, a self-retaining retractor is placed. The right colon and small intestine are carefully packed into the epigastrium with three moist lap pads, followed by a moistened towel rolled to the width of the abdomen. The descending and sigmoid colon are not packed and remain as free as possible, providing the necessary mobility required for the ureteral and pelvic lymph node dissection.

Successful packing of the intestinal contents is an art and prevents their annoying spillage into the operative field. Packing begins by sweeping the right colon and small bowel under the surgeon's left hand along the right sidewall gutter. A moist open lap pad is then swept with the right hand along the palm of the left hand, under the viscera along the retroperitoneum and sidewall gutter. In similar fashion, the left sidewall gutter is packed, ensuring not to incorporate the descending or sigmoid colon. The central portion of the small bowel is packed with a third lap pad. A moist rolled towel is then positioned horizontally below the lap pads, but cephalad to the bifurcation of the aorta.

Occasionally, prior to placement of the first moist lap pad, a mobile greater omental apron can be used to facilitate packing of the intestinal viscera in a fashion similar to that with lap pad. After the bowel has

been packed, a wide Deaver retractor is placed with gentle traction on the previously placed packing to provide cephalad exposure.

Ureteral dissection

The ureters are most easily identified in the retroperitoneum just cephalad to the common iliac vessels. They are carefully dissected into the deep pelvis (several centimeters beyond the iliac vessels) and divided between two large hemoclips. A section of the proximal cut ureteral segment (distal to the proximal hemoclip) is sent for frozen section analysis to ensure the absence of carcinoma in situ or overt tumor. The ureter is then slightly mobilized in a cephalad direction and tucked under the rolled towel to prevent inadvertent injury. Frequently, an arterial branch from the common iliac artery or the aorta needs to be divided to provide adequate ureteral mobilization. In addition, the rich vascular supply emanating laterally from the gonadal vessels should remain intact and undisturbed. These attachments are an important blood supply to the ureter, which ensure an adequate vascular supply for the ureteroenteric anastomosis at the time of diversion. This is particularly important in irradiated patients. Leaving the proximal hemoclip on the divided ureter during the exenteration allows for hydrostatic ureteral dilation and facilitates the ureteroenteric anastomosis. In women, the infundibulopelvic ligaments are ligated and divided at the level of the common iliac vessels.

Pelvic lymphadenectomy

A meticulous pelvic lymph node dissection is routinely performed with radical cystectomy. The extent of the lymphadenectomy may vary depending on the patient and surgeon preference. An accumulating body of evidence suggests that a more extended lymphadenectomy may be beneficial in patients undergoing cystectomy for high-grade, invasive bladder cancer.[12-16] When performing a salvage procedure following definitive radiation treatment (greater than 5000 cGy), a more limited pelvic lymphadenectomy may be performed or even abandoned if there appears to be a significant risk of iliac vessel and obturator nerve injury.[32]

For a combined common and pelvic iliac lymphadenectomy, the lymph node dissection is initiated at the IMA (superior limits of dissection), and extends laterally over the inferior vena cava to the genitofemoral nerve, representing the lateral limits of dissection. Distally, the lymph node dissection extends to the lymph node of Cloquet medially (on Cooper's ligament) and the circumflex iliac vein laterally.

The cephalad portion (at the level of the IMA) of the lymphatics is ligated with hemoclips to prevent lymphatic leak, while the caudal (specimen) side is ligated only when a blood vessel is encountered. Frequently, small anterior tributary veins originate from the vena cava just above the bifurcation. These should be clipped and divided. In men, the spermatic vessels are retracted laterally and spared. In women the infundibulopelvic ligament, along with the corresponding ovarian vessels, has been ligated previously and divided at the pelvic brim as described earlier.

All fibroareolar and lymphatic tissues are dissected caudally off the aorta, vena cava, and common iliac vessels over the sacral promontory into the deep pelvis. The initial dissection along the common iliac vessels is performed over the arteries, skeletonizing them. As the common iliac veins are dissected medially, care is taken to control small arterial and venous branches coursing along the anterior surface of the sacrum. Electrocautery is helpful at this location and allows the adherent fibroareolar tissue to be swept off the sacral promontory down into the deep pelvis with the use of a small gauze sponge. Significant bleeding from these presacral vessels can occur if not properly controlled. Hemoclips are discouraged in this location as they can be easily dislodged from the anterior surface of the sacrum, and troublesome bleeding can occur.

Once the proximal portion of the lymph node dissection is completed, a finger is passed from the proximal aspect of dissection under the pelvic peritoneum (anterior to the iliac vessels), distally toward the femoral canal. The opposite hand can be used to strip the peritoneum from the undersurface of the transversalis fascia and connects with the proximal dissection from above. This maneuver elevates the peritoneum and defines the lateral limit of peritoneum to be incised and removed with the specimen. The peritoneum is divided medial to the spermatic vessels in men, and lateral to the infundibulopelvic ligament in women. The only structure encountered is the vas deferens in the male or round ligament in the female; these structures are clipped and divided.

A large right-angled rake retractor (e.g. Israel) is used to elevate the lower abdominal wall, including the spermatic cord or remnant of the round ligament, to provide distal exposure in the area of the femoral canal. Tension on the retractor is directed vertically toward the ceiling, and care is taken to avoid injury to the inferior epigastric

vessels. This approach provides excellent exposure to the distal external iliac vessels. The distal limits of the dissection are then identified: the circumflex iliac vein crossing anterior to the external iliac artery distally, the genitofemoral nerve laterally, and Cooper's ligament medially. The lymphatics draining the ipsilateral leg, particularly medial to the external iliac vein, are carefully clipped and divided to prevent lymphatic leakage. This includes the lymph node of Cloquet (also known as Rosenmuller), which represents the distal limit of the lymphatic dissection at this location. The distal external iliac artery and vein are then circumferentially dissected and skeletonized, with care being taken to ligate an accessory obturator vein (present in 40% of patients) originating from the inferomedial aspect of the external iliac vein.

Following completion of the distal limits of dissection, the proximal and distal dissections are joined. The proximal external iliac artery and vein are skeletonized circumferentially to the origin of the hypogastric artery (Figure 9.5). Care should be taken to clip and divide a commonly encountered vessel arising from the lateral aspect of the proximal external iliac vessels coursing to the psoas muscle. The external iliac vessels (artery and vein) are then retracted medially, and the fascia overlying the psoas muscle is incised medial to the genitofemoral nerve. On the left side, branches of the genitofemoral nerve often pursue a more medial course and may be intimately related to the iliac vessels, in which case they are excised.

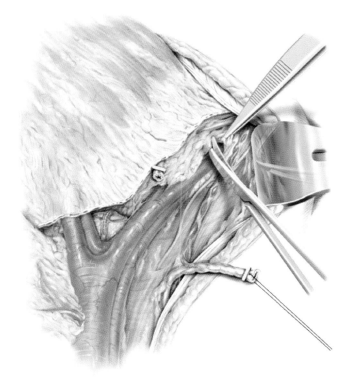

Figure 9.5
Skeletonizing the external iliac artery and vein. Note that the vessels are dissected completely free up to the level of the origin of the hypogastric artery. This allows for the vessels to be carefully retracted medially and the psoas fascia incised to allow passage of a gauze sponge. Reproduced with permission from BJU International 2004; 94: 197–221; © Stephan Spitzer.

At this point, the lymphatic tissues surrounding the iliac vessels are composed of a medial and a lateral component attached only at the base within the obturator fossa. The lateral lymphatic compartment (freed medially from the vessels and laterally from the psoas) is bluntly swept into the obturator fossa by retracting the iliac vessels medially, and passing a small gauze sponge lateral to the vessels along the psoas and pelvic sidewall (Figure 9.6). This sponge should be passed anterior and distal to the hypogastric vein and directed caudally into the obturator fossa. The external iliac vessels are then elevated and retracted laterally, and the gauze sponge carefully withdrawn from the obturator fossa with gentle traction using the left hand (Figure 9.7). This maneuver effectively sweeps all lymphatic tissue into the obturator fossa, and facilitates identification of the obturator nerve deep to the external iliac vein. The obturator nerve is best identified proximally, and carefully dissected free from all lymphatics. The obturator nerve is then retracted laterally along with the iliac vessels (Figure 9.8). At this point, the obturator artery and vein should be carefully entrapped between the index finger (medial to the obturator nerve) laterally and the middle finger medially with the left hand. This isolates the obturator vessels exiting the obturator canal along the pelvic floor. These vessels are then carefully clipped and divided, making certain to stay medial to the obturator nerve. The obturator lymph node packet is then swept medially toward the sidewall of the bladder, and small tributary vessels and lymphatics from the pelvic sidewall and ligated. The nodal packet will be removed en bloc with the cystectomy specimen.

Ligation of the lateral vascular pedicle to the bladder

Following dissection of the obturator fossa and division of the obturator vessels, the lateral vascular pedicle to the bladder is isolated and divided. Developing this plane isolates the lateral vascular pedicle to the bladder; a critical maneuver in performing a safe cystectomy with proper vascular control. Isolation of the lateral vascular pedicle is performed with the left hand. The bladder is retracted toward the pelvis, placing traction and isolating the anterior branches of the hypogastric artery. The left index finger is passed medial to the hypogastric artery, posterior to the anterior visceral branches, and lateral to the previously transected ureter. The index finger is directed caudally toward the endopelvic fascia, parallel to the sweep of the sacrum. This maneuver defines the two major vascular pedicles to the anterior pelvic organs: the lateral pedicle anterior to the index finger, composed of the visceral branches of the anterior hypogastric vessel, and the posterior pedicle posterior to the index finger, composed of the visceral branches between the bladder and rectum.

With the lateral pedicle entrapped between the left index and middle fingers, firm traction is applied vertically and caudally. This facilitates identification and isolation of individual branches off the anterior portion of the hypogastric artery (Figure 9.9). The posterior division of the hypogastric artery, including the superior gluteal, iliolumbar, and lateral sacral arteries, is preserved in order to avoid

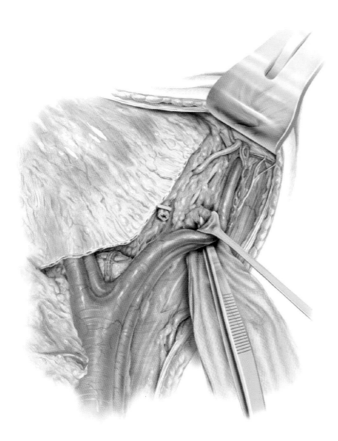

Figure 9.6
Passing a small gauze sponge lateral to the external iliac vessels and medial to the psoas muscle. Reproduced with permission from BJU International 2004; 94: 197–221; © Stephan Spitzer.

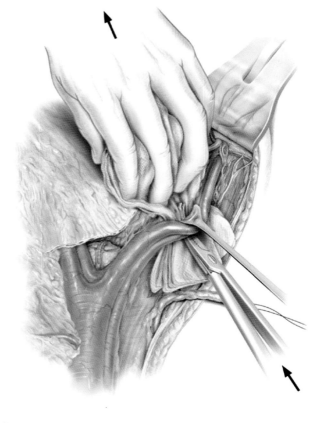

Figure 9.7
Withdrawing the gauze sponge with the left hand. This aids in dissecting and clearing the obturator fossa, sweeping all fibroareolar and lymphatic tissue toward the bladder.
Reproduced with permission from BJU International 2004; 94: 197–221; © Stephan Spitzer.

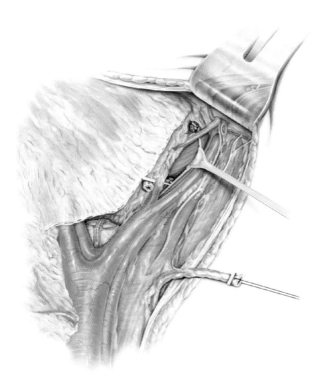

Figure 9.8
Obturator fossa cleaned. This allows proper identification of the obturator nerve passing deep to the external iliac vein. Reproduced with permission from BJU International 2004; 94: 197–221; © Stephan Spitzer.

gluteal claudication. Distal to this posterior division, the hypogastric artery may be ligated for vascular control, but should not be divided since the lateral pedicle is easier to dissect if left in continuity. The largest and most consistent anterior branch to the bladder, the superior vesical artery, is usually isolated and individually ligated and divided easily. The remaining anterior branches of the lateral pedicle are then isolated and divided between hemoclips down to the endopelvic fascia, or as far as is technically possible. With blunt dissection the index finger of the left hand helps identify this lateral pedicle, and protects the rectum as it is pushed medially. Right-angle hemoclip appliers are ideally suited for proper placement of the clips. Hemoclips are positioned as far apart as possible to ensure that 0.5–1 cm of tissue projects beyond each clip when the pedicle is divided. This prevents the hemoclips from being dislodged and thus causing unnecessary bleeding. Occasionally, in patients with an abundance of pelvic fat, the lateral pedicle may be thick and require division into two manageable pedicles. The inferior vesicle vein serves as an excellent landmark because the endopelvic fascia is just distal to this structure. Incision of the endopelvic fascia just lateral to the prostate may help to identify the distal limit of the lateral pedicle.

Ligation of the posterior pedicle to the bladder

Following division of the lateral pedicles, the bladder specimen is retracted anteriorly, exposing the cul-de-sac (pouch of Douglas).

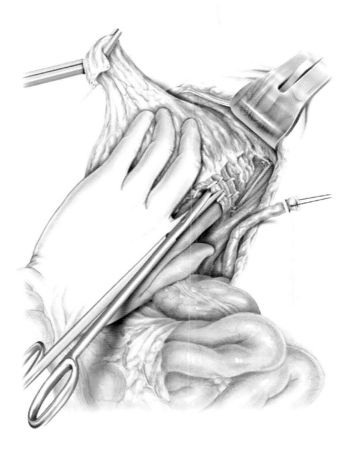

Figure 9.9
Isolation of the lateral vascular pedicle. The left hand is used to define the right lateral pedicle, extending from the bladder to]the hypogastric artery. This plane is developed by the index finger (medial) and the middle finger (lateral), exposing the anterior branches of the hypogastric artery. This vascular pedicle is clipped and divided down to the endopelvic fascia. Traction with the left hand defines the pedicle, allows direct visualization, and protects the rectum from injury. Reproduced with permission from BJU International 2004; 94: 197–221; © Stephan Spitzer.

The surgeon elevates the bladder with a small gauze sponge under the left hand, while the assistant retracts the peritoneum of the rectosigmoid colon in a cephalad direction. This provides excellent exposure to the recess of the cul-de-sac and places the peritoneal reflection on traction, facilitating the proper division. The peritoneum lateral to the rectum is incised and extended anteriorly and medially across the cul-de-sac to join the incision on the contralateral side (Figure 9.10).

An understanding of the fascial layers is critical for the appropriate dissection of this plane. The anterior and posterior peritoneal reflections converge in the cul-de-sac to form Denonvillier's fascia, which extends caudally to the urogenital diaphragm (Figure 9.11, arrow). This important anatomic boundary in the male separates the prostate and seminal vesicles anterior to the rectum posterior. The plane between the prostate and seminal vesicles and the anterior sheath of Denonvillier's fascia will not develop easily. However, the plane between the rectum and the posterior sheath of Denonvillier's (fascia) so called Denonvillier's space should develop easily with blunt and sharp dissection. Therefore, the peritoneal incision in the

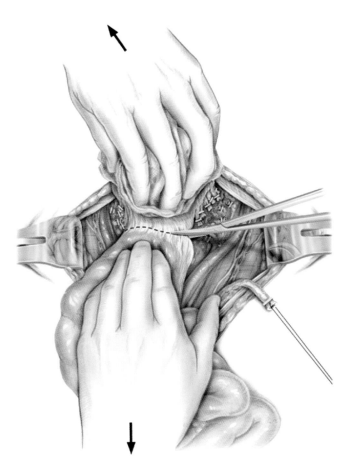

Figure 9.10
The peritoneum lateral to the rectum is incised down into the cul-de-sac, and carried anteriorly over the rectum to join the opposite side. Note that the incision should be made precisely so the proper plane behind Denonvillier's fascia can be developed safely. Reproduced with permission from BJU International 2004; 94: 197–221; © Stephan Spitzer.

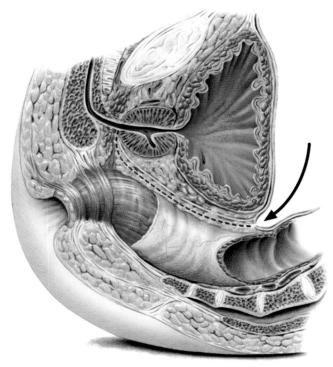

Figure 9.11
The formation of Denonvillier's fascia. Note that it is derived from a fusion of the anterior and posterior peritoneal reflections. Denonvillier's space lies behind the fascia. To successfully enter this space and facilitate mobilization of the anterior rectal wall off Denonvillier's fascia, the incision in the cul-de-sac is made close to the peritoneal fusion on the anterior rectal wall side, and not on the bladder side. Reproduced with permission from BJU International 2004; 94: 197–221; © Stephan Spitzer.

cul-de-sac must be made slightly on the rectal side rather than the bladder side. This allows proper and safe entry and development of Denonvillier's space between the anterior rectal wall and the posterior sheath of Denonvillier's fascia (Figure 9.12). With a posterior sweeping motion of the fingers, the rectum can be carefully swept off of Denonvillier's fascia (with the seminal vesicles, prostate, and bladder anteriorly in men), and off of the posterior vaginal wall in women. This sweeping motion, when extended laterally, helps to thin and develop the posterior pedicles, which appear like a collar emanating from the lateral aspect of the rectum. Care should be taken when developing this posterior plane more caudally because the anterior rectal fibers reflect anteriorly, are often adherent to the specimen, and can offer resistance to blunt dissection. In this region, just cephalad (proximal) to the urogenital diaphragm, sharp dissection may be required to dissect the anterior rectal fibers off the apex of the prostate in order to prevent rectal injury at this location.

Several situations may impede the proper development of this posterior plane. Most commonly, when the incision in the cul-de-sac is made too far anteriorly, proper entry into Denonvillier's space is prevented. Improper entry can occur between the two layers of Denonvillier's fascia, or even anterior to this, making the posterior dissection difficult and increasing the risk of rectal injury.

Furthermore, posterior tumor infiltration or previous high-dose pelvic irradiation can obliterate this plane, making the posterior dissection difficult. To prevent injury to the rectum in these situations, sharp dissection should be performed under direct vision. In order to prevent a rectal injury it is important to avoid blunt dissection with the finger in areas where normal tissue planes have been obliterated by previous surgery or radiation. Sharp dissection under direct vision will dramatically reduce the potential for rectal injury. If a rectotomy occurs, a two- or three-layer closure is recommended. A diverting proximal colostomy is not routinely required unless gross contamination occurs, or if the patient has received previous pelvic radiation therapy. If orthotopic diversion or vaginal reconstruction is planned, an omental interposition is recommended in order to help prevent fistulization.

Once the posterior pedicles have been defined, they are clipped and divided to the endopelvic fascia in the male patient. The endopelvic fascia is then incised adjacent to the prostate, medial to the levator ani muscles (if not done previously), to facilitate the apical dissection. In the female patient, the posterior pedicles, including the cardinal ligaments, are divided 4–5 cm beyond the cervix. With cephalad pressure on a previously placed vaginal sponge stick, the apex of the vagina can be identified, and incised posteriorly just distal to the cervix. The vagina is then circumscribed anteriorly with the cervix attached to the cystectomy specimen. If concern exists regarding an adequate surgical margin at the posterior or base of the wall, prostate, and undersurface of the pubic symphysis are divided. The endopelvic fascia is incised adjacent to the prostate, and the levator muscles are carefully swept off the lateral and apical portions of the prostate. The superficial dorsal vein is identified, ligated, and divided. With tension placed posteriorly on the prostate, the puboprostatic ligaments are identified, and only slightly divided just beneath the pubis, lateral to the dorsal venous complex that courses between these ligaments. Extensive dissection in this region along the pelvic floor should be carefully avoided. The puboprostatic ligaments need to be incised only enough to allow for a proper apical dissection of the prostate. The apex of the prostate and the membranous urethra now become palpable.

Several methods can be used to control the dorsal venous plexus. One may carefully pass an angled clamp beneath the dorsal venous complex, anterior to the urethra (Figure 9.13). The venous complex can then be ligated with a 2-0 absorbable suture and divided close to the apex of the prostate. If any bleeding occurs from the transected venous complex, it can be oversewn with an absorbable (2-0 polyglycolic acid) suture. In a slightly different fashion, the dorsal venous complex may be gathered at the apex of the prostate with a long Allis clamp (Figure 9.14). This may help better define the plane between the dorsal venous complex and the anterior urethra. A figure-of-eight 2-0 absorbable suture can then be carefully placed under direct vision anterior to the urethra (distal to the apex of the

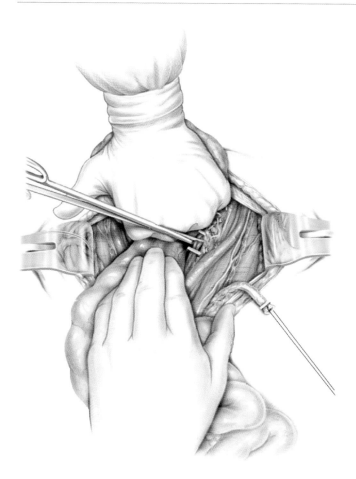

Figure 9.12
After the peritoneum of the cul-de-sac has been incised, the anterior rectal wall can be swept off the posterior surface of the Denonvillier's fascia. This effectively defines the posterior pedicle that extends from the bladder to the lateral aspect of the rectum on either side. Reproduced with permission from BJU International 2004; 94: 197–221; © Stephan Spitzer.

bladder, then the anterior vaginal wall should be removed en bloc with the bladder specimen; vaginal reconstruction will be required if sexual function is desired. It is our preference to spare the anterior vaginal wall if orthotopic diversion is planned. This eliminates the need for vaginal reconstruction, helps to maintain the complex musculofascial support system, and helps to prevent injury to the pudendal innervation to the rhabdosphincter and proximal urethra, both important components to the continence mechanism in women. The anterior vaginal wall is then sharply dissected off the posterior bladder down to the region of the bladder neck (vesicourethral junction), which is identified by palpating the Foley catheter balloon. At this point, the specimen remains attached only at the apex in men and vesicourethral junction in women.

Anterior apical dissection in the male patient

Only after the cystectomy specimen is completely freed and mobile posteriorly is attention directed anteriorly to the pelvic floor and urethra. All fibroareolar connections between the anterior bladder

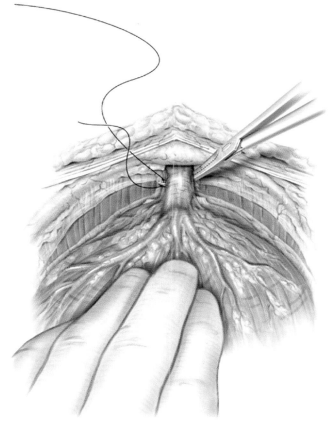

Figure 9.13
Control of the dorsal venous complex. A right-angled clamp can be passed posterior to the venous complex and anterior to the urethra. An absorbable suture can be passed to ligate the complex distal to the apex of the prostate. Reproduced with permission from BJU International 2004; 94: 197–221; © Stephan Spitzer.

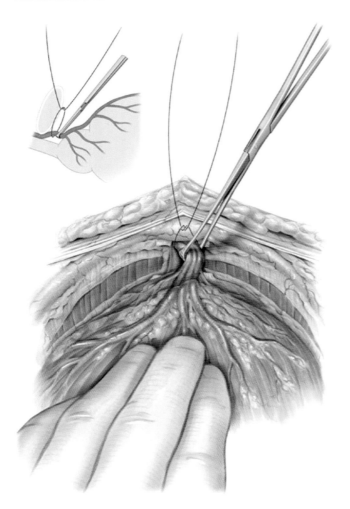

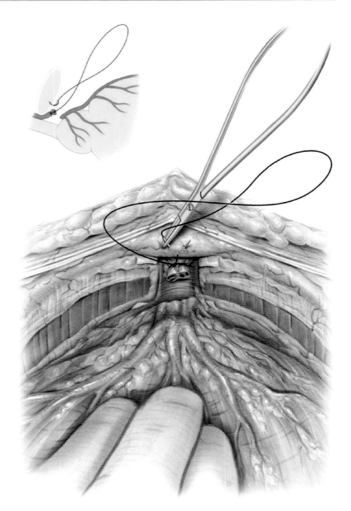

Figure 9.14
The dorsal venous complex is gathered with an Allis clamp distal to the apex of the prostate. This maneuver defines the plane between the dorsal venous complex and urethra. Reproduced with permission from BJU International 2004; 94: 197–221; © Stephan Spitzer.

Figure 9.15
An absorbable suture is carefully passed in a figure-of-eight fashion anterior to the urethra around the gathered dorsal venous complex to control the vascular structure. The dorsal venous complex is completely divided. The previously placed suture is then used to further secure the venous complex. The complex is then fixed anteriorly to the periosteum. Reproduced with permission from BJU International 2004; 94: 197–221; © Stephan Spitzer.

prostate) around the gathered venous complex. This suture is best placed with the surgeon facing the head of the table and holding the needle driver perpendicular to the patient. The suture is then tagged with a hemostat. This maneuver avoids the passage of any instruments between the dorsal venous complex and rhabdosphincter, which could potentially injure these structures and compromise the continence mechanism. After the complex has been ligated, it can be sharply divided with excellent exposure to the anterior surface of the urethra. Once the venous complex has been severed, the suture can be used to further secure the complex. The suture is then used to suspend the venous complex anteriorly to the periosteum to help reestablish anterior fixation of the dorsal venous complex and puboprostatic ligaments and thus possibly enhance continence recovery (Figure 9.15). The anterior urethra is now exposed.

Regardless of the aforementioned technique to control the dorsal venous complex, the urethra is then incised 270° just beyond the apex of the prostate. Six 2-0 polyglycolic acid sutures are placed in the anterior urethra, carefully incorporating only the mucosa and submucosa of the striated urethral sphincter muscle anteriorly. Next, two posterior urethral sutures are placed incorporating the rectourethralis muscle or the caudal extent of Denonvillier's fascia.

The posterior urethra can then be divided and the specimen removed after dividing the Foley catheter between clamps in order to avoid spillage of bladder contents.

Alternatively, the dorsal venous complex can simply be sharply transected prior to securing vascular control of the dorsal venous complex. Cephalad traction on the prostate elongates the proximal and membranous urethra and allows the urethra to be skeletonized laterally by dividing the so-called 'lateral pillars', extensions of the rhabdosphincter. Again, a section comprising the anterior two-thirds of the urethra is divided, exposing the urethral catheter. The urethral sutures are then placed. Six 2-0 polyglycolic acid sutures are placed, equally spaced, into the urethral mucosa and lumen anteriorly. The rhabdosphincter, the edge of which acts as a hood overlying the dorsal venous complex, is included in these sutures if the dorsal venous complex was sharply incised. This maneuver compresses the dorsal vein complex against the urethra for hemostatic purposes. The urethral catheter is then drawn through the urethrotomy, clamped on the bladder side, and divided. Cephalad traction on the bladder side with the clamped catheter occludes the bladder neck, prevents tumor spill from the bladder, and provides exposure to the posterior urethra. Two additional sutures are placed in the posterior urethra, again incorporating the rectourethralis muscle or distal Denonvillier's fascia. The posterior urethra is then divided and the specimen removed. Bleeding from the dorsal vein is usually minimal at this point. If additional hemostasis is required, one or two anterior urethral sutures can be tied to stop the bleeding. Regardless of the technique, frozen section analysis of the distal urethral margin of the cystectomy specimen is then performed in order to exclude tumor involvement.

If a cutaneous form of urinary diversion is planned, urethral preparation is slightly modified. Once the dorsal venous complex is secured and divided, the anterior urethra is identified. The urethra is mobilized from above as far distally as possible into the pelvic diaphragm. With cephalad traction, the urethra is stretched above the urogenital diaphragm, a curved clamp is placed as distal on the urethra as feasible and divided distal to the clamp. Care must be taken to avoid rectal injury with this clamp. This is prevented by placing gentle posterior traction with the left hand or index finger on the rectum and ensuring the clamp is passed anterior. The specimen is then removed. Mobilization of the urethra as distally as possible facilitates secondary urethrectomy should it be necessary. The levator musculature can then be reapproximated along the pelvic floor to facilitate hemostasis.

Anterior dissection in the female

The wide female pelvis allows for better anterior exposure in a woman, particularly at the vesicourethral junction. However, urologists may be less familiar with pelvic surgery in women than in men. In addition, paravaginal vascular control may be troublesome in women, and the venous plexus anterior to the urethra is less well defined in women. When orthotopic diversion is considered in female patients undergoing cystectomy, several technical issues critical to the procedure must be addressed in order to maintain the continence mechanism in these women.

When the posterior pedicles are developed in women, the posterior vagina is incised at the apex just distal to the cervix (Figure 9.16). This incision is carried anteriorly along the lateral and anterior vaginal walls forming a circumferential incision. The anterior lateral vaginal wall is then grasped with curved Kocher clamps. This provides countertraction and facilitates dissection between the anterior vaginal wall and the bladder specimen. Careful dissection of the proper plane will prevent entry into the posterior bladder and also reduce the amount of bleeding in this vascular area (Figure 9.17). Development of this posterior plane and vascular pedicle is best performed sharply and carried just distal to the vesicourethral junction. Palpation of the Foley catheter balloon assists in identifying this region. This dissection effectively maintains a functional vagina.

In the case of a deeply invasive posterior bladder tumor in a woman, with concern of an adequate surgical margin, the anterior vaginal wall should be removed en bloc with the cystectomy specimen. After dividing the posterior vaginal apex, the lateral vaginal wall subsequently serves as the posterior pedicle and is divided distally. This leaves the anterior vaginal wall attached to the posterior bladder specimen. The Foley catheter balloon again facilitates identification of the vesicourethral junction. The surgical plane between the vesicourethral junction and the anterior vaginal wall is then developed distally at this location. A 1 cm length of proximal urethra is mobilized while the remaining distal urethra is left intact with

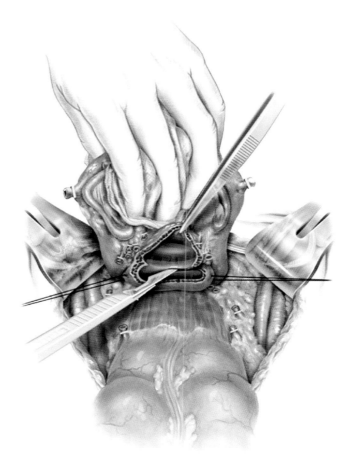

Figure 9.16
In women, the vagina is incised distal to the cervix. Note that cephalad traction on the posterior aspect of the vagina facilitates the incision of the anterior vaginal wall. Slight dissection of the posterior vaginal wall off the rectum provides mobility to the vaginal cuff. Reproduced with permission from BJU International 2004; 94: 197–221; © Stephan Spitzer.

the anterior vaginal wall. Vaginal reconstruction by a clam shell (horizontal) or side-to-side (vertical) technique is required. Other means of vaginal reconstruction may include a rectus myocutaneous flap, detubularized cylinder of ileum, a peritoneal flap, or an omental flap.

It is emphasized that no dissection should be performed anterior to the urethra along the pelvic floor. The endopelvic fascia should remain undisturbed and not be opened in women considering orthotopic diversion. This prevents injury to the rhabdosphincter region and corresponding innervation, which is critical in maintaining the continence mechanism. Anatomic studies have demonstrated that the innervation of this rhabdosphincter region in women arises from branches off the pudendal nerve that course along the pelvic floor posterior to the levator muscles.[33,34] Any dissection performed anteriorly may injure these nerves and compromise the continence status.

When the posterior dissection is completed (with care to dissect just distal to the vesicourethral junction), a Satinsky vascular clamp is placed across the bladder neck. The Satinsky vascular clamp placed across the catheter at the bladder neck prevents any tumor

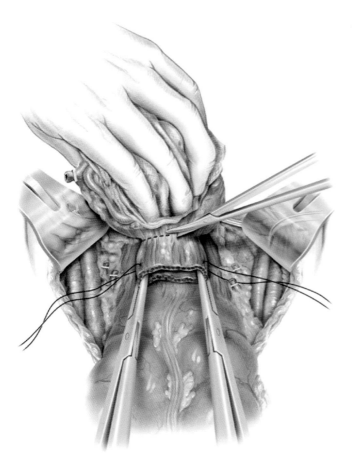

Figure 9.17
Dissection of the anterior vaginal wall off of the bladder. Note caudal traction of the cystectomy specimen with countertraction applied to the vagina in a cephalad direction. Dissection continues only slightly distal to the level of the vesicourethral junction. This can be identified by palpation of the Foley balloon in the bladder (not shown). Reproduced with permission from BJU International 2004; 94: 197–221; © Stephan Spitzer.

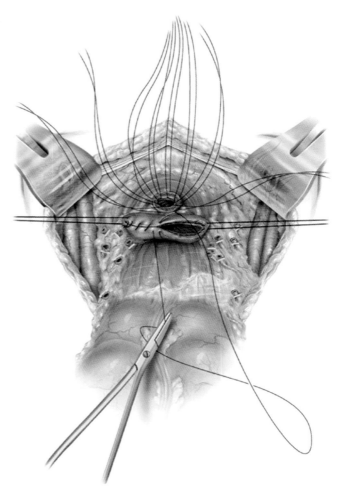

Figure 9.18
View of the female pelvis from above with the partially opened vaginal cuff and the urethral sutures placed. Reproduced with permission from BJU International 2004; 94: 197–221; © Stephan Spitzer.

spill from the bladder. With gentle traction the proximal urethra is completely divided anteriorly, distal to the bladder neck and clamp. The urethra is situated more anteriorly in women than in men, and the urethral sutures can be placed easily after the specimen is completely removed (Figure 9.18). Ten to 12 sutures are placed. Frozen section analysis is performed on the distal urethral margin of the cystectomy specimen in order to exclude tumor. Once hemostasis is obtained, the vaginal cuff may be closed in two layers with absorbable sutures. The vaginal cuff is then anchored via a colposacralpexy using a strut of Marlex mesh to the sacral promontory. This fixates the vagina without angulation or undue tension. Note that at the terminal portions of the surgical procedure, a well-vascularized omental pedicle graft is placed between the reconstructed vagina and neobladder, and secured to the levator ani muscles to separate the suture lines and prevent fistulization (Figure 9.19).

If a cutaneous diversion is planned in the female patient, the posterior pedicles are developed as previously mentioned. Attention is then directed anteriorly, and the pubourethral ligaments are divided. A curved clamp is placed across the urethra, and the ante-

rior vaginal wall is opened distally and incised circumferentially around the urethral meatus. The vaginal cuff is closed as previously described and suspended. Alternatively, a perineal approach may be used for this dissection with complete removal of the entire urethra.

Following removal of the cystectomy specimen, the pelvis is irrigated with warm sterile water. The presacral nodal tissue previously swept off the common iliac vessels and sacral promontory into the deep pelvis is collected and sent separately for pathologic evaluation. Nodal tissue in the presciatic notch bilaterally, anterior to the sciatic nerve, is also sent for histologic analysis. Hemostasis is obtained and the pelvis is packed with a lap pad while attention is directed to the urinary diversion.

The use of various tubes and drains postoperatively is important. The pelvis is drained with a 1-inch Penrose drain for urine or lymph leak for 3 weeks, and a large suction hemovac drain for the evacuation of blood for 24 hours. A gastrostomy tube with an 18 Fr. Foley catheter is placed routinely, utilizing a modified Stamm technique that incorporates a small portion of omentum (near the greater curvature of the stomach) interposed between the stomach and the abdominal wall.[35] This provides a simple means of draining the stomach and prevents the need for an uncomfortable nasogastric tube while the postoperative ileus resolves.

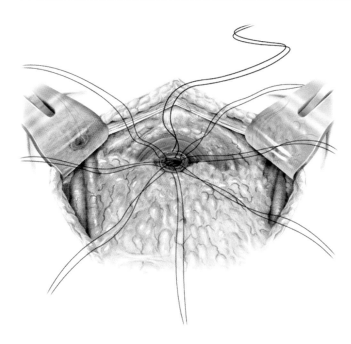

Figure 9.19
View of the female pelvis. Note a vascularized omental pedicle graft is situated anteriorly covering the reconstructed vagina/vaginal cuff. The urethra and sutures will be placed into the neobladder (not shown). The omental graft is secured to the pelvic floor to prevent fistulization between the neobladder and vaginal cuff. Reproduced with permission from BJU International 2004; 94: 197–221; © Stephan Spitzer.

Postoperative care

A meticulous, team-oriented approach to the care of these generally elderly patients undergoing radical cystectomy helps reduce perioperative morbidity and mortality. Patients are best monitored in the surgical intensive care unit (ICU) for at least 24 hours or until stable. Careful attention to fluid management is imperative as third-space fluid loss in these patients can be tremendous and deceiving. Patients with compromised cardiac or pulmonary function may require invasive cardiac monitoring with a pulmonary artery catheter placed prior to surgery to precisely ascertain the cardiac response to fluid shifts. A combination of crystalloid and colloid fluid replacement is given on the night of surgery, and converted to crystalloid on postoperative day 1. Prophylaxis against stress ulcer is initiated with a histamine receptor (H_2) blocker. Intravenous broad-spectrum antibiotics are continued in all patients and subsequently converted to oral antibiotics as the diet progresses. Pulmonary toilet is encouraged with incentive spirometry, deep breathing, and coughing.

Prophylaxis against deep vein thrombosis is important in patients undergoing extensive pelvic operations for malignancies. The anticoagulation is initiated in the recovery room with 10 mg of sodium warfarin via a nasogastric or the gastrostomy tube. The daily dose is adjusted to maintain a prothrombin time in the range of 18–22 seconds. If the prothrombin time exceeds 22–25 seconds, 2.5 mg of vitamin K is administered intramuscularly to prevent possible bleeding. Pain control by a patient-controlled analgesic (PCA) system provides comfort and enhances deep breathing and early ambulation. If digoxin was given preoperatively, it is continued until

discharge. The gastrostomy tube is generally removed on postoperative day 7, or later if bowel function is delayed. The catheter and drain management is specific to the form of urinary diversion. Some patients may develop a prolonged ileus or some other complication that delays the quick return of oral intake. In such circumstances, total parenteral nutrition (TPN) is wisely instituted earlier rather than later, so that the patient will not become farther behind nutritionally.

Discussion

Understanding that invasive bladder cancer can be a lethal disease, we have adopted an early and aggressive surgical approach.[3,4] This includes a radical cystectomy with a meticulous and extended bilateral pelvic iliac lymph node dissection. We firmly believe radical cystectomy provides the best local pelvic control of the disease. In addition, radical cystectomy provides accurate evaluation of the primary bladder tumor (p stage), along with the regional lymph nodes. This pathologic evaluation allows the application of adjuvant treatment strategies based on clear histopathologic determination, not clinical staging, which has been associated with significant errors in 30% to 50% of patients.[3,27,28,36,37] This, coupled with the evolution and application of orthotopic lower urinary tract reconstruction in both men and women, has provided patients with a more acceptable means to store and eliminate urine.[7]

Generally, most invasive TCCs are high-grade tumors. These bladder tumors originate in the bladder mucosa, and progressively invade the lamina propria and, sequentially, the muscularis propria, perivesical fat, and contiguous pelvic structures, with an increasing incidence of lymph node involvement with disease progression (Table 9.1).[4,16,38,39] In over 2200 patients undergoing radical cystectomy from four large contemporary cystectomy series, the cumulative incidence of node-positive bladder cancer at the time of surgery was 25%. Radical cystectomy with an appropriate lymphadenectomy effectively removes the primary bladder tumor and the regional lymph nodes that may contain metastases in a significant number of patients undergoing the procedure. In the USC series of 1054 patients undergoing radical cystectomy for TCC, the incidence of lymph node metastases correlated with the primary bladder tumor stage.[4] Patients with nonmuscle-invasive tumors demonstrated a 5% incidence of node-positive disease, compared with 18% in patients with superficial muscle-invasive bladder tumors (P2A), 27% with deep muscle-invasive bladder tumors (P2B), and approximately 45% of patients with extravesical tumor extension of the primary bladder tumor (P3 and P4) (Table 9.1).

Morbidity and mortality of radical cystectomy and lymphadenectomy

The early clinical results and outcomes with regard to the morbidity and mortality of radical cystectomy were disappointing. Lack of universal acceptance of this procedure was attributed to the considerable complication rate and the need for improvements in urinary diversion. Prior to 1970, the perioperative complication rate of radical cystectomy was approximately 35%, with a mortality rate of nearly 20%. However, with contemporary medical, surgical, and anesthetic techniques, along with better patient selection, the

Table 9.1 Incidence of lymph node metastasis following radical cystectomy in contemporary series: correlation to primary bladder tumor

Lead author	Period	No. pts	No (%) lymph node metastases	Bladder tumor stage* No. (%)				
				P0, Pis, Pa, P1	P2A	P2B	P3	P4
Poulsen[16]	1990–1997	191	50 (26%)	2 (3%)	4 (18%)	7 (25%)	33 (51%)	4 (44%)
Vieweg†[38]	1980–1990	686	193 (28%)	10 (10%)	12 (9%)	22 (23%)	97 (43%)	52 (41%)
Leissner‡[39]	1999–2002	290	81 (28%)	1 (2%)	5 (13%)	12 (22%)	53 (44%)	10 (50%)
Stein[4]	1971–1997	1054	246 (24%)	19 (5%)	21 (18%)	35 (27%)	113 (45%)	58 (43%)
Totals		2221	570 (25%)					

*TNM staging system: 1997 AJCC.[50]
†6 patients with carcinoma in situ of prostatic ducts with lymph node positive disease classified as Pis.
‡Multicenter trial.

Table 9.2 Perioperative mortality and early complication rate following cystectomy at USC

		No. pts	Perioperative mortality*	Early complication†
Form of urinary diversion	Conduit‡	278 (26%)	8 (3%)	83 (30%)
	Continent§	776 (74%)	19 (2%)	209 (27%)
Preoperative adjuvant therapy	None	884 (84%)	26 (3%)	247 (28%)
	Radiation only	108 (10%)	1 (1%)	30 (30%)
	Chemotherapy only	49 (5%)	0	12 (25%)
	Radiation and chemotherapy	13 (1%)	0	3 (23%)
Totals		1054	27 (3%)	292 (28%)

*Any death within 30 days of surgery or prior to discharge.
†Any complications within the first 3 months postoperative.
‡Including ileal and colon conduits.
§Including continent cutaneous, orthotopic, and rectal reservoirs.

mortality and morbidity from radical cystectomy have dramatically decreased. We reported a 3% mortality rate in the USC series (Table 9.2),[4] which is similar to that in other contemporary series of radical cystectomy.[5,16,36–39] Importantly, we found that the administration of preoperative therapy (radiation and/or chemotherapy), and the form of urinary diversion performed (continent or incontinent) did not appear to increase the mortality rate of patients undergoing radical cystectomy.[4]

The early complication rate following radical cystectomy often associated with significant comorbidities should not be underestimated in this elderly group of patients. The median age of patients undergoing cystectomy in our series was 66 years (range 22–93 years). In this series of 1054 patients, 28% developed an early complication within the first 3 months of surgery (Table 9.2).[4] These early complications included all those related to the cystectomy, perioperative care, and urinary diversion. The administration of preoperative therapy (radiation and/or chemotherapy) and the form of urinary diversion did not significantly alter the early complication rate in these cystectomy patients. Most early complications following radical cystectomy are unrelated to the urinary diversion (85% diversion unrelated), and can be managed conservatively without the need for reoperation in approximately 90% of patients.[40] In our experience, the most common early, diversion-unrelated complication is dehydration, while the most common early, diversion-related complication following radical cystectomy is urinary leakage.

Although we have found that preoperative treatment with chemotherapy and/or radiation therapy does not increase the peri-

operative morbidity or mortality, neoadjuvant treatment strategies have not been routinely employed in our patients prior to radical cystectomy for invasive bladder cancer. Preoperative radiation therapy is considered only in those patients with a history of a previous partial cystectomy or those that have experienced extravesical tumor spill at the time of endoscopic management of the primary bladder tumor.[41] Furthermore, although there has been a recent interest in the application of neoadjuvant chemotherapy in patients with muscle-invasive bladder cancer,[42] the routine administration of this is clearly a debatable issue.[43] We have been, and continue to be, strong advocates of postoperative adjuvant chemotherapy when given to high-risk patients, on the basis of accurate pathologic evaluation of the primary bladder tumor and regional lymph nodes.[4,44]

We have also evaluated the clinical outcomes of radical cystectomy in elderly patients (80 years of age or more) requiring therapy for bladder cancer.[45] We found that in appropriately selected individuals the perioperative morbidity and mortality of elderly patients is similar to that of younger patients undergoing the same operation. Our data are similar to those in other reports.[46,47] Collectively, this suggests that an aggressive surgical approach is a viable treatment strategy for properly selected elderly individuals who are in generally good health and require definitive management for bladder cancer. It is clear that physiologic age may be more important than chronologic age when determining who is an appropriate candidate for radical cystectomy. Proper patient selection, and strict attention to perioperative details, along with a dedicated and meticulous surgical approach, are all critical components to minimize the morbidity and mortality of surgery, and to ensure the best clinical outcomes in patients following radical cystectomy (see also Chapter 43 for additional discussion of patient preparation and perioperative management).

Pathologic stage and subgroups

The pathologic stage of the primary bladder tumor and the presence of lymph node metastases are perhaps the most important survival determinants in patients undergoing cystectomy for bladder cancer

(Table 9.3).[4] These pathologic determinants may also be categorized into certain pathologic subgroups that provide risk stratification. It is this pathologic evaluation and subgroup stratification that most precisely directs the need for adjuvant therapy in the appropriately selected individual. The pathologic subgroups are defined as organ-confined, lymph node-negative tumors (P0, Pa, Pis, P1, P2A, P2B), nonorgan-confined (extravesical) lymph node-negative tumors (P3, P4), and lymph node-positive disease (N+). The recurrence-free and overall survival for the entire 1054 patients in the USC series at 5 years was 68% and 66%, and 60% and 43%, respectively, at 10 years (Table 9.3, Figure 9.20). In this cohort, most deaths occurring within the first 3 years after radical cystectomy are

Table 9.3 Recurrence-free and overall survival after radical cystectomy

| | | Probability of surviving and remaining recurrence-free (P $\pm$ SE) | | | |
| | | Recurrence-free | | Overall survival | |
Pathologic stage*	No. pts	5 years	10 years	5 years	10 years
P0, Pa, Pis					
N–	208	0.89 $\pm$ 0.02	0.85 $\pm$ 0.03	0.85 $\pm$ 0.03	0.67 $\pm$ 0.04
N+	5	0.60 $\pm$ 0.22	0.60 $\pm$ 0.22	0.40 $\pm$ 0.22	0.40 $\pm$ 0.22
All pts P0, Pa, Pis	213	0.88 $\pm$ 0.02	0.85 $\pm$ 0.03	0.84 $\pm$ 0.03	0.67 $\pm$ 0.04
P1					
N–	194	0.83 $\pm$ 0.03	0.78 $\pm$ 0.04	0.76 $\pm$ 0.03	0.52 $\pm$ 0.04
N+	14	0.43 $\pm$ 0.13	0.43 $\pm$ 0.13	0.50 $\pm$ 0.13	0.42 $\pm$ 0.13
All pts P1	208	0.80 $\pm$ 0.03	0.75 $\pm$ 0.04	0.74 $\pm$ 0.03	0.51 $\pm$ 0.04
P2A					
N–	94	0.89 $\pm$ 0.03	0.87 $\pm$ 0.04	0.77 $\pm$ 0.04	0.57 $\pm$ 0.06
N+	21	0.50 $\pm$ 0.11	0.50 $\pm$ 0.11	0.52 $\pm$ 0.11	0.52 $\pm$ 0.11
All pts P2A	115	0.81 $\pm$ 0.04	0.80 $\pm$ 0.04	0.72 $\pm$ 0.04	0.56 $\pm$ 0.05
P2B					
N–	98	0.78 $\pm$ 0.05	0.76 $\pm$ 0.05	0.64 $\pm$ 0.05	0.44 $\pm$ 0.06
N+	35	0.41 $\pm$ 0.09	0.37 $\pm$ 0.09	0.40 $\pm$ 0.08	0.26 $\pm$ 0.08
All pts P2B	133	0.68 $\pm$ 0.04	0.65 $\pm$ 0.05	0.58 $\pm$ 0.04	0.39 $\pm$ 0.05
P3					
N–	135	0.62 $\pm$ 0.05	0.61 $\pm$ 0.05	0.49 $\pm$ 0.04	0.29 $\pm$ 0.05
N+	113	0.29 $\pm$ 0.05	0.29 $\pm$ 0.05	0.24 $\pm$ 0.04	0.12 $\pm$ 0.04
All pts P3	248	0.47 $\pm$ 0.04	0.46 $\pm$ 0.04	0.38 $\pm$ 0.03	0.22 $\pm$ 0.03
P4					
N–	79	0.50 $\pm$ 0.06	0.45 $\pm$ 0.07	0.44 $\pm$ 0.06	0.23 $\pm$ 0.06
N+	58	0.33 $\pm$ 0.07	0.33 $\pm$ 0.07	0.26 $\pm$ 0.06	0.20 $\pm$ 0.05
All pts P4	137	0.44 $\pm$ 0.05	0.41 $\pm$ 0.05	0.33 $\pm$ 0.04	0.22 $\pm$ 0.04
Organ-confined†					
N–	594	0.85 $\pm$ 0.02	0.82 $\pm$ 0.02	0.78 $\pm$ 0.02	0.56 $\pm$ 0.0
N+	75	0.46 $\pm$ 0.06	0.44 $\pm$ 0.06	0.45 $\pm$ 0.06	0.37 $\pm$ 0.06
All pts	669	0.80 $\pm$ 0.02	0.77 $\pm$ 0.02	0.74 $\pm$ 0.02	0.54 $\pm$ 0.02
Extravesical‡					
N–	214	0.58 $\pm$ 0.04	0.55 $\pm$ 0.04	0.47 $\pm$ 0.04	0.27 $\pm$ 0.04
N+	171	0.30 $\pm$ 0.04	0.30 $\pm$ 0.04	0.25 $\pm$ 0.04	0.17 $\pm$ 0.03
All pts	385	0.46 $\pm$ 0.03	0.44 $\pm$ 0.03	0.37 $\pm$ 0.03	0.22 $\pm$ 0.03
LN– pts	808	0.78 $\pm$ 0.02	0.75 $\pm$ 0.02	0.69 $\pm$ 0.02	0.49 $\pm$ 0.02
LN+ pts	246	0.35 $\pm$ 0.03	0.34 $\pm$ 0.03	0.31 $\pm$ 0.03	0.23 $\pm$ 0.03
Total group	1054	0.68 $\pm$ 0.02	0.66 $\pm$ 0.02	0.60 $\pm$ 0.02	0.43 $\pm$ 0.02

LN–, without lymph node involvement (node-negative); LN+, with lymph node involvement (node-positive); pts, patients.
*1997 TNM staging system.[50]
†Organ confined, including P0, Pa, Pis, P1, P2, and P2B bladder tumors.
‡Extravesical, including P3 and P4 bladder tumors.

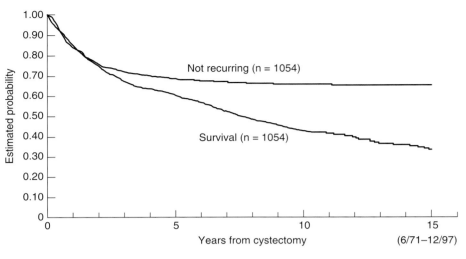

Figure 9.20
Recurrence-free and overall survival for the entire cohort of 1054 patients following radical cystectomy.

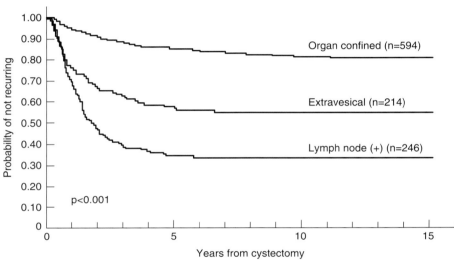

Figure 9.21
Recurrence-free survival in 1054 patients stratified by pathologic subgroups following radical cystectomy. Reproduced with permission from Stein et al.[4]

attributed to bladder cancer recurrences. However, with continued follow-up (after 3 years), most deaths in this elderly group of patients are primarily related to other comorbid diseases, unrelated to bladder cancer.

Organ-confined, lymph node-negative tumors

In the USC series, 56% of patients demonstrated pathologically organ-confined, lymph node-negative bladder tumors.[4] The survival results in this pathologic subgroup of patients are excellent (Table 9.3, Figure 9.21). The recurrence-free survival in this subgroup of organ-confined, lymph node-negative bladder tumors was 85% at 5 years and 82% at 10 years. Importantly, we found no significant survival differences among superficially noninvasive (Pis, Pa), lamina propria invasive (P1), and muscle-invasive (P2A, P2B) tumors—as long as the tumor was confined to the bladder and there was no evidence of lymph node tumor involvement. Similar outcomes for patients with pathologic superficial bladder tumors following cystectomy have been previously reported.[5,37] These data support the notion that the ideal outcome for patients with high-grade, invasive bladder cancer occurs when the primary bladder tumor is confined to the bladder, without evidence of extravesical extension or lymph node metastases. Significant delays in treatment

of patients with invasive bladder cancer obviously should be avoided. There is evidence to suggest that prolonged delays may lead to more advanced pathologic stages and decreased survival in patients with muscle-invasive bladder cancer.[48] Furthermore, it should be emphasized that care should be taken in delaying a more definitive therapy in patients with high-risk superficial bladder tumors, or those tumors that are superficial but have not responded appropriately to conservative forms of therapy.[3]

Extravesical, lymph node-negative tumors

Nonorgan-confined (extravesical) lymph node-negative tumors were found in approximately 20% of our patients undergoing cystectomy (Table 9.3, Figure 9.21).[4] In this pathologic subgroup, no obvious survival differences between extravesical P3 and P4 tumors were observed. The recurrence-free survival in this pathologic subgroup of extravesical, nonorgan-confined, lymph node-negative tumors was 58% at 5 years, and 55% at 10 years. Clearly, patients with these locally advanced tumors have higher recurrence rates and lower survival rates than the subgroup of patients with organ-confined tumor and lymph node-negative tumors.[49] Consequently, adjuvant treatment strategies may be considered for the latter.

In 1997, the TNM (tumor, node, metastases) staging system for bladder cancer was modified by the American Joint Committee on

Cancer (AJCC) and the UICC.[50] The revised TNM classification stratifies extravesical tumor involvement (previously defined as pT3B) into microscopic (pT3A) and gross (pT3B) extravesical tumor extension. In order to determine the clinical significance of this new pathologic subgrouping, we evaluated the clinical outcomes following radical cystectomy in our group of patients with pathologic pT3 disease stratified by microscopic and gross extravesical tumor involvement.[49] We found no significant difference in the recurrence-free and overall survival in patients when evaluating for pT3A and pT3B extravesical tumor extension. The incidence of lymph node involvement was not different between the groups (approximately 45%). However, as one would expect, the presence of lymph node involvement was associated with a higher risk of recurrence and worse overall survival. Because no differences were observed between the clinical outcomes for patients with pT3A and pT3B disease, we believe they should be treated similarly. Furthermore, the fact that future staging systems may classify these tumors collectively may also facilitate comparisons with historical cystectomy series.

Lymph node-positive disease

Despite our aggressive treatment philosophy and approach to bladder cancer, 24% of our patients demonstrated lymph node-positive disease at the time of cystectomy (Table 9.1, Figure 9.21).[4] This underscores the virulent and metastatic capabilities of high-grade, invasive bladder cancer. Although patients with lymph node tumor involvement are a high-risk group of patients, nearly one-third of these patients in our series are alive at 5 years, and 23% at 10 years. It is possible that the surgical approach (with an extended pelvic–iliac lymph node dissection) may provide some advantage with long-term survival in selected individuals with lymph node-positive disease. The impact of adjuvant therapy in this group of patients, although difficult to assess and subject to selection bias, may also play a role in the outcomes of patients with lymph node-positive disease.[4] In fact, in a separate analysis of lymph node-positive patients, we found that the administration of adjuvant chemotherapy was a significant and independent predictor for recurrence and overall survival.[13]

The prognosis in patients with lymph node-positive disease can be stratified by the number of lymph nodes involved (tumor burden), and by the p stage of the primary bladder tumor.[4] In our cystectomy series, patients with fewer than five positive lymph nodes had better survival rates than patients with five or more lymph nodes involved. A significant difference was also observed when patients were stratified by their primary bladder stage. Patients with lymph node-positive disease and organ-confined bladder tumors had a significantly better recurrence-free survival than those with nonorgan-confined, lymph node-positive tumors. Similar results with lymph node-positive tumors following cystectomy have been reported previously.[5,38]

We believe that the number of lymph nodes involved with tumor and the extent of the lymph node dissection are both important variables for patients undergoing cystectomy for bladder cancer. We recently reexamined our 246 patients with lymph node tumor involvement following radical cystectomy,[13] to evaluate other prognostic factors in this high-risk group of patients. This reevaluation subsequently stimulated the concept of 'lymph node density'—an important prognostic factor that better stratifies lymph node-positive patients following radical cystectomy. Lymph node density (defined as the total number of positive lymph nodes divided by the total number of lymph nodes removed) accounts for the extent of

the lymph node dissection (number of lymph nodes removed) and the tumor burden (number of positive lymph nodes) following radical cystectomy for patients with lymph node-positive disease. Lymph node density incorporates these concepts simultaneously.

If lymph tumor burden and the extent of the lymphadenectomy are important variables in patients with lymph node-positive disease, it is only logical that lymph node density is also important. In fact, we found lymph node density to be a significant and independent prognostic variable in patients with lymph node metastases and that it may best stratify this high-risk group of patients (Figure 9.22).[13] It is possible that future staging systems, and the application of adjuvant therapies in clinical trials, should consider applying these concepts to better stratify this high-risk group of patients after radical cystectomy. Regardless, patients with any lymph node involvement remain at high risk for disease recurrence and should be considered for adjuvant treatment strategies.

Recurrence following cystectomy

Recurrence following radical cystectomy for bladder cancer is not unusual and correlates directly to the pathologic stage and subgroup. In our report of 1054 patients with long-term follow-up (median 10 years), recurrences were classified as local (pelvic), distant, and urethral. Local recurrences, by definition, are those tumor recurrences that occur within the soft tissue field of exenteration. Distant recurrences are defined as those that occur outside the pelvis, while urethral tumors are classified as a new primary tumor that occurs in the retained urethra. Overall, 30% of the 1054 patients in the USC series experienced a local or distant tumor recurrence. The median time to any recurrence was 12 months, with 86% of all patients developing their recurrence within the first 3 years postoperatively. Of the 311 patients in our series that developed a recurrence, 75% of all recurrences were distant (median time to distant recurrence, 12 months), and 25% of all recurrences were only local (median time to local recurrence, 18 months).

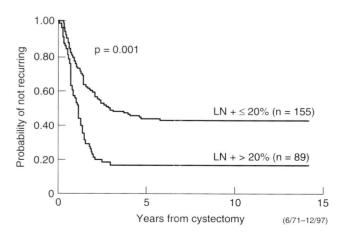

Figure 9.22

Recurrence-free survival in 244 patients with lymph node positive disease stratified by lymph node density (20% or less and greater than 20%). (Reproduced with permission from Stein et al.[13])

Pelvic (local) recurrence

Radical cystectomy clearly provides the best local (pelvic) control of the disease. Of the 311 patients in our series that developed a recurrence, the median time to distant recurrence was 12 months while the median time to local recurrence was 18 months.[4] The use of a high-dose, short course of preoperative radiation therapy does not reduce the risk of pelvic recurrence.[41] Nearly all patients suffering a pelvic recurrence following cystectomy will die of their disease despite additional and even aggressive therapeutic efforts.

Metastatic (distant) recurrence

Recurrences following radical cystectomy are most commonly found at distant sites. Distant recurrences can also be stratified by pathologic subgroups. In our series, patients with organ-confined, lymph node-negative tumors demonstrated a 13% recurrence rate, which increased to 32% for those with extravesical lymph node-negative tumors, and 52% for patients with lymph node-positive tumors.[4] Patients at high risk for tumor recurrence clearly should be considered for adjuvant chemotherapy protocols.

Urethral recurrence

It is generally believed that urethral tumors, in patients with a history of bladder cancer following radical cystectomy, represent a second manifestation of the multicentric defect of the primary transitional cell mucosa that led to the original bladder tumor. The term 'urethral recurrence' may therefore be somewhat misleading, suggesting a failure of definitive treatment of the bladder cancer as the etiology of the urethral lesion. Rather, most urethral tumors probably represent simply another occurrence of the TCC in the remaining urothelium. As radical cystectomy has emerged as the most effective therapy for invasive bladder cancer, and as orthotopic diversion to the native intact urethra has increasingly been performed, the fate of the retained urethra has become an increasingly important oncologic issue.

The advent of orthotopic lower urinary tract reconstruction has arguably improved the quality of life in patients following radical cystectomy for bladder cancer. Approximately 90% of all patients undergoing cystectomy for TCC of the bladder at our institution receive an orthotopic neobladder substitute. From an oncologic perspective, only those patients found to have a positive margin at the proximal urethra (distal to the apex of the prostate in men and just distal to the bladder neck in women) on intraoperative frozen section are absolutely excluded from orthotopic reconstruction. This enthusiasm to preserve the native urethra following radical cystectomy and allow for orthotopic reconstruction has rightfully increased concerns for the potential for urethral recurrence in these patients.

Prior to the orthotopic era in women, urethral tumor recurrence was not considered an important oncologic issue, as the entire urethra was routinely removed at the time of cystectomy. With a better understanding of female pelvic anatomy and the innervation of the rhabdosphincter and continence mechanism in women,[33] along with the identification of various pathologic risk factors for urethral tumor involvement in these patients, orthotopic diversion has now become a commonly performed form of urinary diversion in women following cystectomy.[51] We have demonstrated that tumor involving the bladder neck is the most important risk factor

for urethral tumor involvement in women.[52,53] Although bladder neck involvement is a significant risk factor for urethral tumors, not all women with tumor involving the bladder neck will have urethral tumors. Approximately 50% of women with tumor at the bladder neck will have a urethra free of tumor. In this situation, the patient may potentially be considered an appropriate candidate for orthotopic diversion. Furthermore, we have shown that intraoperative frozen-section analysis of the distal surgical margin provides an accurate and reliable means to evaluate the proximal urethra, and currently is the primary pathologic factor that determines appropriate candidacy for orthotopic diversion.[53] With this selection process, we have not, to date, had a female urethral recurrence.[51]

A growing number of male patients with the urethra reconstructed following cystectomy exist today, and longer follow-up will expose them to a greater risk for a urethral recurrence. The historical incidence of second primary tumors in the retained urethra following cystectomy for bladder cancer ranges from 6% to 10%.[54] Specific clinical and pathologic risk factors may include multifocal tumors, carcinoma in situ, tumor involvement of the prostate (particularly invasion of the prostatic stroma), and the form of urinary diversion performed (orthotopic or cutaneous).[54–60]

We recently evaluated our clinical experience regarding the incidence and associated risk factors for urethral tumors in a large group of male patients undergoing radical cystectomy and urinary diversion for TCC of the bladder with long-term follow-up.[61] We analyzed the clinical and pathologic results of 768 consecutive male patients undergoing radical cystectomy with the intent to cure for high-grade, invasive bladder cancer (median follow-up 13 years); 397 men (52%) underwent an orthotopic urinary diversion (median follow-up 10 years) and 371 men (48%) underwent a cutaneous urinary diversion (median follow-up 19 years). Overall, a total of 45 patients (7%) developed a urethral recurrence, with an overall median time to occurrence of 2 years (range 0.2–13.6 years): 16 men (5%) with an orthotopic, and 29 men (9%) with a cutaneous form of urinary diversion.

In this cohort of male patients, multiple risk factors were analyzed with regard to second primary tumors of the urethra.[61] In a multivariable analysis, two important variables were identified that significantly increased the risk of a urethral tumor recurrence following cystectomy, including any prostate tumor involvement and the form of urinary diversion. The estimated 5-year probability of a urethral recurrence was 5% without any prostate involvement, and increased to 12% and 18% with superficial (prostatic urethra and ducts) and invasive (stroma) prostate involvement, respectively. Furthermore, patients undergoing an orthotopic diversion demonstrated a significantly lower risk of urethral recurrence than those undergoing a cutaneous form of urinary diversion.

The overall management of the urethra in male patients treated for high-grade invasive bladder cancer is an important issue. This concern has become even more critical from an oncologic perspective since the advent of orthotopic diversion. The indications and timing of a prophylactic urethrectomy in those undergoing cystectomy and a cutaneous diversion are debatable. This may include urethrectomy at the time of cystectomy, based on preoperative clinical parameters or the intraoperative frozen-section analysis of the urethral margin, or a delayed urethrectomy based on final pathologic evaluation of the cystectomy specimen.

Our long-term findings provide some insight regarding the issue of management of the retained urethra in both men and women following cystectomy for bladder cancer. We believe that intraoperative frozen-section analysis of the proximal urethra by an experienced pathologist is a reliable and accurate means to determine candidacy for orthotopic diversion in all patients. It has been our practice to construct an orthotopic neobladder in men and women whose intraoperative frozen section of the proximal urethra is without tumor. Our data suggest that this approach does not appear to increase the risk of a urethral recurrence in these patients.[53,54,61] Male patients with known prostatic tumor involvement should not necessarily be excluded from receiving an orthotopic substitute if the intraoperative biopsy is normal. Similarly, female patients with bladder neck involvement should not necessarily be excluded from having an orthotopic neobladder if the intraoperative biopsy is normal. All patients should be carefully counseled regarding the careful follow-up, the long-term risks of a urethral recurrence, and the possible need for urethrectomy following cystectomy for TCC of the bladder.

Importance of surgical technique

The dedication of the surgeon and technical commitment to a properly performed cystectomy and adequate lymphadenectomy are important to the success and clinical outcomes in patients with high-grade bladder cancer. The importance of surgical technique is well illustrated in the role this may have played in a recently reported randomized multi-institutional cooperative group trial.[42] In this prospective study, 270 patients underwent cystectomy with half of the patients receiving neoadjuvant chemotherapy. In a separate analysis of this trial, various surgical factors were subsequently analyzed.[43] Of these 270 patients, 24 had no lymph node dissection, 98 had a limited dissection of the obturator lymph nodes only, and 146 patients had a so-called standard (not extended) pelvic lymph node dissection. The 5-year survival rates for these groups were 33%, 46%, and 60%, respectively. The median number of lymph nodes removed for the entire cohort was 10. As expected, the survival rate for patients with <10 lymph nodes removed was significantly lower than in patients with >10 lymph nodes removed (44% versus 61%, respectively). In a multivariate analysis, the extent of the lymph node dissection, number of lymph nodes removed, and the number of cases performed by the individual surgeon were the most significant factors influencing survival in patients undergoing cystectomy for bladder cancer.[43] It is emphasized that, although this well-publicized study was not intended to analyze the surgical approach and/or technical differences in the treatment of bladder cancer, it was the surgical factors and not neoadjuvant chemotherapy that were most critical as predictors in the outcomes of these patients.[40]

Although the current standard for high-grade, invasive bladder cancer remains radical cystectomy, a current trend in urologic oncology has been to minimize the surgical approach, attempting organ preservation without compromising the cancer outcomes. So-called sexual-function-preserving cystectomy has recently been advocated for some patients with bladder cancer to improve clinical outcomes including continence, potency, and fertility. This surgical (modified cystectomy) approach generally includes sparing the prostate, vasa deferentia, and seminal vesicles while resecting the prostatic adenoma (in some cases) and reconstructing the lower urinary tract to the prostate. In appropriately selected young men who require cystectomy, and for whom potency and fertility remain relevant issues, this may be an important technique that will preserve erectile function, improve voiding, and maintain the ability to reproduce. In fact, our group at USC was one of the first to describe and promote a modified, prostate-sparing cystectomy in carefully selected male patients, with nonurothelial malignancies or nonmalignant bladder diseases, that necessitated cystectomy but not neces-

sarily prostatectomy.[62] We continue to emphasize that this modified technique can be performed in certain appropriately selected young men requiring cystectomy but must not let it compromise the control of cancer.

Recently, various prostate-sparing techniques have been reported in patients with TCC of the bladder undergoing radical cystectomy.[63–67] The rationale for this technique includes improvement in urinary continence results (compared with continence following orthotopic diversion to the urethra), enhancement in erectile preservation and function, and maintenance of fertility in younger patients. Several important oncologic issues must be considered, including the risks of adenocarcinoma of the prostate in nearly 40% of men and TCC involving the prostate in patients undergoing cystectomy for bladder cancer. In addition, it could be argued that the functional and clinical results with orthotopic reconstruction are indeed very good and, in the properly selected patient, nerve-sparing techniques can also be performed to preserve erectile function. Until we better define the long-term oncologic risks associated with prostate-sparing techniques, all patients considering these procedures should provide proper informed consent and be advised that radical cystectomy remains the standard therapy for high-grade, invasive bladder cancer.

Conclusion

Unlike other therapies, radical cystectomy pathologically stages the primary bladder tumor and regional lymph nodes. This histologic evaluation provides important prognostic information and identifies high-risk patients who may benefit from adjuvant therapy. Our data suggest that patients with extravesical tumor extension, or with lymph node-positive disease, appear to be at increased risk for recurrence and may be considered for adjuvant chemotherapy strategies.[4] Additionally, the recent application of molecular markers, based on pathologic staging and analysis, may also serve to identify patients at risk for tumor recurrence who may benefit from adjuvant forms of therapy.[68]

The clinical results and outcomes following radical cystectomy demonstrate good survival, with excellent local recurrence rates for high-grade, invasive bladder cancer. These results provide sound data, and a standard to which other forms of therapy for invasive bladder cancer can be compared. Furthermore, improvements in orthotopic urinary diversion have improved the quality of life in patients following cystectomy. Continence rates following orthotopic diversion are good and provide patients with a more natural voiding pattern per urethra. Contraindications to orthotopic urinary diversion are the presence of tumor within the urethra or extending to the urethral margin as determined by frozen-section analysis of the distal surgical margin at the time of cystectomy, compromised renal function (creatinine >2.5 ng/ml), or the presence of inflammatory bowel disease. Even in patients with locally advanced disease, orthotopic diversion can be employed without concern over subsequent tumor-related reservoir complications.

The question whether patients have a better quality of life following cystectomy or following bladder-sparing protocols, which require significant and prolonged treatment to the bladder with the potential for tumor recurrence, has not been elucidated. Currently, orthotopic diversion should be considered the diversion of choice in all cystectomy patients, and the urologist should have a specific reason why an orthotopic diversion is *not* performed. Patient factors such as frail general health, motivation, or comorbidity, and the cancer factor of a positive urethral margin, may disqualify some patients. Nevertheless, the option of lower urinary tract reconstruction to the intact urethra has been shown to decrease physician reluctance and increase patient acceptance to undergo earlier cystectomy when the disease may be at a more curable stage.[8]

In conclusion, a properly performed radical cystectomy with an appropriate lymphadenectomy provides the best survival rates, with the lowest reported local recurrence rates for high-grade, invasive bladder cancer. The surgical technique is critical to optimize the best clinical and technical outcomes in patients undergoing this procedure. Advances in lower urinary tract reconstruction provide a reasonable alternative for patients undergoing cystectomy, and have improved the quality of life of those patients requiring removal of their bladders.

References

1. Jemal A, Thomas A, Murray T, Thun M. Cancer statistics 2002. CA Cancer J Clin 2002; 52: 23–47.
2. Prout G, Marshall VF. The prognosis with untreated bladder tumors. Cancer 1956; 9: 551–8.
3. Stein JP. Indications for early cystectomy. Urology 2003; 62: 591–5.
4. Stein JP, Lieskovsky G, Cote R, et al. Radical cystectomy in the treatment of invasive bladder cancer: long-term results in 1054 patients. J Clin Oncol 2001; 19: 666–75.
5. Ghoneim MA, El-Mekresh MM, El-Baz MA, El-Attar IA, Ashamallah A. Radical cystectomy for carcinoma of the bladder: critical evaluation of the results in 1,026 cases. J Urol 1997; 158: 393–9.
6. Montie JE. Against bladder sparing: surgery. J Urol 1999; 162: 452–5.
7. Stein JP, Skinner DG. Orthotopic bladder replacement. In Walsh PC, Retik AB, Vaughan ED, Wein AJ (eds): Campbell's Urology, 8th ed. Philadelphia: WB Saunders, 2002, pp 3835–64.
8. Hautmann RE, Paiss T. Does the option of the ileal neobladder stimulate patient and physician decision toward earlier cystectomy? J Urol 1998; 159: 1845–50.
9. Stein JP, Skinner DG. Radical cystectomy in the female. Atlas Urol Clin North Am 1997; 5(20): 37–64.
10. Stein JP, Skinner DG, Montie JE. Radical cystectomy and pelvic lymphadenectomy in the treatment of infiltrative bladder cancer. In Droller MJ (ed): Bladder Cancer: Current Diagnosis and Treatment. Totowa, NJ: Humana Press, 2001, pp 267–307.
11. Stein JP, Quek MD, Skinner DG. Contemporary surgical techniques for continent urinary diversion: continence and potency preservation. Atlas Urol Clin North Am 2001; 9: 147–73.
12. Stein JP. The role of lymphadenectomy in bladder cancer. Am J Urol Rev 2003;1:146–8.
13. Stein JP, Cai J, Groshen S, Skinner DG. Risk factors for patients with pelvic lymph node metastases following radical cystectomy with en bloc cystectomy: the concept of lymph node density. J Urol 2003; 170: 35–41.
14. Herr HW, Bochner BH, Dalbagni G, Donat SM, Reuter VE, Bajorin DF. Impact of the number of lymph nodes retrieved on outcome in patients with muscle invasive bladder cancer. J Urol 2002; 167: 1295–8.
15. Leissner J, Hohenfellner R, Thuroff JW, Wolf HK. Lymphadenectomy in patients with transitional cell carcinoma of the urinary bladder; significance for staging and prognosis. Br J Urol Int 2000; 85: 817–23.
16. Poulsen AL, Horn T, Steven K. Radical cystectomy; extending limits of pelvic lymph node dissection improves survival for patients with bladder cancer confined to the bladder wall. J Urol 1998; 160: 2015–19.
17. Freeman JA, Esrig D, Stein JP, et al. Radical cystectomy for high risk patients with superficial bladder cancer in the era of orthotopic urinary reconstruction. Cancer 1995; 76: 833–9.
18. Anderstrom C, Johansson S, Nilsson S. The significance of lamina propria invasion on the prognosis of patients with bladder tumors. J Urol 1980; 124: 23–6.
19. Heney NM, Ahmed S, Flanagan MJ, Frable W, Corder MP, Hafermann MD, Hawkins IR. Superficial bladder cancer: progression and recurrence. J Urol 1983; 130: 1083–6.
20. Dalesio O, Schulman CC, Sylvester R, et al. Prognostic factors in superficial bladder tumors. A study of the European Organization for Research on Treatment of Cancer: Genitourinary Tract Cancer Cooperative Group. J Urol 1983; 129: 730–3.
21. Herr HW, Jakse G, Sheinfeld J. The T1 bladder tumor. Semin Urol 1990; 8: 254–61.
22. Fitzpatrick JM. The natural history of superficial bladder cancer. Semin Urol 1993; 11: 127–36.
23. Malkowicz SB, Nichols P, Lieskovsky G, Boyd SD, Huffman J, Skinner DG. The role of radical cystectomy in the management of high grade superficial bladder cancer (PA, P1, PIS and P2). J Urol 1990; 144: 641–5.
24. Schellhammer PF, Bean MA, Whitmore WF Jr. Prostatic involvement by transitional cell carcinoma: pathogenesis, patterns, and prognosis. J Urol 1977; 118: 399–403.
25. Prout GR Jr, Griffin PP, Daly JJ, Henery NM. Carcinoma in situ of the urinary bladder with and without associated vesical neoplasms. Cancer 1983; 52: 524–32.
26. Utz DC, Farrow DM. Management of carcinoma in situ of the bladder: a case for surgical management. Urol Clin North Am 1980; 7: 533–40.
27. Voges GE, Tauschke E, Stockle M, Alken P, Hohenfellner R. Computerized tomography: an unreliable method for accurate staging of bladder tumors in patients who are candidates for radical cystectomy. J Urol 1989; 142: 972–4.
28. Pagano F, Bassi P, Galetti TP, Meneghini A, Milani C, Artibani W, Garbeglio A. Results of contemporary radical cystectomy for invasive bladder cancer: a clinicopathologic study with an emphasis on the inadequacy of the tumor, nodes and metastases classification. J Urol 1991; 145: 45–50.
29. Nichols RL, Broido P, Condon RE, Gorbach SL, Nyhus LM. Effect of preoperative neomycin–erythromycin intestinal preparation on the incidence of infectious complications following colon surgery. Ann Surg 1973; 178: 453–62.
30. Pinaud MLJ, Blanloeil YAG, Souron RJ. Preoperative prophylactic digitalization of patients with coronary artery disease—a randomized echocardiographic and hemodynamic study. Anesth Analg 1983; 62: 685–9.
31. Burman SO. The prophylactic use of digitalis before thoracotomy. Ann Thorac Surg 1972; 14: 359–68.
32. Crawford ED, Skinner DG. Salvage cystectomy after radiation failure. J Urol 1980; 123: 32–4.
33. Colleselli K, Stenzl A, Eder R, Strasser H, Poisel S, Bartsch G. The female urethral sphincter: a morphologic and topographical study. J Urol 1998; 160: 49–50.
34. Grossfeld GD, Stein JP, Bennett CJ, Ginsberg DA, Boyd SD, Lieskovsky G, Skinner DG. Lower urinary tract reconstruction in the female using the Kock ileal reservoir with bilateral ureteroileal urethrostomy: update of continence results and fluorodynamic findings. Urology 1996; 48: 383–8.
35. Buscarini M, Stein JP, Lawrence MA, Skinner DG. Tube gastrostomy following radical cystectomy and urinary diversion: surgical technique and experience in 709 patients. Urology 2000; 56: 150–2.
36. Frazier HA, Robertson JE, Dodge RK, and Paulson DF. The value of pathologic factors in predicting cancer-specific survival among patients treated with radical cystectomy for transitional cell carcinoma of the bladder and prostate. Cancer 1993; 71: 3993–4001.
37. Amling CL, Thrasher JB, Frazier HA, Dodge RK, Robertson JE, Paulson DF. Radical cystectomy for stages Ta, Tis and T1 transitional cell carcinoma of the bladder. J Urol 1994; 151: 31–5.
38. Viewig J, Gschwend JE, Herr HW, Fair WR. The impact of primary stage on survival in patients with lymph node positive bladder cancer J Urol 1999; 161: 72–6.
39. Leissner J, Ghoneim MA, Abol-Enein H, et al. Extended radical lymphadenectomy in patients with urothelial bladder cancer: results of a prospective multicenter study. J Urol 2004; 171: 139–44.

40. Stein JP, Dunn MD, Quek ML, Miranda G, Skinner DG. The orthotopic T-pouch ileal neobladder: experience with 209 patients. J Urol 2004; 172: 584–7.
41. Skinner DG, Lieskovsky G. Contemporary cystectomy with pelvic node dissection compared to preoperative radiation therapy plus cystectomy in management of invasive bladder cancer. J Urol 1984; 131: 1069–72.
42. Grossman HB, Natale RB, Tangen CM, et al. Neoadjuvant chemotherapy plus cystectomy compared with cystectomy alone for locally advanced bladder cancer. N Engl J Med 2003; 349: 859–66.
43. Herr HW. Surgical factors in bladder cancer: more (nodes) + more (pathology) = less (mortality). BJU Int 2003; 92: 187–8.
44. Skinner DG, Daniels JA, Russell CA, et al. The role of adjuvant chemotherapy following cystectomy for invasive bladder cancer: a prospective comparative trial. J Urol 1991; 145: 459–67.
45. Figueroa AJ, Stein JP, Dickinson M, et al. Radical cystectomy for elderly patients with bladder carcinoma. An updated experience with 404 patients. Cancer 1998; 83: 141–7.
46. Koch MO, Smith JA Jr. Influence of patient age and co-morbidity on outcome of a collaborative care pathway after radical prostatectomy and cystoprostatectomy. J Urol 1996; 155: 1681–4.
47. Chang SS, Alberts G, Cookson MS, Smith JA Jr. Radical cystectomy is safe in elderly patients at high risk. J Urol 2001; 166: 938–41.
48. Sanchez-Ortiz RF, Huang WC, Mick R, Van Arsdalen KN, Wein AJ, Malkowicz SB. An interval longer than 12 weeks between the diagnosis of muscle invasion and cystectomy is associated with worse outcome in bladder carcinoma. J Urol 2003; 169: 110–15.
49. Quek ML, Stein JP, Clark PE, et al. Microscopic and gross extravesical extension in pathologic staging of bladder cancer. J Urol 2004; 171: 640–5.
50. AJCC Cancer Staging Manual, 5th ed. Philadelphia: Lippincott-Raven, 1997, pp 241–3.
51. Stein JP, Ginsberg DA, Skinner DG. Indications and technique of the orthotopic neobladder in women. Urol Clin North Am 2002; 29: 725–34.
52. Stein JP, Cote RJ, Freeman JA, et al. Indications for lower urinary tract reconstruction in women after cystectomy for bladder cancer: a pathological review of female cystectomy specimens. J Urol 1995; 154: 1329–33.
53. Stein JP, Esrig D, Freeman JA, et al. Prospective pathologic analysis of female cystectomy specimens: risk factors for orthotopic diversion in women. Urology 1998; 51: 951–5.
54. Freeman JA, Esrig D, Stein JP, Skinner DG. Management of the patient with bladder cancer. Urethral recurrence. Urol Clin North Am 1994; 21: 645–51.
55. Freeman JA, Tarter TA, Esrig D, et al. Urethral recurrence in patients with orthotopic ileal neobladders. J Urol 1996; 156: 1615–19.
56. Stenzl A, Bartsch G, Rogatsch H. The remnant urothelium after reconstructive bladder surgery. Eur Urol 2002; 41: 124–31.
57. Levinson AK, Johnson DE, Wishnow KI. Indications for urethrectomy in an era of continent urinary diversion. J Urol 1990; 144: 73–5.
58. Hardeman SW, Soloway MS. Urethral recurrence following radical cystectomy. J Urol 1990; 144: 666–9.
59. Stockle M, Gokcebay E, Riedmiller H, Hohenfellner R. Urethral tumor recurrences after radical cystoprostatectomy: the case for primary cystoprostatourethrectomy? J Urol 1990; 143: 41–42; discussion 43.
60. Tobisu K, Tanaka Y, Mizutani T, Kakizoe T. Transitional cell carcinoma of the urethra in men following cystectomy for bladder cancer: multivariate analysis for risk factors. J Urol 1991;146:1551–1553; discussion 1553–4.
61. Stein JP, Clark, P, Miranda G, Cai J, Groshen S, Skinner DG. Urethral tumor recurrence following cystectomy and urinary diversion: clinical and pathologic characteristics in 768 male patients. J Urol 2005; 173(4): 1163–8.
62. Spitz A, Stein JP, Lieskovsky G, Skinner DG. Orthotopic urinary diversion with preservation of erectile and ejaculatory function in men requiring radical cystectomy for nonurothelial malignancy: a new technique. J Urol 1999; 161: 1761–4.
63. Vallancien G, El Fettouh HA, Cathelineau X, Baumert H, Fromont G, Guillonneau B. Cystectomy with prostate sparing for bladder cancer in 100 patients: 10-year experience. J Urol 2002; 168: 2413–17.
64. Ghanem AN. Experience with 'capsule sparing' cystoprostadenectomy for orthotopic bladder replacement: overcoming the problems of impotence, incontinence and difficult urethral anastomosis. BJU Int 2002; 90: 617–20.
65. Horenblas S, Meinhardt W, Ijzerman W, Moonen LFN. Sexuality preserving cystectomy and neobladder; initial results. J Urol 2001; 166: 837–40.
66. Colombo R, Bertini R, Salonia A, et al. Nerve and seminal sparing radical cystectomy with orthotopic urinary diversion for selected patients with superficial bladder cancer: an innovative surgical approach. J Urol 2001; 165: 51–5.
67. Colombo R, Bertini R, Salonia A, et al. Overall clinical outcomes after nerve and seminal sparing radical cystectomy for the treatment of organ confined bladder cancer. J Urol 2004; 171: 1819–22.
68. Stein JP, Grossfeld GD, Ginsberg DA, et al. Prognostic markers in bladder cancer: a contemporary review of the literature. J Urol 1999; 160: 645–59.

10

Cystectomy in the female

Aristotelis G Anastasiadis, Susan Feyerabend, Markus A Kuczyk, Arnulf Stenzl

Introduction

The Czech surgeon Pawlik reported the first cystectomy in a female more than a century ago.[1] He described an implantation of the ureters into the vagina with a good postoperative result regarding continence as well as a survival of 16 years. Other physicians could not achieve similar results and therefore this technique of urinary diversion was subsequently abandoned. Until recently, women undergoing cystectomy for bladder cancer received urinary diversion either into the intact rectosigmoid or into the abdominal skin.[2–6] Despite increasing popularity for orthotopic neobladders after cystectomy in men with bladder cancer during the last decade, a similar approach for female patients was thought not to be appropriate because of the need for a concomitant total urethrectomy.[7]

However, results of a combined series from two institutions have indicated that selected women with transitional cell cancer (TCC) undergoing radical cystectomy can safely be spared a portion of their urethra.[8,9] The remaining urethral segment would be sufficient for a continence mechanism when anastomosed to a low-pressure intestinal reservoir. Important aspects which have to be taken into consideration in female patients with TCC prior to cystectomy and urinary diversion are discussed in this chapter. These aspects include anatomical considerations, patient selection, and surgical techniques, as well as oncologic and functional outcome.

Incidence of urethral tumors in bladder cancer of the female—is urethra-sparing cystectomy oncologically safe?

An important question when considering urethra-sparing cystectomy in female patients is whether there is a risk of compromising oncologic outcome. In order to use the urethra for bladder reconstruction, about 80% of the urethra should be preserved.[10] Within the urethra, the level of transition between transitional and squamous epithelium varies considerably. With increasing age, the transition zone moves cranially and can even cover the whole urethra, bladder neck, and part of the trigone, probably due to the influence of estrogen.[11,12] Since the bladder neck and a small portion of the proximal urethra are resected during surgery, only a very short segment, in

some patients even none, of the remnant urethra will be covered by transitional cell epithelium, whereas the major part of the urethral mucosa will consist of either regular or metaplastic squamous epithelium. Therefore, often only squamous metaplasia is found at the level of urethral dissection. To the authors' knowledge, no data describe a TCC recurrence on squamous epithelium after removal of the entire urothelium of the bladder during cystectomy.

Several studies have tried to address the risk of urethral tumors in the remnant female urethra after cystectomy. In retrospective analyses, Stein et al[13] and Coloby et al[14] step-sectioned urethrocystectomy specimens of female bladder cancer patients and found urethral tumor involvement in 7 of 65 (10.7%) and 3 of 47 (6.4%) patients, respectively. A strong correlation with cancer at the bladder neck and/or the trigone was found in both studies, and a subtotal urethrectomy was suggested. On the other hand, De Paepe et al[15] found carcinoma in situ or papillary tumors in the urethra in 8 of 22 (36%) patients and suggested that a urethrectomy should be performed in all women undergoing radical cystectomy for TCC of the bladder. It should be borne in mind, however, that there were only 22 patients included in this report and that no details about the localization of either primary tumor in the bladder or secondary tumors in the urethra were provided.

Ashworth[16] and Stenzl et al[17] also evaluated the incidence of secondary urethral tumors of more than 600 patients treated for bladder cancer. In these series, the incidence of secondary urethral tumors was 1.4% and 2%, respectively. Interestingly, women showed a lower incidence of urethral involvement than male patients from the same institution.[18]

Anatomy of the female urethra

The sphincter system of the female urethra consists of smooth muscle layers, which are controlled by autonomic nerves, and striated muscle layers innervated by somatic nerves. The autonomic nerve branches for the smooth muscle portion of the urethral sphincter originate from the pelvic plexus.[19,20] The innervation of the voluntary sphincter system is controversial: although most authors suggest that branches of the pudendal nerve provide the nerve supply to this sphincter,[21,22] others have suggested that the autonomic nervous system is responsible for its innervation.[23]

Women treated with distal partial urethrectomy, for example for complicated diverticula or tumors, remain continent unless a major portion of the middle third of the urethra is resected.[24]

It is, therefore, generally accepted that the bladder neck, together with an adequate proximal urethral segment, is sufficient for urinary continence in women. Fetal and adult cadaver studies have demonstrated that the entire rhabdosphincter, which is innervated by the pudendal nerve caudally, is located in the caudal half of the urethra and merges approximately halfway with the mid-layer of the proximal smooth musculature.[25] Smooth muscle fibers of the outer and inner layer, innervated by the autonomic nervous system, however, are present throughout the whole length of the urethra.

Nerve fibers originating from the pelvic plexus located dorsolaterally from the rectum have been traced on their route to the bladder neck and urethra to run dorsal to the distal ureter, underneath the lateral vesical pedicle and along the lateral walls of the vagina.[26] An anterior exenteration with complete resection of the vagina with the caudal margin below the bladder neck would therefore result in the dissection of the majority, if not all, of the autonomic nerves to the female urethra. As a consequence, a careful dissection of the lateral vaginal walls, bladder neck, and proximal urethra would leave the majority of plexus fibers to the urethra intact, thus preserving the sphincter mechanism.[27–29]

The suspensory fascial reinforcements of the remnant urethra will not be compromised if a nerve-sparing cystectomy is performed, since care is taken to stay as close as possible to the urethra proximally and to avoid any dissection caudal to the level of the urethral division.

Another important aspect is the lymphatic drainage of the remnant urethra after cystectomy. Bladder tumors which are close to, but not adjacent to, the bladder neck and show grossly enlarged lymph nodes preoperatively may cause reverse lymphatic tumor cell drainage to the external inguinal lymph nodes. This could increase the risk of periurethral tumor cell nests in the remnant urethra. One should therefore consider the status of the pelvic and inguinal nodes in addition to the location of the primary tumor in selecting female patients for orthotopic reconstruction. If preoperatively performed biopsies of these areas are positive for cancer, this is a relative contraindication for orthotopic urinary diversion.

Patient selection criteria

Female candidates for creation of an orthotopic neobladder to the urethra should be selected according to tumor extension, urethral competence, performance status, and motivation (Box 10.1).[10] Preoperatively, bimanual and endoscopic tumor evaluation, a computed tomography (CT) scan of the abdomen and thorax, and a bone scan, as well as biopsies of the bladder neck, should be performed. Urethral competence should be assessed by the patient's history, endoscopy, radiography, and intraluminal urethra pressure profile (UPP).

Patients with an orthotopic neobladder need strength and motivation for continence training and should be able to adhere to simple rules, for example, a certain micturition pattern in the early postoperative period. An acceptable performance status and motivation are therefore necessary. This includes the understanding and handling of specific problems, such as possible urinary retention or increased post void residuals that may require intermittent catheterization, or nocturnal and diurnal incontinence.

Surgical technique

The technique of anterior exenteration and concomitant lymphadenectomy has been described elsewhere in the literature.

Box 10.1 Exclusion criteria for an orthotopic reconstruction of the lower urinary tract to the urethra in women with bladder or other pelvic malignancies

1. Tumor extension
   - Tumor/carcinoma in situ at bladder neck
   - Urethral tumor
   - Any positive surgical margin on frozen section
   - ≥N2
   - Any tumor involvement of inguinal nodes
   - M+
2. Urethral competence
   - History of stress incontinence ≥Grade II due to sphincteric incompetence
   - Marked urethral hypermobility
   - P_{rest} <30 cm H2O in the intraluminal urethra pressure profile (UPP)
   - Full dose radiation to the urethra
3. Performance status and motivation
   - Any reduced performance status, e.g. Karnofsky index ≤90%
   - No motivation to undergo intensive continence training if necessary
   - No motivation to wear pads if necessary
   - No motivation or dexterity for clean intermittent catheterization if necessary

---

Therefore, in the present chapter we will describe only those variations which are relevant for female patients undergoing an orthotopic reconstruction of the lower urinary tract. All our patients receive an ileal low-pressure reservoir with an antireflux protection for the upper urinary tract and direct anastomosis of the pouch to the remnant urethra. To facilitate intraoperative catheterization of the pouch after dividing the Foley catheter during cystectomy, the patient can be placed in a low lithotomy position. In most cases, however, we place the patient in a simple supine position to avoid possible complications related to positioning.

During pelvic lymphadenectomy care is taken to minimize dissection in the region of the upper hypogastric nerve crossing the common iliac artery. Special attention is then directed towards dissection and resection of the inner genitalia. After mobilization of the ovaries, tubes and uterus, only the vaginal fundus and the anterior vaginal wall down to the level of the subsequent urethral dissection are resected (Figure 10.1). The dorsal half of the vaginal fundus is incised circumferentially around the cervical insertion or scar from a previous hysterectomy. The line of incision is continued ventrally and caudally to include an approximately 2 cm wide segment of the ventral wall of the vagina. The bladder neck and proximal urethra are then carefully 'peeled' out of the surrounding connective tissue and fascia. Care is taken to incise the endopelvic fascia medially, where it leaves the bladder surface. The dissection of the proximal urethra is performed by incising the fascia longitudinally in the midline and staying as close to the urethral wall as possible in order to avoid damage to the nerve fibers coursing to the remnant urethra (Figure 10.2). The proximal urethra with its Foley catheter is clamped with a strong Overholt clamp and dissected approximately 0.5–1 cm distal to the bladder neck (Figure 10.3). The specimen is then removed and a transverse frozen section of the urethra is sent for intraoperative pathologic evaluation.

Squamous metaplasia was present in all our specimens, but no tumor or dysplasia was diagnosed at the level of urethral dissection. In obese patients, a ureteral catheter placed in an antegrade fashion may be an additional help in guiding the final pouch catheter

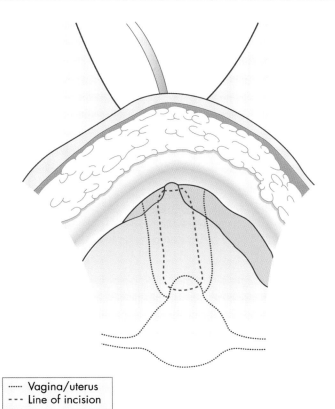

| ..... | Vagina/uterus |
| - - - | Line of incision |

Figure 10.1
Incision line during nerve-sparing cystectomy in order to preserve autonomic nerve fibers to the remnant urethra. Adapted from Stenzl A, Draxl H, Posch B, Colleselli K, Falk M, Bartsch G. The risk of urethral tumors in female bladder cancer: can the urethra be used for orthotopic reconstruction of the lower urinary tract? J Urol 1995; 153: 950–5.

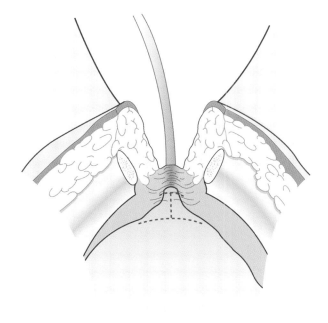

Figure 10.2
Adult anatomic specimen of the bladder neck and urethra with part of the pubic bone removed. When following the dashed line of incision (- - -) during dissection and staying close to the urethra and bladder neck respectively, neither the majority of the autonomic nerves to the remnant urethra nor the urethral suspensory system will be damaged. Adapted from Stenzl A, Draxl H, Posch B, Colleselli K, Falk M, Bartsch G. The risk of urethral tumors in female bladder cancer: can the urethra be used for orthotopic reconstruction of the lower urinary tract? J Urol 1995; 153: 950–5.

transurethrally prior to closure of the urethroileal anastomosis. The vaginal defect is closed transversely with a running 0 polyglycolic acid (PGA) suture (Figure 10.4). If necessary, continence training devices may be introduced into the resulting small vaginal pouch. If the patient is sexually active, the vaginal defect might also be closed with a small-detubularized ileal patch.

Any low-pressure reservoir can be anastomosed to the remnant urethra with preferably six 2-0 synthetic absorbable sutures. We have observed that caudal migration of the pouch into the pelvis may result in intestinal folds that may cause intermittent obstructive valves at the ileourethral anastomosis. Instead of anastomosing the spout-like residual opening, which is connected to the urethra in the hemi-Kock or T-pouch, we therefore now employ a technique used in other pouches, in which a circular ileal opening close to the mesentery at the lowest part of the pouch is anastomosed to the urethra.[30]

At the end of the procedure, a J-shaped omentum flap is brought down and around the bottom of the pouch.[17] Alternatively, portions of the ileal pouch adjacent to this anastomosis can be sutured to the anterior and lateral pelvic walls as well as the remnant vaginal stump to avoid both the formation of obstructive folds over the urethral anastomosis and the formation of a 'pouchocele' due to a postoperative descensus of the reservoir. Initial attempts to perform a 'neobladder neck suspension' to improve early continence were not

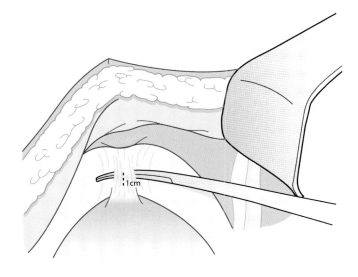

Figure 10.3
The urethra is clamped and dissected approximately 0.5–1 cm caudal of the bladder neck. Adapted from Stenzl A, Draxl H, Posch B, Colleselli K, Falk M, Bartsch G. The risk of urethral tumors in female bladder cancer: can the urethra be used for orthotopic reconstruction of the lower urinary tract? J Urol 1995; 153: 950–5.

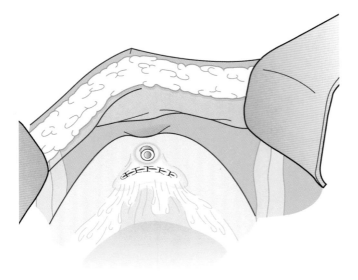

Figure 10.4
After removal of the specimen, the vagina is closed transversely. Any low-pressure reservoir can now be anastomosed to the remnant urethra. A J-shaped omentum flap or additional attachment sutures of the pouch to the pelvic wall are advocated to improve postoperative micturition results. Adapted from Stenzl A, Draxl H, Posch B, Colleselli K, Falk M, Bartsch G. The risk of urethral tumors in female bladder cancer: can the urethra be used for orthotopic reconstruction of the lower urinary tract? J Urol 1995; 153: 950–5.

successful because of urinary retention. Suspension of the vaginal vault with remnant portions of the round ligaments or fascial strips to prevent kinking of the pouch and subsequent retention have been suggested recently, but long-term results are not yet available.

Both ureteroileal anastomoses are stented with 7 Fr. single J-shaped ureteral catheters, which are brought out either transurethrally along the urethral catheter or through the lower abdominal wall. Pelvic drains are removed on the fifth postoperative day, ureteral catheters after approximately 8–10 days, and the 20 Fr. urethral catheter after 14 days, if a previous pouchogram shows no extravasation.

Results

Oncologic results

In a multicenter study, the combined data of 102 women aged 28–79 (mean 59) years who underwent a urethra-sparing cystectomy and orthotopic urinary diversion were reviewed.[31] Surgery was performed for bladder cancer (n=96), cervical cancer (n=2), vaginal cancer (n=1), cancer of the fallopian tube (n=1), uterine sarcoma (n=1), or rectal cancer (n=1). The histology of the 96 bladder cancers was TCC in 81, adenocarcinoma in 8, squamous cell cancer in 5, small cell carcinoma in 1, and unclassified in 1 patient. The mean follow-up time was 26 months. At completion of the study, 88/102 patients were alive and 83/102 patients were alive and disease free.

The bladder neck was free of tumor in all patients. The bladder neck and up to 1 cm of the proximal urethra were removed with the

specimen. An ileal orthotopic neobladder was performed if staging biopsies of the bladder neck and intraoperative frozen section of the urethral margin revealed no tumor. No perioperative deaths were reported, and early and late complications requiring secondary interventions occurred in 5% and 12% of patients, respectively. With 88 of 102 patients alive and 83 of 102 patients disease free, a disease-specific survival of 74% and a disease-free survival of 63% could be estimated at 5 years. The remnant urethra was monitored via voided cytology and endoscopically. Three pelvic recurrences occurred in patients with gynecologic tumors and one in a patient with adenocarcinoma of the bladder, but none of them in the area of the urethra or its supplying autonomic nerves.

The incidence of concomitant secondary malignant involvement of gynecologic organs in female cystectomy specimens has been evaluated in a recent study.[32] Overall gynecologic organ involvement was documented in 16 of 609 patients (2.6%). Although the majority of these women were diagnosed with squamous cell bladder carcinoma, which may not be representative for many geographic areas, first evidence is provided that the risk of secondary malignant involvement of genital organs in female cystectomy specimens is low. Therefore, the routine removal of involved gynecologic organs during radical cystectomy in women may be an issue of discussion in the future.

Functional outcome

Voiding pattern

A routine postoperative urodynamic evaluation of the pouch and remaining urethra is not necessary, but was performed in 15 patients.[10] The voiding pattern, including volumes at each micturition, was evaluated by a detailed questionnaire. To obtain the maximum pouch volume, the average of three maximum volumes was calculated and was used as a value up to which the pouch was filled during urodynamic testing. The calculated bladder capacity in these women ranged from 400 to 750 (mean 560) cc. Post void residuals ranged from 0 to 150 cc.

The intraluminal pouch pressures at rest were below 30 cm H_2O in all patients except one, who showed intermittent peak pressures of up to 38 cm H_2O after 6 months. Maximum intraluminal urethral pressures in the UPP ranged from 30 to 35 (mean 32) cm H_2O, which was virtually unchanged, from preoperative values with an average of 33.4 (range 28–42) cm H_2O.

Diurnal and nocturnal continence

For the evaluation of diurnal and nocturnal continence we used definitions from the literature.[7] In patients followed for more than 6 months postoperatively, daytime and nocturnal continence could be achieved in 85.5% and 79%, respectively. Interestingly, only 25% of preoperatively irradiated patients for gynecologic malignancies have regained diurnal continence, whereas all other patients have Grade I–II stress incontinence. We therefore consider a full course of preoperative radiation a relative contraindication for this surgical procedure. Urodynamic results from patients included in the multicenter study mentioned above are also available.[31] Daytime and nocturnal continence rates with maximally one pad for safety were 82% and 72%, respectively. Twelve patients (12%) were unable to empty their bladders completely and needed some form of catheterization.

Urinary retention or unacceptably large post void residuals in patients with an ileal valve obstructing the neobladder outlet partially or completely could be treated successfully. This entity, first described in 1997,[10] can be observed endoscopically when positioning the cystoscope just below the bladder neck and draining the pouch. This problem can be resolved completely by incising these valves carefully.

Sexual function

Another important aspect of nerve-preserving surgery is that of sexual function. Similar to male erectile physiology, nitric oxide (NO) plays a major role in vasodilation in clitoral tissues.[33] Autonomic nerves are responsible not only for NO-mediated changes in the clitoris, but also for vasoactive intestinal polypeptide (VIP) mediated vasodilation and secretion of the vaginal mucosa. The latter plays a major role during the phase of sexual arousal. Neurotransmitters, in turn, are able to modulate the sensitivity of sensory nerve fibers to central or peripheral stimuli.[34] Similar to erectile dysfunction in men, female sexual dysfunction (FSD) can be a sequela of pelvic surgery with a major impact on quality of life, relationships, and psychosocial function.

Although sexual function may play only a minor role for many cancer patients, for a subset of patients it represents an important aspect of quality of life. Unfortunately, data on sexual function of cancer patients remain scant in the literature. In addition, FSD in cancer patients is extremely difficult to evaluate because of its complexity due to somatic and psychological aspects, which are often intertwined.[35] More studies are needed in this field to further optimize surgical techniques and to improve patients' quality of life.

Conclusion

Recent larger series confirm our initial results, showing that sparing the urethra after cystectomy will not compromise oncologic outcome and can be used satisfactorily for orthotopic reconstruction of the lower urinary tract in female patients. Diurnal and nocturnal continence rates of 87.5% and 79%, respectively, and clean intermittent catheterization in 10% after 6 months are comparable to results in larger male series and justify the use of orthotopic neobladders as a procedure of choice in selected females.

We now know that urinary continence of any bladder substitution can be maintained despite removal of the bladder neck and the adjacent proximal urethra. In our anatomic studies as well as those of others, no prominent sphincteric structure was present in either the female bladder neck or the cranial urethra. The bulk of the striated intrinsic sphincter ('rhabdosphincter') is located in the mid to caudal third of the urethra and will not be removed with proximal urethrectomy, as described above. Its innervation via the pudendal nerve will not be compromised during the surgical procedure.

Controversy still exists as to whether dissecting autonomic nerves to the urethra when performing a subtotal colpectomy and resection of the bladder neck including a wide margin of surrounding tissue will compromise long-term results. As yet, we do not know if these autonomic nerves are needed for satisfactory function of the urethral smooth muscles, nor can we determine to what extent these nerves can be spared at each individual surgery. Based on available anatomic and functional studies, however, it is suggested that most of the autonomic innervation of the remnant urethra should stay intact postoperatively to preserve both muscular resistance and continence despite removal of a safe segment of the proximal urethra for oncologic reasons.[19,36]

Over the years, it was possible to further improve postoperative functional results by:

1. leaving the posterior and lateral vaginal walls intact when performing a nerve-sparing anterior exenteration—this can be achieved by carefully dissecting out the bladder neck and the proximal urethra;
2. removing 0.5–1 cm of the cranial urethra en bloc with the cystectomy specimen and obtaining a frozen section of the whole urethral circumference;
3. using previous experience with low-pressure reservoirs in male patients;
4. preventing complications related to a downward migration of the pouch by using either a J-shaped omentum flap or stay sutures between the pouch wall and the surrounding pelvic structures.[37,38]

References

1. Pawlik K. Extirpace mechyre mocoveho, Lekaru Ceskych 1890; 29: 705–6.
2. Bricker E. Bladder substitution after pelvic evisceration. Surg Clin North Am 1950; 30: 1511–21.
3. Clarke B, Leadbetter W. Ureterosigmoidostomy: collective review of results in 2,897 reported cases. J Urol 1955; 73: 999–1008.
4. Fisch MWR, Müller SC, Hohenfellner R. The sigma-rectum pouch (Mainz pouch II). Scand J Urol Nephrol (Suppl) 1992; 142: 187–8.
5. Ghoneim M. The modified rectal bladder: a bladder substitute controlled by the anal sphincter. Scand J Urol Nephrol 1992; 142: 89–91.
6. Gilchrist R, Merricks J, Hamlin H. Construction of a substitute bladder and urethra. Surg Gynecol Obstet 1950; 90: 752–60.
7. Skinner DG, Boyd SD, Lieskovski G, Bennett C, Hopwood B. Lower urinary tract reconstruction following cystectomy: experience and results in 126 patients using the Kock ileal reservoir with bilateral ureteroileal urethrostomy. J Urol 1991; 146: 756–60.
8. Cancrini A, de Carli P, Fattahi H, Pompeo V, Cantiani R, von Heland M. Orthotopic ileal neobladder in female patients after radical cystectomy: 2-year experience. J Urol 1994; 153: 956–8.
9. Stein J, Stenzl A, Esrig D, et al. Lower urinary tract reconstruction following cystectomy in women using the Kock ileal reservoir with bilateral utereroileal urethrostomy: initial clinical experience. J Urol 1994; 152: 1404–8.
10. Stenzl A, Colleselli K, Bartsch G. Update of urethra-sparing approaches in cystectomy in women. World J Urol 1997;15:134–138.
11. Packham D. The epithelial lining of the female trigone and urethra. Br J Urol 1971; 43: 201–8.
12. Wiener D, Koss L, Salaby B, Freed S. The prevalence and significance of Brunn's nests, cystitis cystica, and squamous metaplasia in normal bladders. J Urol 1979; 122: 317–23.
13. Stein J, Cote R, Freeman J, et al. Indications for lower urinary tract reconstruction in women following cystectomy for bladder cancer: a pathologic review of female cystectomy specimens. J Urol 1995; 154: 1329–33.
14. Coloby P, Kakizoe T, Tobisu KI. Urethral involvement in female bladder cancer patients: mapping of 47 consecutive cysto-urethrectomy specimens. J Urol 1994; 152: 1438–42.
15. De Paepe M, Andre R, Mahadevia P. Urethral involvement in female patients with bladder cancer. A study of 22 cystectomy specimens. Cancer 1990; 65: 1237–42.
16. Ashworth A. Papillomatosis of the urethra. Br J Urol 1956; 28: 3–11.

17. Stenzl A, Colleselli K, Poisel S, Feichtinger H, Bartsch G. The use of neobladders in women undergoing cystectomy for transitional cell cancer. World J Urol 1996; 14: 15–21.

18. Erckert M, Stenzl A, Falk M, Bartsch G. The incidence of urethral tumor involvement in male bladder cancer patients. World J Urol 1996; 14: 3–8.

19. Baader B, Baader SL, Herrmann M, Stenzl A. Anatomical bases of the autonomic innervation of the female pelvis. Urologe A 2004; 43: 133–49.

20. Wein A, Levin R, Barrett D. Voiding function: relevant anatomy, physiology, and pharmacology. In Gillenwater J, Grayhack J, Howards S, Duckett J (eds): Adult and Pediatric Urology, 2nd ed. Chicago: Year Book, 1991, pp 933–999.

21. Gosling JA, Dixon JS, Critchley HO, Thompson SA. A comparative study of the human external sphincter and periurethral levator ani muscles. Br J Urol 1981; 53: 35–41.

22. Tanagho EA, Meyers FH, Smith DR. Urethral resistance: its components and implications. II. Striated muscle component. Invest Urol 1969; 7: 195–205.

23. Donker P, Droes J, Van Ulden B. Anatomy of the musculature and innervation of the bladder and the urethra. In Williams D, Chisholm G (eds): Scientific Foundations of Urology, vol II. London: Heinemann, 1976, p 32.

24. Neuwirth H, Stenzl A, de Kernion J. Urethral cancer. In Haskell C (ed): Cancer Treatment. Philadelphia: Saunders, 1990, pp 762–64.

25. Strasser H, Ninkovic M, Hess M, Bartsch G, Stenzl A. Anatomic and functional studies of the male and female urethral sphincter. World J Urol 2000; 18: 324–9.

26. Colleselli K, Stenzl A, Eder R, Strasser H, Poisel S, Bartsch G. The female urethral sphincter: a morphological and topographical study. J Urol 1998; 160: 49–54.

27. De Petriconi R, Kleinschmidt K, Flohr P, Paiss T, Hautmann R. Ileal neobladder with anastomosis to the female urethra. Urologe A 1996; 35: 284–90.

28. Mills RD, Studer UE. Female orthotopic bladder substitution: a good operation in the right circumstances. J Urol 2000; 163: 1501–4.

29. Stenzl A, Draxl H, Posch B, Colleselli K, Falk M, Bartsch G. The risk of urethral tumors in female bladder cancer: can the urethra be used for orthotopic reconstruction of the lower urinary tract? J Urol 1995; 153: 950–5.

30. Studer U, Ackermann D, Casanova G, Zingg E. Three years experience with an ileal low pressure bladder substitute. Br J Urol 1989;63:43–52.

31. Stenzl A, Jarolim L, Coloby P, et al. Urethra-sparing cystectomy and orthotopic urinary diversion in women with malignant pelvic tumors. Cancer 2001; 92: 1864–71.

32. Ali-El-Dein B, Abdel-Latif M, Mosbah A, Eraky I, Shaaban AA, Taha NM, Ghoneim MA. Secondary malignant involvement of gynecologic organs in radical cystectomy specimens in women: is it mandatory to remove these organs routinely? J Urol 2004; 172: 885–7.

33. Burnett AL, Calvin DC, Silver RI, Peppas DS, Docimo SG. Immunohistochemical description of nitric oxide synthase isoforms in the human clitoris. J Urol 1997; 158: 75–8.

34. McKenna KE. The neurophysiology of female sexual dysfunction. World J Urol 2002; 20: 93–100.

35. Anastasiadis AG, Davis AR, Sawczuk IS, et al. Quality of life aspects in kidney cancer patients: data from a national registry. Supp Care Cancer 2003; 11: 700–6.

36. Stenzl A, Anastasiadis AG, Corvin S, Feil G, Strasser H, Kuczyk M. Advantages of nerve sparing pelvic surgery—results of experimental and clinical studies. Urologe A 2004; 43: 141–9.

37. Stenzl A, Höltl L. Orthotopic bladder reconstruction in women—what we have learned over the last decade? Crit Rev Oncol Hematol 2003; 47: 147–54.

38. Stenzl A. Current concepts for urinary diversion in women. EAU Update Series 2003; 1: 91–9.

11

Nerve-sparing radical cystectomy

Marc S Chuang, Gary D Steinberg, Mark P Schoenberg

Introduction

Bladder cancer is the second most common genitourinary malignancy, with transitional cell carcinoma (TCC) comprising nearly 90% of all primary bladder cancers. Although the majority of patients present with superficial bladder tumors, 20% to 40% either present with or develop invasive disease.[1]

The first cystectomy was performed in the late 1800s.[2] However, early techniques were associated with high rates of morbidity and mortality. Young and Davis[3] indicated that high mortality rates and poor success rates made cystectomy unjustifiable. In 1939, Hinman[4] reported a mortality rate of 34.5% in a series of 250 cystectomies. More recently, improvements in surgical anesthetic techniques as well as perioperative care have reduced the mortality rate of radical cystectomy to 1% to 3%.[1,5,6]

During the 1960s and 1970s, various regimes of preoperative radiation were used in an attempt to improve survival after cystectomy; however, these failed to demonstrate any additional benefit.[7] In the largest series to date, Stein et al[1] evaluated their long-term experience with 1054 patients diagnosed with invasive bladder cancer. They were able to demonstrate excellent long-term, recurrence-free survival in patients with organ-confined, lymph-node-negative disease. Patients with lymph node involvement or extravesical extension had a significantly higher probability of recurrence. Patients could also be stratified by the extent of lymph node involvement. The overall recurrence rate was 30%. These data and data from similar studies support aggressive surgical management of invasive bladder carcinoma.[8,9] Thus, radical cystectomy is currently considered the gold standard for muscle invasive disease.[10]

With improved survival following radical cystectomy, increased emphasis was placed on quality of life issues. In 1982, Walsh and Donker demonstrated that impotence following radical prostatectomy arises from injury to the pelvic nerve plexus that provides autonomic innervation to the corpora cavernosa.[11] The technique for radical prostatectomy and cystoprostatectomy was therefore modified to avoid injury to these cavernous nerves and preserve potency. In 1985, Lepor and associates reported a detailed three-dimensional model of the course of the cavernous nerves in the region of the prostate based on microscopic step-sections taken from a human cadaver.[12] In 1987, Schlegel and Walsh demonstrated the exact relationship of the cavernous nerves to the seminal vesicles and bladder (Figure 11.1).[13] This study demonstrated that the pelvic plexus is located retroperitoneally on the lateral wall of the rectum, 5–11 cm from the anal verge with its midpoint related to the tip of the seminal vesicle. The cavernous branches travel in a direct route from the pelvic plexus toward the posterolateral base of the prostate. Because the bulk of the pelvic plexus and its important branches are located lateral and posterior to the seminal vesicles, these vesicles

can be used as an intraoperative landmark to avoid injury to the pelvic plexus when ligating the posterior pedicle of the bladder. Using this technique in 25 patients, the authors reported an 83% potency rate among patients undergoing cystectomy without urethrectomy.

Pritchett et al[14] questioned the cancer control of the nerve-sparing technique when they were able to demonstrate lymph nodes in the tissue left behind during the preservation of the neurovascular bundle. As these lymph nodes were thought to potentially represent the first site of metastasis, the authors cautioned against using this technique. Brendler et al[15] reviewed their results using the nerve-sparing technique in 76 men, and demonstrated a 5-year actuarial local recurrence rate of 7.5%; 64% of patients that underwent cysto-prostatectomy alone were potent at follow-up. Therefore it was concluded that the nerve-sparing technique did not compromise cancer control, and had the added benefit of preserving potency in most men. Schoenberg et al[16] reviewed the long-term follow-up in the same cohort of patients. They demonstrated a disease-specific 10-year survival rate for all stages of bladder cancer of 69%, and a 10-year survival rate free of local recurrence of 94%. The overall potency rate was 42%. Recovery of sexual function following nerve-sparing cystectomy correlated with patient age: 62% in men aged 40–49 years old, 47% in men 50–59 years old, 43% in men 60–69 years old, and 20% in men 70–79 years old. Marshall et al[17] were able to demonstrate a 71% potency rate in patients that underwent total ileocolic neobladder reconstruction following nerve-sparing cystectomy for transitional cell carcinoma.

Despite the encouraging potency results reported by some investigators, sexuality after urinary diversion remains a significant patient concern. After cystectomy there is an overall decrease in sexual desire, interaction with one's partner, and sexual activities. Hart et al[18] found that concerns with sexual function were one of the most common complaints following radical cystectomy and urinary diversion. Moderate to severe sexual dissatisfaction was noted in 47% of patients compared to 16% prior to surgery. However, men with severe postoperative erectile dysfunction demonstrated a statistically significant improvement in sexual function and satisfaction following penile prosthesis implantation. Henningsohn and colleagues[19] reported that 94% of men had some degree of erectile dysfunction following radical cystectomy compared to 48% in age-matched controls. Importantly, in this cohort of patients no attempt was made at nerve sparing.

In properly selected patients, nerve-sparing cystectomy can be performed safely. It offers long-term survival and recurrence rates similar to the standard radical cystectomy, and can preserve potency in the majority of patients. Nevertheless, patients should be counseled preoperatively regarding the possibility of permanent sexual dysfunction.

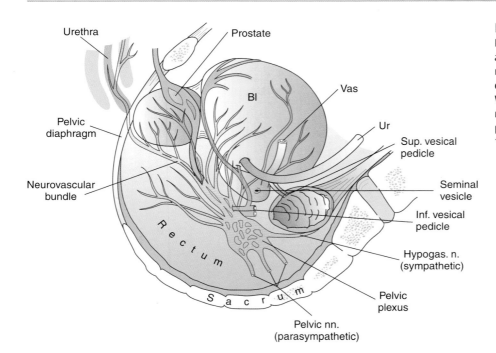

Urethra · Prostate · Vas · Ur · Sup. vesical pedicle · Pelvic diaphragm · Bl · Neurovascular bundle · Seminal vesicle · Inf. vesical pedicle · Hypogas. n. (sympathetic) · Rectum · Sacrum · Pelvic plexus · Pelvic nn. (parasympathetic)

Figure 11.1
Left lateral view of pelvic organs and neuroanatomy in man as reconstructed based on cadaveric dissections. Adapted from Schlegel PN, Walsh PC. Neuroanatomical approach to radical cystoprostatectomy with preservation of sexual function. J Urol 1987;138:1402–1406.

Preoperative preparation

Prior to surgery, patients meet with an enterostomal therapist to learn about urinary diversion and to become familiar with various stomal appliances. Most patients are understandably anxious about having a stoma, and discussion with a trained enterostomal therapist preoperatively and perhaps meeting with other ostomy patients greatly reduces psychological stress before surgery. An optimal stomal site is selected by examining the patient in various positions (sitting, reclining, and standing). This ensures that placement will be away from any sites that might affect proper seating of the urinary appliance, such as bony prominences, skin creases, scars, and clothing. The proper site is marked indelibly so that during preoperative skin preparation the marking will not wash away. This is helpful even in patients in whom urinary tract reconstruction without a stoma is planned because operative findings may make a stoma necessary. However, the majority of patients today should have a continent urinary diversion.

The day prior to surgery patients are started on a low residue diet and instructed to drink 3–4 liters of Go-Lytely. One gram of a second-generation cephalosporin is given intravenously on call to the operating room and every 8 hours for the next 24 hours. Thromboembolism-deterrent (TED) hose compression stockings are placed prior to induction of anesthesia, and subcutaneous heparin is administered for deep vein thrombosis prophylaxis.

Surgical technique
Position

Patients are positioned supine with the umbilicus positioned over the break of the table. The table is tilted into slight Trendelenburg position.

Incision and exposure

A 22 Fr. catheter with a 30 cc balloon is passed into the bladder and the balloon is inflated with 40–50 cc of saline.

A midline abdominal incision is made from the symphysis pubis to just below the umbilicus. The anterior rectus fascia is incised, and the rectus muscles parted bluntly in the midline, exposing the transversalis fascia, which is incised from the symphysis pubis up to the semilunar line of Douglas. It is important to incise the transversalis fascia before developing the space of Retzius to avoid injuring the inferior epigastric vessels.

The space of Retzius is then developed and the peritoneum is mobilized on either side of the bladder by blunt finger dissection. Careful cranial mobilization of the peritoneum along the pelvic sidewall exposes the iliac vessels and vas deferens. The vas deferens is used as a tractor on each side to complete the mobilization of the peritoneum above the bifurcation of the common iliac vessels and to develop a pocket in the retroperitoneum over the psoas muscle just medial to the spermatic vessels. The vas deferens is divided, the ureter is identified, and a vessel loop is placed around the ureter. This is performed bilaterally, typically by opening the peritoneum and dividing the urachus as well as the lateral peritoneal 'wings' of the bladder. The peritoneal incision is then extended downward obliquely on each side towards the internal inguinal ring. This dissection is facilitated by having first mobilized the peritoneum from the pelvis on each side as previously described, enabling the surgeon to place one hand in the pelvis behind the mobilized peritoneum to provide traction and exposure while the peritoneal incision is extended from above. Care should be taken not to incise the peritoneum too close to the bladder; by incising the peritoneum directly against the surgeon's hand, inadvertent injury to the bladder is avoided. A self-retaining retractor is positioned in the abdomen and the intestines are packed out of the pelvis.

Pelvic lymphadenectomy

Pelvic lymphadenectomy is performed, removing all fibroareolar tissue along the external iliac vessels and obturator fossa bilaterally. The limits of this dissection are:

- lateral—genitofemoral nerve;
- medial—bladder;
- cephalad—bifurcation of common iliac artery;
- caudad—circumflex iliac vein.

The lymph node dissection is begun by opening the fibroareolar tissue sheath surrounding the external iliac artery from the femoral canal up to and above the common iliac bifurcation. After all nodal tissue is circumferentially swept off the external iliac artery, the sheath overlying the external iliac vein is incised. This dissection is often aided by the use of a large vein retractor to elevate the external iliac artery and vein. In dissecting the distal portion of the external iliac vein, care should be taken not to injure the accessory obturator vein which exists in about 25% of patients; it courses from the distal external iliac vein into the obturator canal. The lymphatic channels at the distal extent of the dissection are secured with large hemoclips, particularly those draining into the node of Cloquet, and then divided.

The lateral extent of dissection is performed by blunt finger dissection along the psoas muscle, carefully lifting the nodal package medially off the genitofemoral nerve, thus allowing the package to drop behind the iliac vessels. Lifting the package medially allows the fibroareolar tissue to be bluntly freed off the pelvic sidewall into the obturator fossa. Frequently, small perforator vessels can be coagulated and divided to prevent subsequent inadvertent tearing and bleeding.

The proximal portion of the lymph node dissection is completed by gently lifting the package with caudal traction and teasing out the lymphatic channels which are fulgurated and divided. Great care must be utilized at the proximal extent of the dissection to prevent accidental transection of the obturator nerve. The nodal package is fractured off of the obturator nerve and attachments to the bladder. Typically the entire nodal package can be removed in toto.

Bleeding is usually minimal during this dissection, and small vessels are usually easily controlled with fulguration. Occasionally, the hypogastric vein may be injured as the lymph node package is being removed, and bleeding can be quite profuse and difficult to control. In this situation, it is best to simply place a small sponge over the vein and leave it for 10–15 minutes. The bleeding will almost always tamponade spontaneously, and attempts at suture ligation or fulguration are more likely to worsen bleeding than control it.

Opening and packing of the abdomen

Once the peritoneal incisions have been carried to the level of the hypogastric arteries, they are extended cephalad about 10 cm along the colic gutters bilaterally. Attachments of the sigmoid colon to the peritoneum are dissected sharply to facilitate mobilization of the colon.

One of the most critical steps in radical cystoprostatectomy is proper packing of the intestines out of the operative field. This must be done precisely and requires practice. Three moistened Mikulicz pads and a rolled moist towel are used to pack the small bowel and right colon into the epigastrium. An opened moist lap pad is packed cephalad into each colic gutter and a third lap pad is used to pack the central small bowel. A rolled moist towel is then placed horizontally over the lower edge of the Mikulicz pads with the open edges placed cephalad into each pericolic gutter.

Transection of ureters and division of proximal vesical pedicles

Once pelvic lymphadenectomy is completed, the ureters are identified bilaterally as they cross the external iliac arteries. The ureters are encircled with vessel loops and dissected distally under mild traction. If a continent urinary reconstruction which requires greater ureteral length is planned, it may be necessary to dissect the ureters, particularly the left, almost to the level of the bladder.

Precise identification, ligation, and division of the vascular pedicles to the bladder are facilitated by understanding that the pedicles to the bladder cross anterolateral to the ureter. Dissecting over the ureters prior to ureteral transection allows the individual vesical vascular pedicles to be identified and ligated close to the hypogastric vessels. This avoids mass ligation of the pedicles that frequently results in avulsion and considerable bleeding. The ureters should be traced almost to the ureterovesical junction before transection, allowing division of the obliterated umbilical, superior, and middle vesical pedicles.

After the vascular pedicles have been divided and the ureters mobilized distally, the ureters are dissected proximally for an appropriate distance to allow subsequent anastomosis to the intestinal reservoir. On the left side, it may be necessary to carry this dissection almost to the lower pole of the kidney, particularly in obese patients. However, additional mobilization risks devascularization of the ureter. Once the ureters have been mobilized both caudad and cephalad, a right-angled clamp is placed distally on each ureter, and they are divided. Frozen sections are obtained of the distal margins to ensure there is no dysplasia or carcinoma. If there is, the ureters must be sectioned higher until normal margins are obtained. The distal ureteral stumps are ligated with a 2-0 silk suture.

Mobilization of the bladder from the rectum

The peritoneum overlying the dome of the bladder is incised transversely about 2 cm above the rectum. It is important to incise the peritoneum since this will allow the plane between the bladder and rectum to be developed properly; however, care should be taken not to incise too deeply as this may cause inadvertent injury to the bladder. Once the peritoneum has been incised, a plane behind the bladder is developed, initially by sharp dissection; the dissection is then continued bluntly. The surgeon places one hand behind the bladder palm up and sweeps the fingers backward to dissect the rectum from the bladder. Usually this plane develops quite easily unless the patient has had previous radiotherapy or surgery. It is important to continue the sharp dissection until the seminal vesicles have been exposed. The seminal vesicles can be visualized by elevating the posterior wall of the bladder with a Deaver retractor (Figure 11.2).

Once the seminal vesicles have been identified, the remaining vascular pedicles to the bladder are ligated and divided immediately lateral to the seminal vesicle on each side. Visualization of the seminal vesicles allows these pedicles to be transected anterior to the neurovascular bundle but posterior to the bladder. However, in cases

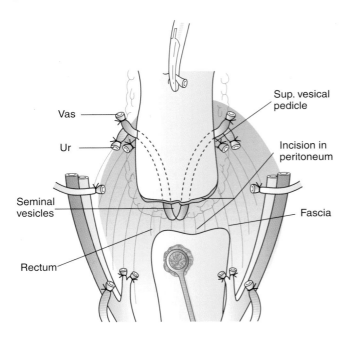

Figure 11.2
Peritoneal reflection in rectovesical cul-de-sac has been incised and bladder is elevated from rectum. Tips of seminal vesicles are seen. Adapted from Schlegel PN, Walsh PC. Neuroanatomical approach to radical cystoprostatectomy with preservation of sexual function. J Urol 1987;138:1402–1406.

where there is induration or the possibility of extravesical disease, one must widely excise the lateral tissue and neurovascular bundle.

In dividing the vascular pedicles to the bladder, there may be significant venous bleeding that is difficult to control with suture ligation. In such cases, it may be helpful to open the endopelvic fascia bilaterally, transect the puboprostatic ligaments, and ligate the deep dorsal vein of the penis.

Division of puboprostatic ligaments and control of dorsal vein

The dissection from above is continued until the pedicles adjacent to the seminal vesicles have been ligated and divided. At this point, the inferior vesical pedicles are the only remaining vessels to the bladder as in a nerve-sparing radical prostatectomy. However, in some patients, visualization of the seminal vesicles may be difficult and in those cases the dissection should cease and begin anteriorly.

The catheter balloon is positioned under the malleable blade and drawn cephalad to expose the prostate, taking care not to tear the bladder. The fat overlying the prostate is dissected away using a forceps. This dissection should start on the anterolateral surface of the prostate, avoiding dissecting in the midline which may injure the superficial branch of the deep dorsal vein of the penis. It is important, however, to remove as much fat as possible in order to properly expose the puboprostatic ligaments.

The endopelvic fascia is then wiped with a moist sponge stick on each side lateral to the prostate. This exposes the fascia, and frequently a small ovale in the fascia will be seen just lateral to the deep dorsal vein of the penis. Using this opening, the endopelvic fascia is incised sharply about 1 cm lateral to the prostate. Care should be taken to incise only the fascia and to incise lateral to the prostate to

avoid injuring the lateral branches of the dorsal vein complex. The incision is begun sharply and then extended both anteriorly and posteriorly using the index finger. A sponge stick is then used to displace the prostate posteriorly.

If the entire fat lateral to the dorsal vein has been dissected away and the endopelvic fascia has been opened completely, the puboprostatic ligaments will be visualized easily. These ligaments are avascular, but the dorsal vein runs immediately between them, and frequently in continuity. Therefore, before transecting these ligaments, it is important to develop the plane both laterally and medially to the ligaments using sharp dissection. This must be done carefully but completely in order to avoid injuring the dorsal vein when the ligaments are transected. The ligaments should be transected close to the prostate before attempting to ligate the dorsal vein complex.

The dorsal vein is suture ligated distally and proximally. The dorsal vein is transected sharply. Additional bleeders may be suture ligated with a circle-tapered UR needle, using a sponge stick to displace the prostate posteriorly. The dorsal vein must be controlled completely in order to visualize and preserve the neurovascular bundles for potency.

Mobilization of the prostate

The final phase of nerve-sparing cystoprostatectomy is dissection of the prostate and ligation and division of the inferior vesical pedicles. Dissection of the prostate is done as in a nerve-sparing radical prostatectomy. Following division of the dorsal vein, the urethra is dissected just distal to the prostate. Care should be taken not to injure the neurovascular bundles which lie immediately lateral to the urethra at this point. An umbilical tape then is passed around the urethra and gentle traction is exerted cephalad. Using a Kitner dissector, the urethra is dissected from the urogenital diaphragm, removing only urethral mucosa and smooth muscle, leaving the striated muscle of the urogenital diaphragm behind. This dissection continues until the membranous urethra has been liberated completely from the urogenital diaphragm. Even in patients in whom nerve sparing is not a consideration, pelvic dissection of the membranous urethra greatly facilitates the perineal dissection if a urethrectomy is subsequently required. The anterior urethra is then gently pulled out of the urogenital diaphragm and transected distal to the urogenital diaphragm. The catheter is transected, the posterior wall of the urethra divided, and the catheter drawn cephalad into the wound.

In patients in whom an orthotopic continent diversion is planned, the urethra must be handled similar to a nerve-sparing radical prostatectomy. In brief, the anterior wall of the urethra is transected just distal to the prostate until the Foley catheter comes into view. A right-angled clamp pulls the catheter into the pelvis and the catheter is transected. With use of a right-angled clamp, the space between the rectum, striated urethral sphincter, rectourethralis muscle, and posterior wall of the urethra is developed. The neurovascular bundles are posterolateral at this point. The tissue on top of the clamp is then transected sharply to free the prostate from the rectum. This is a critical step in all nerve-sparing radical pelvic operations, and must be done carefully and precisely to avoid injuring the underlying neurovascular bundles which lie immediately posterolateral to the rectourethralis. Elevating the rectourethralis muscle before incising it allows preservation of the underlying neurovascular bundles and avoids injuring the rectum.

The lateral pelvic fascia on each side of the prostate is then incised; this allows the neurovascular bundles to drop posteriorly.

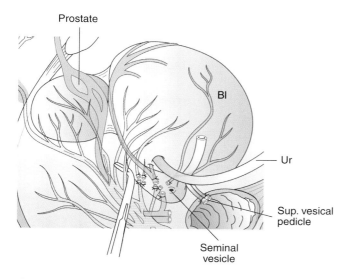

Prostate

BI

Ur

Sup. vesical pedicle

Seminal vesicle

Figure 11.3
Schematic illustration of division of left posterior pedicle along lateral edge of left seminal vesicle. Note that cavernous nerves are preserved posteriorly. Adapted from Schlegel PN, Walsh PC. Neuroanatomical approach to radical cystoprostatectomy with preservation of sexual function. J Urol 1987;138:1402–1406.

The small vascular branches to the apex of the prostate are then gently mobilized with a fine right-angled clamp, secured proximally with small metal clips, and divided. Following division of the apical vascular branches, the neurovascular bundles fall laterally, allowing the larger lateral pedicles to be ligated and divided (Figure 11.3). When the prostate has been mobilized cranially to the level of the seminal vesicles, Denonvilliers' fascia overlying the seminal vesicles is incised transversely. Once the seminal vesicles have been exposed from below, a plane of communication between the cranial and caudal dissection is formed, allowing the remaining vascular pedicles to the prostate and bladder to be divided immediately lateral to the seminal vesicles. The bladder, prostate, and seminal vesicles are removed en bloc, and the intact neurovascular bundles can be visualized in the pelvis. Urinary tract reconstruction is then performed.

Wide excision of the neurovascular bundle

The primary goal of radical cystoprostatectomy must be eradication of cancer. Whenever the tumor encroaches upon the posterior pedicle, the neurovascular bundle should be widely excised to ensure adequate surgical margins. The anatomic radical cystoprostatectomy allows mobilization of the neurovascular bundles off the rectum, permitting wider surgical margins that incorporate all perivesical tissues lateral to the hypogastric vessels. Thus, improved surgical margins can be achieved while still preserving potency in the majority of patients, even when only a single neurovascular bundle is preserved.

Postoperative care

TED hose compression stockings remain on for at least 48 hours and subcutaneous heparin is administered until the patient is ready for

discharge. Ambulation is begun the day following surgery. Intravenous antibiotics are administered for 24 hours postoperatively; usually, a second-generation cephalosporin is given. Ureteral stents are left in place for 7–10 days to allow healing of the ureterointestinal anastomoses. Drains are left in the pelvis until the ureteral stents have been removed. Patients are usually discharged between the sixth and eighth postoperative day.

References

1. Stein JP, Lieskovsky G, Cote R, et al. Radical cystectomy in the treatment of invasive bladder cancer: long-term results in 1,054 patients. J Clin Oncol 2001; 19(3): 666–75.
2. Jimenez VK, Marshall FF. Surgery of bladder cancer. In Walsh PC et al (eds): Campbell's Urology, 8th ed. Philadelphia: WB Saunders, 2002, pp 2819–44.
3. Young HH, Davis DM. Young's Practice of Urology, vol 12. Philadelphia: WB Saunders, 1926.
4. Hinman F. The technique and late results of ureterointestinal implantation and cystectomy for cancer of the bladder. Int Soc Urol Rep 1939; 7: 464–524.
5. Bracken RB, McDonald MW, Johnson DE. Complications of single stage radical cystectomy and ileal conduit. Urology 1981; 27: 141–6.
6. Hendry WF. Morbidity and mortality of radical cystectomy (1971–1978 and 1978–1985). J Roy Soc Med 1981; 79: 395–400.
7. Skinner DG, Lieskovsky G (eds). Management of invasive and high grade bladder cancer. In Diagnosis and Management of Genitourinary Cancer. Philadelphia: WB Saunders, 1988, pp 295–312.
8. Quek ML, Stein JP, Clark PE, et al. Natural history of surgically treated bladder carcinoma with extravesical tumor extension. Cancer 2003; 98(5): 955–61.
9. Skinner DG, Stein JP, Lieskovsky G, et al. 25-year experience in the management of invasive bladder cancer by radical cystectomy. Eur Urol 1998; 33(Suppl 4): 25–6.
10. Stein JP, Ginsberg DA, Skinner DG. Indications and technique of the orthotopic neobladder in women. Urol Clin North Am 2002; 29: 725–34.
11. Walsh PC, Donker PJ. Impotence following radical prostatectomy: insight into etiology and prevention. J Urol 1982; 128: 492.
12. Lepor H, Gregerman M, Crosby R, Mostofi FK, Walsh PC. Precise localization of the autonomic nerves from the pelvic plexus to the corpora cavernosa: a detailed anatomical study of the adult male pelvis. J Urol 1985; 133: 207–12.
13. Schlegel PN, Walsh PC. Neuroanatomical approach to radical cystoprostatectomy with preservation of sexual function. J Urol 1987; 138: 1402–6.
14. Pritchett TR, Schiff WM, Klatt E, Lieskovsky G, Skinner DG. The potency-sparing radical cystectomy: does it compromise the completeness of the cancer resection? J Urol 1988; 140: 1400–3.
15. Brendler CB, Steinberg GD, Marshall FF, Mostwin JL, Walsh PC. Local recurrence and survival following nerve-sparing radical cystoprostatectomy. J Urol 1990; 144: 1137–41.
16. Schoenberg MP, Walsh PC, Breazeale DR, Marshall FF, Mostwin JL, Brendler CB. Local recurrence and survival following nerve sparing radical cystoprostatectomy for bladder cancer: 10-year followup. J Urol 1996; 155: 490–4.
17. Marshall FF, Mostwin JL, Radebaugh LC, Walsh PC, Brendler CB. Ileocolic neobladder post-cystectomy: continence and potency. J Urol 1991; 145: 502–4.
18. Hart S, Skinner EC, Meyerowitz BE, Boyd S, Lieskovsky G, Skinner DG. Quality of life after radical cystectomy for bladder cancer in patients with an ileal conduit, or cutaneous or urethral Koch pouch. J Urol 1999; 162: 77–81.
19. Henningsohn L, Steven K, Kallestrup EB, Steineck G. Distressful symptoms and well-being after radical cystectomy and orthotopic bladder substitution compared with a matched control population. J Urol 2002; 168: 168–75.

12

Laparoscopic radical cystectomy and urinary diversion

Inderbir S Gill, Ingolf Tuerk

Introduction

Ongoing technical and technologic developments have refined various laparoscopic procedures such that they have become viable alternatives to their conventional open surgical counterparts. With the worldwide acceptance of laparoscopic techniques, initially in the management of upper urinary tract pathology, and more recently for laparoscopic radical prostatectomy, a natural progression has been made to applying these techniques to bladder surgery. In the United States in 2004, bladder cancer was diagnosed in 44,640 men and 15,600 women, leading to 8780 and 3930 deaths, respectively.[1] Radical cystectomy is currently the accepted standard of treatment for patients with localized muscle invasive bladder cancer. Since the initial report of laparoscopic radical cystectomy (LRC) with bilateral pelvic lymphadenectomy/ileal conduit urinary diversion performed entirely intracorporeally by Gill and colleagues[2] in 2000, more than 225 cases from over 20 institutions worldwide have been reported[3] (Table 12.1).[2,4-20] In this chapter, we review the current worldwide experience with LRC and urinary diversion, focusing on historical background, laboratory experience, surgical technique, current controversies and future directions.

Historical background

In early 1992, Parra et al described the initial report of laparoscopic simple cystectomy in a female patient suffering from pyocystis of a retained bladder.[21] This patient had previously undergone open surgical supravesical diversion for management of neurogenic bladder; accordingly, urinary diversion was not performed as part of the laparoscopic procedure. In 1995, Sanchez et al described the first report of laparoscopic-assisted radical cystectomy with an ileal conduit formed extracorporeally in a 64-year-old woman with invasive bladder cancer.[22] Puppo et al reported the first small series of laparoscopic-assisted transvaginal radical cystectomies in five females, wherein the ileal conduit was created via a mini-laparotomy incision after completion of the LRC.[23] In another publication, the same group reported cutaneous ureterostomies in nine patients with advanced pelvic cancer.[24]

While these early studies established the technical feasibility of LRC, it was not until 2000 that LRC and ileal conduit were performed completely intracorporeally in the initial two clinical cases after successful pilot studies in animals had been performed at the Cleveland Clinic.[2] To date, the ileal conduit, the orthotopic ileal neobladder (Studer), and the sigmoid–rectum pouch (Mainz II) have all been created purely laparoscopically with exclusively intracorporeal suturing techniques.[4,8]

Experimental laparoscopic urinary diversion in animal models

Experimental studies of urinary diversion have formed the basis for the subsequent clinical experience. Anderson et al investigated the feasibility of laparoscopic-assisted Mainz II (sigmoid–rectum) pouch in nine mini pigs.[25] The cystectomy and dissection of ureter and large bowel were performed laparoscopically, and the Mainz II pouch was created extracorporeally by open techniques. Forty-four percent of animals developed stones across metallic staple lines used to create the Mainz II pouch.

The major technical difficulty encountered in performing a laparoscopic urinary diversion remains the performance of intracorporeal reconstruction. Reconstructive techniques have been performed by three different approaches: performing the entire procedure intracorporeally, performing extracorporeal suturing and returning the diversion into the abdomen for intracorporeal completion, or performing urinary diversion through a mini-laparotomy. Investigators at the Cleveland Clinic were the first to demonstrate the feasibility of creating urinary diversion following cystectomy with ileal loop (in 10 surviving pigs) and orthotopic ileal neobladder (Studer) (in 12 surviving pigs) using completely intracorporeal laparoscopic techniques.[26,27] These laparoscopic procedures duplicated principles of open surgery and demonstrated that reconstruction of bowel could be performed with purely intracorporeal freehand suturing techniques without complications such as ileoureteral or ileourethral anastomotic strictures or leakage.

Indications and contraindications

Proper patient choice/identification is crucial during the early learning experience for any emerging technique. Currently, we offer

Table 12.1 World experience with laparoscopic radical cystectomy (LC) and urinary diversion

Technique	Lead author	Institution/location	No. pts	Comment on abstract/manuscript or technique
Purely laparoscopic	Gill IS2,[4–7]	Cleveland, USA	30	Purely laparoscopic reconstruction of the urinary diversion
	Tuerk, I[8,9]	Massachusetts, USA and Berlin, Germany	15	Mainz II continent sigmoid–rectum pouch
Laparoscopic assisted	Van Velthoven R[5]	Brussels, Belgium	22	Extracorporeal reconstruction, variety of diversions
	Basillote JB[10]	Irvine, USA	13	Comparison between LC and open radical cystectomy, extracorporeal reconstruction
	Hemal AK[11]	New Delhi, India	11	Emphasis on complications of the initial experience with LC, extracorporeal ileal conduit
	Simonato A[12]	Milan, Italy	10	Detailed steps of LC with illustrations. A variety of diversions including intracorporeal and extracorporeal reconstruction
	Denewer A[13]	Mnsoura, Egypt	10	Salvage cystectomy after radical radiotherapy. A modified ureterosigmoidostomy diversion through a mini-laparotomy (8 cm)
	Abdel-Hakim AM[14]	Cairo, Egypt	9	Extracorporeal reconstruction of ileal neobladder
	Castillo O[5]	Santiago, Chile	7	Extracorporeal reconstruction, Studer neobladder
	Paz A[5]	Ashkelon, Israel	7	Comparison between LC and open radical cystectomy, extracorporeal reconstruction
	Popken G[5]	Berlin, Germany	7	Extra/intracorporeal reconstruction with a variety of diversions
	Puppo P[7]	Pietra Ligure, Italy	5	First transvaginal and laparoscopic approach for bladder cancer. Ileal conduit was accomplished through a mini-laparotomy at the stoma site
	Xiao LC[5]	Guangzhou, China	5	Extracorporeal reconstruction, Indiana pouch
	Huan SK[5]	Chi Mei, Taiwan	4	Extracorporeal reconstruction, Indiana pouch
	Sung GT[5]	Pusan, Korea	4	Extracorporeal ileal conduit
	Guazzoni G[15]	Milan, Italy	3	Nerve sparing LC with extracorporeal W-shaped neobladder
	Pedraza R[5]	New York, USA	2	Patients underwent LC with total ureterectomy and creation of pyelocutaneous ileal conduit intracorporeally
Hand assisted	McGinnis DE[16]	Bryn Mawr, USA	7	Hand-assisted LC with extracorporeal ileal conduit
	Fan EW[5]	Chi Mei, Taiwan	6	Hand-assisted laparoscopic bilateral nephroureterectomy with radical cystectomy (end stage renal disease)
	Peterson AC[17]	Tacoma, USA	1	First reported case of hand-assisted LC with extracorporeal ileal conduit
Robotic assisted	Menon M[18]	Detroit, USA	14	Nerve-sparing robotic-assisted LC
	Balaji KC[19]	Omaha, USA	3	LC with robotic assistance for intracorporeal suturing of the ureter–ileal conduit anastomosis (two patients with interstitial cystitis)
	Beecken WD[20]	Frankfurt, Germany	1	First reported case of robotic-assisted LC with intracorporeal orthotopic neobladder
Other	Goharderakhshan R[7]	Harbor City, USA	25	Series focusing on complications associated with LC. Reconstructive technique not detailed
	Vallancien G[7]	Paris, France	20	Prostate-sparing cystectomy. Reconstructive technique not detailed

Adapted from Moinzadeh & Gill.[3]

LRC to patients with organ-confined, non-bulky bladder malignancy as determined by preoperative radiographic and clinical findings. We have no experience with LRC in the presence of prior radiotherapy and neoadjuvant chemotherapy, or morbidly obese patients. These factors currently constitute relative contraindications because of the potential increase in technical challenge. In relatively obese patients, difficulty may be expected in delivering a loop of ileum through an obese abdominal wall to the skin level. Prior abdominal surgery per se is no longer considered as an absolute contraindication to laparoscopic surgery. Attention must be paid to avoid intra-abdominal injury upon insertion of the initial access port at the beginning of the procedure.

Surgical techniques

Laparoscopic radical cystectomy

Surgical technical steps of LRC aim to mirror established open surgical techniques. Typically a five- or six-port transperitoneal technique is employed similar to that for a standard laparoscopic prostatectomy. The retrovesical dissection is performed initially. In the male, a transverse periotomy is created in the rectovesical cul-de-sac, and the vas deferens is divided bilaterally. Dissection is performed towards Denonvilliers' fascia, which is incised horizontally to provide visualization of the yellowish prerectal fat, signifying proper entry into the plane between the rectum posteriorly and the prostate and bladder anteriorly. Unlike the procedure in a laparoscopic radical prostatectomy, the seminal vesicles and vas deferens are not mobilized individually but maintained en bloc with the bladder specimen. The lateral and posterior vascular pedicles of the bladder and prostate are developed with blunt dissection and controlled bilaterally with sequential firings of the endoscopic GIA stapler. Both ureters are clipped and divided close to the bladder, and the distal ureteral margin is sent for frozen section evaluation. The proximal cut end of each ureter is temporarily clip-occluded to facilitate hydrostatic distension.

An inverted V-shaped peritoneotomy is created, starting lateral to the right medial umbilical ligament, proceeding up towards the umbilicus where the urachus is incised, and extending lateral to the left medial umbilical ligament. In this manner, the urachus is divided high, near the umbilicus. The anterior surface of the bladder is mobilized with the entire perivesical fat being maintained with the bladder specimen. The endopelvic fascia is incised bilaterally and the dorsal vein secured with a stitch, similar to that used in a laparoscopic radical prostatectomy. In the male patient the puboprostatic ligaments and the prostatourethral junction are divided sharply, maintaining an adequate stump of sphincter-active urethra. The few remaining prostate attachments are divided, and the specimen immediately entrapped in an Endocatch-II bag. Frozen section biopsy of the cut end of the urethral stump is confirmed to be negative for cancer.

In the female, a sponge stick in the vagina or Koh colpotomiser system allows the vaginal apex to be identified and incised. After complete dissection of the bladder and surrounding structures (uterus/fallopian tube/ovary), the specimen is placed in an impervious, plastic-enclosed bag and retrieved through either the vagina, the rectum, or a midline 5 cm incision. Frozen section of distal ureteral margin and the cut end of the urethral stump are confirmed to be negative for malignancy.

Extended pelvic lymph node dissection (PLND)

Given the absence of pelvic lymphadenopathy on preoperative computed tomography, which is further corroborated by intraoperative laparoscopic inspection, cystectomy is performed initially, followed by PLND. Right lymphadenectomy is carried out first. The patient is tilted 30° up on the right side in the 30° Trendelenburg head-down position. The lateral border of dissection is developed along the genitofemoral nerve by dividing the fibroareolar tissue and exposing the iliopsoas muscle. The lymphatic tissue packet is completely lifted en bloc off of the surface of the iliopsoas muscle and swept medially.

Tissue anterior to the external iliac artery and vein is then individually split longitudinally using J-hook electrocautery, skeletonizing the two vessels circumferentially. It should be noted that the external iliac vein typically appears as a flat ribbon at standard (15 mmHg) pneumoperitoneum pressures. To facilitate identification of the external iliac vein in case of doubt, pneumoperitoneum pressures can be decreased to 5 mmHg to allow redistension of the vein.[6]

Cephalad dissection along the proximal common iliac artery is facilitated by the fact that the transected ureter has already been mobilized away during the cystectomy procedure. The circumferentially mobilized common iliac is retracted with a vessel loop to completely retrieve fatty tissue in the area distal to the aortic bifurcation. The hypogastric artery is mobilized with care taken not to injure the internal iliac vein. The released packet is rolled medially, posterior to the mobilized external iliac artery and vein, and delivered into the pelvis. Dissection along the medial aspect of the packet identifies the obturator nerve. Distally the lymphatics caudal to the node of Cloquet are clipped and transected. To guard against local seeding, care must be taken to avoid cutting into any enlarged lymph node(s). The entire specimen is immediately placed in an Endocatch bag without the specimen touching adjacent tissues. Lymphadenectomy is performed on the left side in similar fashion with the patient tilted 30° up on that side. Bilateral lymphadenectomy specimens are entrapped separately, extracted intact, and submitted separately for analysis.

Laparoscopic-assisted ileal conduit urinary diversion

Informed consent is obtained with a discussion of risks including, but not limited to, adjacent organ and bowel injury, and open conversion. Full mechanical bowel preparation with 4 liters of polyethylene glycol is performed, oral antibiotics are administered, and the patient is admitted on the morning of surgery. Preoperative antibiotic prophylaxis with a second-generation cephalosporin and lower extremity compressive devices are routine. Once general anesthesia is induced, a nasogastric tube is inserted, the abdomen and genitalia are properly draped, and a 16 Fr. Foley catheter is placed from the sterile field.

Pneumoperitoneum is obtained and a five-port transperitoneal technique is employed: a primary 10 mm trocar at the umbilicus, two 10 mm trocars at each lateral pararectal line 10 cm above the pubic symphysis, and two 5 mm trocars 2–3 cm medial and superior to the anterior–superior iliac spines.

Both ureters are dissected proximally, clipped, and transected close to the ureterovesical junction. The cut ends are sent for frozen section analysis. Two 4-0 vicryl holding sutures are placed at the distal ends of the ureters for subsequent identification and atraumatic manipulation. The vascular pedicles of the bladder and prostate are controlled with serial applications of an articulating endoscopic GIA laparoscopic stapler. The urethra is sectioned at the prostate apex, completing the bladder excision. The bladder is placed into a laparoscopic retrieval bag, which in female patients can be retrieved through an opening in the anterior vaginal wall. In males, the specimen bag is retrieved at the end of the operation by extending one of the port sites.

The ureters are dissected for a distance sufficient to reach the proximal end of the loop. Care is taken to preserve periureteral tissue and thus the ureteral vascular supply. Blunt dissection is used to develop a tunnel posterior to the sigmoid mesocolon and anterior to the sacrum. The left ureter is passed under the sigmoid colon using the previously placed holding suture. Ureteral length is once again confirmed to assure that both ureters reach the proximal portion of the ileal segment in order to avoid undue tension on the anastomoses. A previously marked stoma site away from desired trocar sites should not compromise optimal port placement. When the stoma site is separate from all trocars, a 4.5 cm infraumbilical incision is made. The specimen is retrieved. The color-coded ureteral holding sutures are exteriorized. A 15 cm segment of ileum is selected with care to spare 15–20 cm proximal to the ileocecal junction. The segment of bowel is delivered through the incision and isolated with a GIA stapler. The mesentery is appropriately divided with care to preserve the major mesenteric vasculature. The isolated segment is dropped posteriorly.

Applications of a GIA 55 mm stapler are used to create a side-to-side, functional, end-to-end ileoileal anastomosis along the antimesenteric border of the small bowel. The open end of the anastomosis is then closed using a Ta 55 mm stapler. The end staple line is imbricated with interrupted, absorbable suture. The window through the mesentery is then closed with interrupted absorbable suture to prevent internal hernia formation.

Gentle traction on the ureteral holding sutures pulls the distal ureters into the operative field. The ureters are gently spatulated for approximately 1 cm. Bilateral ureteral 6 Fr. single J stents are passed into the renal pelvis. The ureters are sequentially implanted into the proximal end of the ileal segment in a standard Bricker fashion. The proximal end of the ileal conduit is replaced into the abdominal cavity. The ureteral stents are exteriorized through the ileal segment.

The rectus fascia is partially closed, leaving space through which the conduit passes. The ileal segment is secured to the fascia using interrupted 2-0 polyglactin sutures. The stoma is matured in the standard open fashion. In the obese patient, ureteroileal anastomoses performed through an incision may require excessive proximal ureteral mobilization. In these cases, the stoma is matured first, and the ureteroileal anastomoses are performed completely intracorporeally.

Postoperative management is as with the comparable open procedure. Patients receive prophylaxis for deep venous thrombosis, and ambulation is begun on the first postoperative day. The nasogastric tube is removed once bowel function returns, and the diet is advanced accordingly. The drain is removed once output diminishes. The stents are removed between postoperative days 10 and 12 as outpatient procedure.

Pure laparoscopic ileal conduit urinary diversion

A 15 cm segment of ileum is selected while sparing the distal 15–20 cm of ileum. The efferent limb should reach the abdominal wall at the previously marked stoma site without undue tension or mesenteric kinking. The segment of bowel is isolated with an endoscopic GIA stapler by transecting proximally and distally. The mesentery is divided below these areas with care to preserve the major mesenteric vasculature. Endoscopic staplers, the harmonic scalpel, or serial application of laparoscopic clips can be used to transect the mesentery with complete hemostasis. The isolated segment is dropped posteriorly.

The stapled edges of the distal and proximal ileum are removed sharply. Applications of an endoscopic GIA stapler are used to create a side-to-side, functional, end-to-end anastomosis along the antimesenteric border of the small bowel. The open end of the anastomosis is then closed using an endoscopic Ta stapler. The end staple line is imbricated intracorporeally with interrupted, absorbable suture. The window through the mesentery is then closed with interrupted absorbable suture to prevent internal hernia formation.

The previously marked stoma site is matured in the standard everting fashion. The ileal segment is secured to the fascia using interrupted 2-0 polyglactin sutures. A previously marked stoma site away from desired trocar sites should not compromise optimal port placement.

Creating the stoma first greatly facilitates intracorporeal suturing of the ureteroileal anastomosis by providing a point of fixation for the ileal segment. Gentle traction on the ureteral holding sutures pulls the distal ureters to the proximal end of the ileal segment. The ureters are spatulated for approximately 1 cm. Six French single J stents are grasped by a laparoscopic right-angle clamp and inserted though the stoma into the conduit lumen. The right angle clamp tents the ileal loop at the desired ileotomy site. A laparoscopic electrosurgical J-hook is used to create the ileostomy, and the stent is delivered into the abdominal cavity. The ureters are sequentially implanted in a standard Bricker fashion. The apices are fixed to the bowel using three interrupted 4-0 poliglecaprone sutures. The remainder of the ureteral implantation is performed using a running 4-0 poliglecaprone suture. The stent is passed into the renal pelvis on each side when 80% of the anastomosis is complete.

The ureters and ileal diversion are inspected for any undue tension. The abdominal cavity is irrigated with sterile antibiotic solution. Once meticulous hemostasis is assured, a flat Jackson-Pratt drain is placed through a lateral 5 mm trocar site into the pelvis. The port sites are closed in the usual fashion with fascial closure for all sites ≥10 mm under direct vision with 0 polyglactin.

Postoperative management is as with the comparable open procedure. Patients receive prophylaxis for deep venous thrombosis and ambulation is begun on the first postoperative day. The nasogastric tube is removed once bowel function returns, and the diet is advanced accordingly. The drain is removed once output diminishes. The stents are removed between postoperative days 10 and 12.

Pure laparoscopic orthotopic ileal neobladder

Preoperative preparation and LRC are performed as previously described. The left ureter is transposed to the right side posterior to the sigmoid colon.

A 65 cm segment of ileum is selected with care to spare the distal 15–20 cm proximal to the ileocecal junction (Figure 12.1A). The mid-portion of the segment should reach the urethral stump without undue tension or mesenteric kinking. The ileum, with its mesenteric pedicle, is isolated with an endoscopic GIA stapler. Endoscopic staplers, the harmonic scalpel, or serial application of laparoscopic clips can be used to transect the mesentery with complete hemostasis. The isolated segment is dropped posteriorly. An endoscopic GIA stapler is used to create a side-to-side, functional, ileoileal anastomosis along the antimesenteric border. The open end of the anastomosis is closed using an endoscopic Ta stapler. The end staple line is imbricated intracorporeally with interrupted, absorbable suture.

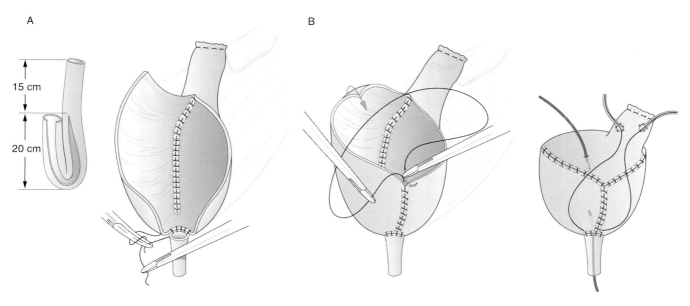

Figure 12.1
(A) Completed posterior neobladder plate and suturing of urethroneovesical anastomosis. (B) Anterior suture line and completed neobladder with drains. (Adapted with permission from The Cleveland Clinic Foundation.)

The staple lines are removed and the bowel lumen is cleansed using a suction-irrigation device. Care is taken to preserve the proximal 10 cm as an afferent Studer limb for the ureteral anastomosis. The remaining 55 cm is incised along its antimesenteric side using monopolar electrocautery, endoshears, and/or harmonic scalpel. The posterior plate of the neobladder is created by suturing the medial edges of the detubularized bowel in a running fashion with 2-0 polyglactin such that the bowel forms a J-shaped configuration (Figure 12.1B).

The anterior plate of the neobladder is partially closed using another running 2-0 polyglactin suture. Before completion of the anterior wall, both ileoureteral stents are delivered into the Studer limb and retrieved into the peritoneal cavity through two separate ileotomy incisions at the proposed site of ureteroileal anastomoses. The anterior enterotomy is left open at its inferior-most portion in order to create the urethroneovesical anastomosis.

The most dependent portion of the ileal plate is delivered to the urethral stump. The anastomosis is started at the 6 o'clock position with two running 2-0 poliglecaprone sutures in a parachute fashion and extended to the 12 o'clock position on either side. The sutures are then tied to each other. Once the anastomosis is complete, a 22 Fr. Foley catheter is placed (Figure 12.2).

The ureters are spatulated for approximately 1 cm. Bilateral ureteral 6 Fr. single J stents are passed into the renal pelvis. The stents are exteriorized through the wall of the neobladder and then through one of the lateral 5 mm port sites. The ureters are sequentially implanted into the proximal portion of the ileal segment in a standard Bricker fashion.

The ureters and ileal neobladder are inspected in situ for any undue tension. A flat Jackson-Pratt drain is placed through a lateral 5 mm trocar site into the small pelvis. The port sites are closed in the usual fashion with fascial closure for all sites ≥10 mm under direct vision with 0 polyglactin.

Postoperative management is as with the comparable open procedure. Patients receive prophylaxis for deep venous thrombosis, and ambulation is begun on the first postoperative day. The nasogastric tube is removed once bowel function returns, and the diet is advanced accordingly. The drain is removed once output diminishes. The stents are removed between postoperative days 10 and 12. The Foley catheter is removed one day following stent removal after absence of leak is confirmed on cystogram.

Clinical studies of laparoscopic radical cystectomy and urinary diversion

Notable advantages of LRC appear to be decreased blood loss, less postoperative pain, and earlier return to activity. The decreased blood loss (approximately 300–400 cc) is likely due to clear visualization and delicate hemostatic handling of the bladder pedicles with linear stapling devices, in addition to the tamponade effects afforded by the CO_2 pneumoperitoneum pressure. Although total operative times in the initially published series were 7–11 hours,[2,4,8] in more recent series the operative times have been reduced to 4.3–8.3 hours.[12]

It is likely that, with further experience, operative times will continue to decrease as, in the authors' experience, the LRC part of the procedure now comprises approximately 2 hours. More recently, a retrospective study of 13 laparoscopically assisted radical cystectomies with ileal neobladder compared with the 11 procedures employing the open approach revealed no statistically significant difference in operative time.[10] It should be noted, however, that in this study, radical cystectomy was performed laparoscopically and the reconstructive portion (ileal orthotopic neobladder) was performed through a 15 cm low Pfannenstiel incision.

Although the initial clinical publications focused on laparoscopic surgical techniques, recent reports have described the use of robotic assistance,[19,20,28] as well as hand assistance.[5,16,17] The perceived advantage of these various assisted laparoscopic techniques (open, robotic, or hand) compared to pure laparoscopic technique is their decreased learning curve for surgeons when transitioning from open to laparoscopic pelvic urologic surgery.[18,29] Surgical robotic systems provide multiangled movement with endo-wrist instruments and three-dimensional stereoscopic visualization. Recently, Balaji et al reported on the feasibility of robot-assisted totally intracorporeal laparoscopic ileal conduit in three patients, although each case took more than 10 hours.[19] The benefits of robotic applications in large series of patients remain unknown.

Seminal and prostate-sparing cystectomy may represent an alternative in young patients in whom preservation of both sexual potency and urinary continence are important.[15] However, from an oncologic point of view, long-term outcomes are the key to confirming whether this surgery can be proposed as a valid option for

treatment of young, fully potent, and socially active patients with organ-confined bladder malignancy.

Oncologic outcomes

A major area of laparoscopic approach for bladder malignancy remains to prove its acceptability for long-term, disease-free survival. So far, most of the publications of LRC reported the institutions' initial experience focusing on technique and perioperative results. Recently Hrouda et al reviewed a total of nine articles on LRC with available follow-up.[30] Among the total of 102 patients described in these nine articles, there were no instances of positive margins or inadvertent incisions in the bladder. However, the small number of patients and the short duration of follow-up (maximum of 2 years) do not permit any conclusions about oncologic outcome (Table 12.2).[6,8,10–14,18,23]

Although reports of oncologic outcomes of LRC are limited, Gupta et al reported 2-year follow-up of five patients having undergone LRC with ileal loop creation with good outcomes.[31] More recently, authors from the same institution added both follow-up and complications data in their initial report of experiences with 11 patients undergoing LRC.[11] One patient had surgical margins positive for tumor and received cisplatin-based chemotherapy; he had no recurrence in their follow-up period. At a mean of 18.4 months follow-up, all patients had normal renal function and preserved upper tracts with no evidence of metastasis and no local recurrence.

Recent emphasis on extended pelvic lymphadenectomy for transitional cell carcinoma of the bladder deserves discussion. Finelli et al reported their analysis of 22 cases of laparoscopic pelvic lymphadenectomy for bladder cancer.[6] The initial 11 patients that underwent a limited dissection were compared with the subsequent 11 consecutive patients that had an extended lymphadenectomy. Bilateral extended lymphadenectomy required approximately 1.5 hours compared to the 30–45 minutes required for the limited template. With a limited lymphadenectomy, the median and mean number of lymph nodes retrieved were 3 and 6 (range 1–15) versus 21 and 18 (range 6–30) for the extended template (p=0.001). The median nodal yield of the extended laparoscopic lymphadenectomy was in keeping with series of open surgical procedures recommending

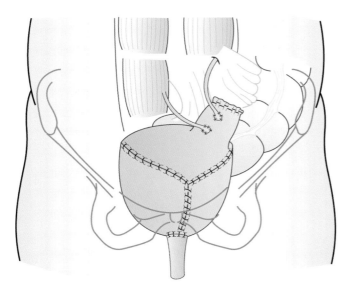

Figure 12.2
Completed neobladder in the pelvis. (Adapted with permission from The Cleveland Clinic Foundation.)

Table 12.2 Oncologic outcomes

Lead author (year)	No. pts	Technique (reconstruction)	Margins	Lymphadenectomy (n node, range)	Mean (range) months at stated follow-up	No. pts overall survival
Puppo (1995)[23]	5	Lap (extra)	Not stated	Limited (not stated)	10.8 (6–18)	5
Denewer (1999)[13]	10	Lap (extra)	Not stated	Limited (not stated)	Not stated	9
Tuerk (2001)[8]	5	Lap (purely intra)	5/5 negative	Limited (not stated)	Not stated	5
Abdel-Hakim (2002)[14]	9	Lap (extra)	9/9 negative	Limited (n=2–4)	Not stated	9
Simonato (2003)[12]	10	Lap (extra)	10/10 negative	Limited (not stated)	12.3 (5–18)	10
Menon (2002)[18]	17	Robot (extra)	17/17 negative	Limited (n=4–27)	Not stated (2–11)	17
Hemal (2004)[11]	11	Lap (extra)	10/11 negative	Limited (not stated)	18.4 (1–48)	10
Basillote (2004)[10]	13	Lap (extra)	12/13 negative	Limited (not stated)	Not stated	13
Gill (2004)[6]	22	Lap (purely intra)	21/22 negative	11/22 Extended (n=21, 6–30)	11 (2–43)	18

Adapted from Hrouda et al.[30]
Extra, extracorporeal; intra, Intracorporeal; Lap, laparoscopic; Robot, robotic-assisted.

that at least 10–15 lymph nodes be removed.[32] No patient developed port-site or local recurrence over the short follow-up of 11 months (range 2–43 months).

Functional outcomes and complications

LRC is a complex procedure and requires advanced laparoscopic expertise. While increasing numbers of publications regarding LRC have demonstrated the technical feasibility of the surgery, a critical appraisal of the attendant complications is essential (Table 12.3).[6,7,10–13,18] Sharp et al[7] reported the outcomes in the Cleveland Clinic of the initial 21 cases of LRC, all with intracorporeally created urinary diversion. Six major (29%) and nine minor (45%) complications were reported. The major complications, all of which required reoperation, were small bowel obstruction (three), and one each of ureteroileal anastomotic leak, urethrovaginal fistula, and bowel perforation with delayed death. Minor complications were related mainly to prolonged ileus.

In the initial experiences since 1999 of 11 patients that underwent LRC and an open-hand sewn ileal conduit, Hemal et al reported one case with positive margin and five others (45%) with procedure-specific complications.[11] There were three intraoperative complications including injury to the external iliac vein in one patient and a small rectal tear in two, all repaired by laparoscopic free-hand suturing. Other laparoscopic-related complications were subcutaneous emphysema in one patient and hypercarbia, necessitating conversion to open surgery in another. The authors concluded that LRC is associated with complications similar to those seen with other laparoscopic and open surgical procedures, especially during the initial period.

A recent retrospective study comparing 11 men that underwent open approach with 13 men that underwent laparoscopically assisted radical cystectomy with ileal neobladder suggested that the laparoscopic approach provided a significant decrease in postoperative pain (parenteral morphine equivalent use: open, 144 versus laparoscopy, 61, $P = 0.042$) and quicker recovery (start of oral liquids: open, 5 versus laparoscopy, 2.8, $P = 0.004$; start of oral solids: open, 6.1 versus laparoscopy, 4.1, $P = 0.002$; hospital stay: open, 8.4 days versus laparoscopy, 5.1 days, $P = 0.0004$; resumption of light work: open, 19 versus laparoscopy, 11, $P = 0.0001$) without a

Table 12.3 Complications in the papers with complication descriptions (n=10 or more)

Lead author (year)	No. pts	No. of complications	Description of complications (Ætreatment and event)
Basillote (2004)[10]	13	8 4 major (31%)	1 ureteral obstruction (→ percutaneous nephrostomy) 1 bladder neck contracture (→reoperation) 1 epididymal abscess (→orchidectomy) 1 wound dehiscence (→reoperation) 1 obturator nerve paresis (→physical therapy) 1 pyelonephritis (→intravenous antibiotics) 1 pouchitis (→intravenous antibiotics) 1 positive margin at prostate apex (prostate cancer)
Simonato (2003)[12]	10	5	2 metabolic acidosis (→sodium bicarbonate administration) 1 Grade 3 bilateral hydronephrosis 1 Grade 2 bilateral hydronephrosis 1 Grade 2 monolateral hydronephrosis
Denewer (1999)[13]	10	6	1 external iliac artery clipped (→vascular resection anastomosis from open part), leading to 1 postoperative deep venous thrombus (→thrombolytics) 1 reactionary hemorrhage (→re-exploration) (→delayed death) 1 urine leak (→conservative drainage) 1 pelvic collection (→ultrasound-guided drainage) 1 pyelonephritis (→parenteral antibiotics) in diabetes patient
Menon (2002)[18]	17	15	13 bilharziasis with periureteric, perivesicular and perivesical scarring 1 bleeding (→re-exploration) 1 for a malfunction of lens (→open conversion)
Hemal (2004)[11]	11	6 3 major (27%)	2 small rectal tear (→laparoscopic suturing) 1 external iliac vein injury (→laparoscopic suturing) 1 subcutaneous emphysema (→resolved over 4 days) 1 hypercarbia (→open) (→delayed death, 4 weeks after surgery) 1 positive margin (→cisplatin-based chemotherapy)
Gill (2004),[6] (2004)[7]	22	16 6 major (27%)	6 prolonged ileus (→conservative management) 3 bowel obstruction (→open conversion) 2 deep venous thrombosis (→thrombolytics) 1 urethrovaginal fistula (→open conversion) 1 bowel perforation (→open conversion) (→delayed death) 1 ureteroileal leak (→open conversion) 1 postoperative bleed (→laparoscopic suturing) 1 deep pelvic vein injury (→laparoscopic suturing)

Table 12.4 Operative outcomes

Lead author (year)	No. pts	Technique (reconstruction)	Urinary diversion	Mean (range) operative duration (h)	Blood loss (ml) (transfusion)	Ileus (days)	Length of stay (days)	Time to oral intake (days)	Time to return to work (days)	Follow-up months (range)	Functional outcomes
Puppo (1995)[23]	5	Transvaginal and lap-assisted (extra)	Ileal conduit, 4 Cutaneous, 1	7.2 (6–9)	(3 transfused 2–6 units)	2.6 (2–4)	10.6 (7–18)	2–4	Not stated	11 (6–16)	4/5 discharged with no postop. complications 1 discharged after 18 days due to obesity and diabetic problems
Denewer (1999)[13]	10	Lap-assisted (extra)	Sigmoid pouch, 10 (extra)	3.6 (3.3–4.1)	(mean 2.2 units, range 2–3)	Not stated	10–13	Not stated	Not stated	Not stated	All continent 1 ureterosigmoid urine leak 1 pyelonephritis
Tuerk (2001)[8]	5	Purely intracorporeal laparoscopic	Sigmoid–rectum pouch, 5 (purely intra)	7.4 (6.9–7.9)	245 (190–300)	Not stated	10 (in all 5)	Liquid 3	Not stated	Not stated	All 5 continent and no obstruction of upper urinary tract in urogram on 10th postop. day
Abdel-Hakim (2002)[14]	9	Lap-assisted (extra)	Orthotopic, 9 (extra)	8.3 (6.5–12)	150–500	Not stated	Not stated	3	Not stated	Not stated	No complications in pouchgram on 10th postop. day
Simonato (2003)[12]	10	Lap-assisted (extra)	Orthotopic, 6 Sigmoid, 2 Cutaneous, 2 (extra)	Orthotopic, 7.1 Sigmoid, 5.8 Cutaneous, 4.7	310 (220–440)	3.3 (1–5)	Orthotopic, 8.1 Sigmoid, 8 Cutaneous, 5	3–6	Not stated	12.3 (5–18)	2 bilateral hydronephrosis and metabolic acidosis 1 monolateral hydronephrosis
Menon (2002)[18]	17	Robotic-assisted (extra)	Orthotopic, 14 Ileal conduit, 3 (extra)	Orthotopic, 5.1 Ileal conduit, 4.3	<150	Not stated	Not stated	Not stated	Not stated	Not stated	13 bilharziasis with periureteric, perivesicular and perivesical scarring
Hemal (2004)[11]	11	Lap-assisted (extra)	Ileal conduit, 11 (extra)	6.1 (4.3–8)	530 (300–900)	Not stated	10.5	Not stated	26	18.4 (1–48)	All had normal renal function and preserved upper urinary tracts
Basillote (2004)[10]	13	Lap-assisted (extra)	Orthotopic, 13 (extra)	8.0 (± 77 min)	1000 ± 414	Not stated	5.1 ± 1.2	Liquid 2.8 Solid 4.1	11.0 ± 1.9	Not stated	1 ureteral obstruction 1 bladder neck contracture 1 obturator nerve paresis
Gill (2004),[6] (2003)[7]	22	Purely intracorporeal laparoscopic	Ileal conduit, 14 Orthotopic, 6 (intra) Indiana, 2 (extra)	8.6	490	6 prolonged ileus 3 bowel obstruction	Not stated	8	Not stated	11 (2–43)	1 ureteroileal leak 1 urethrovaginal fistula

Adapted from Hrouda et al.[30]

Extra, extracorporeal; Intra, intracorporeal; Lap, laparoscopic.

significant increase in operative time and with similar complication rate.[10] The authors concluded that LRC contributes to decreased postoperative pain and quicker recovery with complication rates similar to those of the open approach (Table 12.4).[6–8,10–14,18,23]

At the time of writing, the authors have performed more than 50 laparoscopic radical cystectomies at their respective institutions. LRC is now a well-established technique, typically performed in less than 2 hours with a blood loss of 50–100 cc. Because we have noted neither significant reduction of morbidity nor earlier return of bowel function associated with the entire urinary diversion procedure performed completely intracorporeally, we now perform the urinary diversion part of the procedure through a mini-laparotomy incision. Double-teaming this with a surgeon who performs an open procedure has resulted in time savings of up to 2 hours, with increased confidence in the bowel and ureteral reconstructive parts of the operation. We have noted a considerable reduction in bowel-related complications more recently in contrast to our earlier, completely intracorporeal experience. While requirement for blood transfusion continues to be minimal, hospital stay continues to range from 3 to 6 days, depending on the time it takes for bowel function gradually to return, the rate-limiting part of the procedure. Unquestionably, LRC with urinary diversion is an advanced undertaking, and is best reserved for teams with considerable experience in laparoscopic and open pelvic surgery. To date, more than 241 laparoscopic radical cystectomies have been performed at more than 15 centers worldwide.

Future directions

LRC is being performed in an increasing number of centers that have significant experience with other laparoscopic urologic surgery, particularly prostatectomy. However, the most challenging aspect is the laparoscopic reconstructive part of the procedure. Most laparoscopic surgeons should exercise caution with completely intracorporeal urinary diversion until more experience is gained.

Although there is considerable difference of opinion and clinical practice regarding urinary diversion as well as bladder substitution, currently orthotopic ileal neobladders represent the most physiological bladder substitute after radical cystectomy for malignancy and have been used in both men and women. However, there are considerable disadvantages of using intestinal segments in urinary tract reconstruction including metabolic changes, mucus production, and tumor formation. These disadvantages may be exaggerated in patients with compromised renal function. Consequently, the search for the perfect urinary bladder substitute continues. In the future, novel bladder substitutes such as tissue engineering[33] and ureteral augmentation[34] or the use of absorbable endoscopic staples may decrease the technical difficulty associated with laparoscopic reconstruction.

Conclusion

As growing experience is reported from the major medical centers throughout the world, minimally invasive surgery for bladder malignancy and urinary diversion is gaining acceptance as an alternative to open surgical procedures. Refinements in instrumentation and techniques can only provide additional improvements. Careful prospective evaluations of oncologic and functional outcomes are awaited in order to define LRC as a viable alternative to standard open radical cystectomy.

References

1. Jemal A, Tiwari RC, Murray T, et al. Cancer statistics, 2004. CA Cancer J Clin 2004; 54: 8–29.
2. Gill IS, Fergany A, Klein EA, et al. Laparoscopic radical cystoprostatectomy with ileal conduit performed completely intracorporeally: the initial two cases. Urology 2000; 56: 26–9.
3. Moinzadeh A, Gill IS. Review of laparoscopic radical cystectomy. Cancer 2005; in press.
4. Gill IS, Kaouk JH, Meraney AM, et al. Laparoscopic radical cystectomy and continent orthotopic ileal neobladder performed completely intracorporeally: the initial experience. J Urol 2002; 168: 13–18.
5. Abstracts: 21st World Congress on Endourology and SWL, September 21–24. J Endourol 2003;17(Suppl):A80.
6. Finelli A, Gill IS, Desai MM, Moinzadeh A, Magi-Galluzzi C, Kaouk JH. Laparoscopic extended pelvic lymphadenectomy for bladder cancer: Technique and initial outcomes. J Urol 2004; 172: 1809–12.
7. Abstracts: American Urological Association Annual Meeting, April 26–May 1, 2003, Chicago, IL. 2003, 169(Suppl).
8. Tuerk I, Deger S, Winkelmann B, Schonberger B, Loening SA. Laparoscopic radical cystectomy with continent urinary diversion (rectal sigmoid pouch) performed completely intracorporeally: the initial 5 cases. J Urol 2001; 165: 1863–6.
9. Abstracts: NE-AUA 72th Annual Meeting September 11–14, 2003, Quebec, Canada. 2003, Abstract 42.
10. Basillote JB, Abdelshehid C, Ahlering TE, Shanberg AM. Laparoscopic assisted radical cystectomy with ileal neobladder: a comparison with the open approach. J Urol 2004; 172: 489–93.
11. Hemal AK, Kumar R, Seth A, Gupta NP. Complications of laparoscopic radical cystectomy during the initial experience. Int J Urol 2004; 11: 483–8.
12. Simonato A, Gregori A, Lissiani A, Bozzola A, Galli S, Gaboardi F. Laparoscopic radical cystoprostatectomy: a technique illustrated step by step. Eur Urol 2003; 44: 132–8.
13. Denewer A, Kotb S, Hussein O, El-Maadawy M. Laparoscopic assisted cystectomy and lymphadenectomy for bladder cancer: initial experience. World J Surg 1999;23:608–611.
14. Abdel-Hakim AM, Bassiouny F, Abdel Azim MS, et al. Laparoscopic radical cystectomy with orthotopic neobladder. J Endourol 2002; 16: 377–81.
15. Guazzoni G, Cestari A, Colombo R, et al. Laparoscopic nerve- and seminal-sparing cystectomy with orthotopic ileal neobladder: the first three cases. Eur Urol 2003; 44: 567–72.
16. McGinnis DE, Hubosky SG, Bergmann LS. Hand-assisted laparoscopic cystoprostatectomy and urinary diversion. J Endourol 2004; 18: 383–6.
17. Peterson AC, Lance RS, Ahuja S. Laparoscopic hand assisted radical cystectomy with ileal conduit urinary diversion. J Urol 2002; 168: 2103–5.
18. Menon M, Shrivastava A, Tewari A, et al. Laparoscopic and robot assisted radical prostatectomy: establishment of a structured program and preliminary analysis of outcomes. J Urol 2002; 168: 945–9.
19. Balaji KC, Yohannes P, McBride CL, Oleynikov D, Hemstreet GP 3rd. Feasibility of robot-assisted totally intracorporeal laparoscopic ileal conduit urinary diversion: initial results of a single institutional pilot study. Urology 2004; 63: 51–5.
20. Beecken WD, Wolfram M, Engl T, et al. Robotic-assisted laparoscopic radical cystectomy and intra-abdominal formation of an orthotopic ileal neobladder. Eur Urol 2003; 44: 337–9.
21. Parra RO, Andrus CH, Jones JP, Boullier JA. Laparoscopic cystectomy: initial report on a new treatment for the retained bladder. J Urol 1992; 148: 1140–4.
22. Sanchez de Badajoz E, Gallego Perales JL, Reche Rosado A, Gutierrez de la Cruz JM, Jimenez Garrido A. Laparoscopic cystectomy and ileal conduit: case report. J Endourol 1995; 9: 59–62.

23. Puppo P, Perachino M, Ricciotti G, Bozzo W, Gallucci M, Carmignani G. Laparoscopically assisted transvaginal radical cystectomy. Eur Urol 1995; 27: 80–4.

24. Puppo P, Ricciotti G, Bozzo W, Pezzica C, Geddo D, Perachino M. Videoendoscopic cutaneous ureterostomy for palliative urinary diversion in advanced pelvic cancer. Eur Urol 1995; 28: 328–33.

25. Anderson KR, Fadden PT, Kerbl K, McDougall EM, Clayman RV. Laparoscopic assisted continent urinary diversion in the pig. J Urol 1995; 154: 1934–8.

26. Fergany AF, Gill IS, Kaouk JH, Meraney AM, Hafez KS, Sung GT. Laparoscopic intracorporeally constructed ileal conduit after porcine cystoprostatectomy. J Urol 2001; 166: 285–8.

27. Kaouk JH, Gill IS, Desai MM, et al. Laparoscopic orthotopic ileal neobladder. J Endourol 2001; 15: 131–42.

28. Menon M, Hemal AK, Tewari A, et al. Nerve-sparing robot-assisted radical cystoprostatectomy and urinary diversion. BJU Int 2003; 92: 232–6.

29. Binder J, Jones J, Bentas W, et al. [Robot-assisted laparoscopy in urology. Radical prostatectomy and reconstructive retroperitoneal interventions]. Urologe A 2002; 41: 144–9.

30. Hrouda D, Adeyoju AA, Gill IS. Laparoscopic radical cystectomy and urinary diversion: fad or future? BJU Int 2004; 94: 501–5.

31. Gupta NP, Gill IS, Fergany A, Nabi G. Laparoscopic radical cystectomy with intracorporeal ileal conduit diversion: five cases with a 2-year follow-up. BJU Int 2002; 90: 391–6.

32. Stein JP, Cai J, Groshen S, Skinner DG. Risk factors for patients with pelvic lymph node metastases following radical cystectomy with en bloc pelvic lymphadenectomy: concept of lymph node density. J Urol 2003; 170: 35–41.

33. Atala A. Tissue engineering for the replacement of organ function in the genitourinary system. Am J Transplant 2004; 4(Suppl 6): 58–73.

34. Desai MM, Gill IS, Goel M, et al. Ureteral tissue balloon expansion for laparoscopic bladder augmentation: survival study. J Endourol 2003; 17: 283–93.

13

Role of extended pelvic lymphadenectomy

Bernard H Bochner, Seth P Lerner

Historical perspective and rationale for radical cystectomy and lymphadenectomy

Anatomic studies define the external and internal iliac and the obturator as the primary lymphatic drainage sites of the bladder and the common iliac sites as the secondary. In addition, there are lymphatics which drain the trigone and the posterior wall directly to the presacral lymph node.[1] Following the identification of the primary and secondary lymphatic drainage basins of the bladder within the pelvis, it remained to be determined whether a therapeutic advantage could be gained through their excision at the time of cystectomy. Experience with a similar radical surgical approach for cervical cancer, in which a therapeutic pelvic lymphadenectomy was combined with a total exenterative procedure, demonstrated not only that it could safely be executed but that it also potentially improved outcome.[2]

Early experience with radical cystectomy and regional lymphadenectomy for patients with nodal metastases suggested that, despite a more aggressive surgical approach, most node-positive patients experienced an exceedingly poor long-term outcome. Lymph node metastases thus appear to be surrogate markers for systemic disease. In 1956, Whitmore and Marshall published their experience of 100 consecutive bladder cancer patients undergoing radical cystectomy and a regional pelvic lymphadenectomy.[3] In 32 patients with node-positive disease, only 22% were reported alive at 1 year. Three patients (9%) survived 2 years and only 1 (3%) was alive at 3 years, the majority developing metastatic disease. While these data represented an overall improvement in outcome in node-positive patients, the poor survival in patients with regionally advanced disease led many to question whether radical cystectomy was indicated in the presence of positive regional nodes.

Patients with pelvic node metastases are curable

Supported by reports of success with the Wertheim technique for cervical cancer, which included removal of the external and internal iliac as well as the common iliac lymph nodes, along with a total hysterectomy, Leadbetter and Cooper proposed inclusion of a thorough pelvic lymph node dissection that included the hypogastric, external iliac, presacral, and common iliac lymphatics at cystectomy.[4] Subsequently, Skinner championed the benefits of

a thorough lymph node dissection at the time of cystectomy and presented compelling evidence supporting its therapeutic benefits.[5] Contemporary experience with patients whose bladder cancer has involved the regional pelvic lymph nodes establishes a significantly more favorable outcome following radical cystectomy and pelvic lymphadenectomy than described in earlier reports.

Current reports note that approximately 25–33% of all patients with invasive bladder cancer involving the regional lymph nodes will be rendered disease free following radical cystectomy and a thorough pelvic lymph node dissection (Table 13.1).[6–9] Stein and colleagues reported their updated series of 1054 bladder cancer patients including 246 patients with pathologic evidence of regional lymph node involvement. At 5 and 10 years, 35% and 34% of all lymph node-positive bladder cancer patients, respectively, were found to be free of disease following radical cystectomy and an extended pelvic lymphadenectomy, which included all nodes from the aortic bifurcation distally to the inguinal ligament.[7] The Memorial Sloan-Kettering experience with 193 contemporary node-positive bladder cancer patients that received radical cystectomy and a more limited pelvic lymph node dissection (PLND)—proximal limit at the bifurcation of the common iliac vessels—reported a 31% disease-specific survival and 25% overall survival at 5 years.[8] Ghoneim et al found 188 (18%) node-positive patients among 1026 patients with bladder cancer treated with radical cystectomy and pelvic lymphadenectomy that included the nodes at the distal common iliac vessels. Squamous cell carcinoma accounted for 59% of these patients and 85% were associated with bilharziasis.[9] The 5-year survival was 23.4% in the node-positive patients. Mills et al reported a 29% overall survival in 83 node-positive patients that underwent cystectomy and pelvic lymphadenectomy that included nodes from the bifurcation of the common iliac distally.[6] Other groups have similarly documented that, overall, approximately 25–33% of all patients with regional metastatic bladder cancer can be expected to survive 5 years following radical cystectomy and PLND. These data are confounded to some extent by the fact that many of the patients were treated with perioperative systemic chemotherapy. Pelvic lymphadenectomy is essential to identify patients with node metastases and to accurately stage the cancer, but the true contribution of the node dissection per se to overall survival in patients treated with chemotherapy is difficult to ascertain in these retrospective series.

Morbidity

Several studies have compared the morbidity of a pelvic lymphadenectomy that generally includes the external iliac, hypogastric,

Table 13.1 Outcome following radical cystectomy and pelvic lymphadenectomy for patients with node metastases

Author	No. pts	Median survival (months)	5-yr survival (%)	10-year survival (%)
Mills et al[6]	83	20	29	NS
Stein et al[7]	246	~24	31	23
Vieweg et al[8]	193	~21	25	20.8
Ghoneim et al[9]	188	11	23.4	NS
BCRC	211	24	33	19

BCRC, Bladder Cancer Research Consortium (Baylor College of Medicine, UT Southwestern Johns Hopkins); NS, not significant.

and obturator lymph nodes to an extended node dissection initiated at the aortic bifurcation or the inferior mesenteric artery (IMA), including the common iliac nodes and often the presacral nodes. Poulsen et al reported a similar incidence of lymphoceles of 1.5% versus 1.6%, respectively.[10] In a study comparing two institutions' experience with radical cystectomy and a limited versus extended node dissection, the median operative time was 53 minutes longer in the extended dissection group. There was no difference in 30-day surgical morbidity, with the exception of a higher incidence of pneumonia in the limited dissection group.[11] Leissner et al described detailed lymph node mapping in a multicenter trial involving six centers.[12] Most surgeons felt that a dissection that began at the origin of the IMA added 60 minutes to a cystectomy and node dissection that was initiated distal to the common iliac arteries. They also noted that the extended dissection allowed performance of the cystectomy more rapidly without affecting the blood loss.

Table 13.2 Impact of pathologic tumor stage on incidence and survival in node-positive disease after radical cystectomy

	Overall incidence positive nodes 20–25% in contemporary radical cystectomy series[13]			
	P0–P1	*P2*	*P3*	*P4*
8 series	0–6	6–30	27–59	43–59
	Survival probability impacted by pathologic T stage (p<0.001)[14]			
Path. stage	*No. pts*	*2 years*	*5 years*	*10 years*
P0–P2	43	74	50	37
P3, P4	89	45	18	12

Pathologic stage of the primary tumor and number of positive nodes impacts survival

Incidence

The incidence of nodal metastasis increases with more advanced pathologic tumor stage (Table 13.2).[13] Patients with nodal metastasis but otherwise organ-confined bladder primary tumors have a better prognosis than node-positive patients with non-organ-confined tumors. The number of positive nodes also impacts survival independent of the primary tumor stage. In the original series of 132 patients with node metastases reported from the University of Southern California, the 5-year survival probability of patients with organ-confined cancer was 50% compared to 18% for patients with non-organ-confined cancer (Table 13.2).[14] Stein et al corroborated these findings in a recent update including 246 node-positive patients (Figure 13.1).[7] Vieweg et al reported outcomes from the Memorial Sloan-Kettering Cancer Center series with a 51% 5-year overall survival in 44 P0–P3a, LN+ patients compared to a 17% 5-year survival in 149 patients with P3b–P4, N+ disease.[15]

Volume of disease

A similar stratification of outcome can be observed when considering the volume of disease at the level of the regional lymph nodes. If the number of positive nodes or size of the involved node(s) is considered as a measure of the extent of tumor involvement of the regional nodes, patients with fewer involved nodes or smaller tumor-bearing nodes have been found to have an improved outcome. Vieweg et al reported the 5-year disease-specific survival of 193 node-positive patients that underwent cystectomy based on TNM node staging (1987 system) as 44%, 27%, and 0% for N1, N2, and N3 patients, respectively.[15] The median survival for these three groups was 3.1, 1.9, and 0.9 years, respectively (p=0.0006). Lerner et al noted that patients with fewer than six involved lymph nodes exhibited a significantly improved 5-year survival compared to patients with more than six positive nodes.[14] An update of this series found that eight or fewer nodes involved was an optimized cut-off in that patients with eight or fewer involved nodes (n=193) demonstrated a 41% 5-year recurrence-free survival and 37% overall 5-year survival compared to 10% and 4%, respectively, in patients with more than eight involved nodes (n=51), p<0.001 (see Figure 13.1).[16] Other series have confirmed similar differences in outcome, as noted in a study by Mills et al, in which patients with fewer than five involved lymph nodes did significantly better than those with more involved nodes (5-year survival of approximately 50% versus 10%).[6]

Number of nodes removed

The number of nodes removed is also important in node-negative patients. Herr demonstrated that disease-specific survival was favorably impacted in node-negative patients with an increasing number of nodes removed (Figure 13.2).[17] The presumed explanation for this is that low node counts may lead to decreased sensitivity for detecting node metastases and these patients may in fact be understaged. Higher node counts more accurately identify patients that are true node negative.

Location of nodes

The location of nodal disease may also have an impact. There are lymph nodes embedded in the perivesical tissue and these are frequently identified in radical cystectomy specimens. Bella and

colleagues identified perivesical lymph nodes in 32 of 198 patients treated with radical cystectomy.[18] Metastatic disease in these nodes was identified in 14 of these patients and in 10 of 14 this was the only site of node metastases. These patients had a worse outcome compared to similar staged patients and perivesical node metastasis was an independent predictor of overall and disease-specific survival.

Size of nodes

Additional measurements of the burden of disease, such as the size of the involved nodes or the presence of extracapsular lymph node extension by tumor within the regional lymph nodes, may also prove to be prognostically important. Mills et al reported that patients with involved nodes greater than 0.5 cm or the presence of extracapsular extension within the involved nodes demonstrated a lower survival.[6] Multivariate analysis of the relative importance of the number of positive nodes, size of involved nodes or the presence of extracapsular lymph node perforation demonstrated that only the presence of extracapsular perforation remained independently predictive of outcome, with a hazard ratio of 2.61 (1.69–3.54).[6]

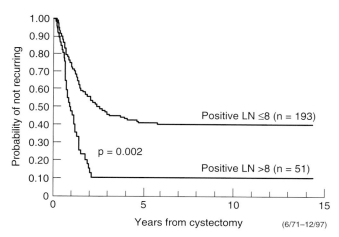

Figure 13.1
Recurrence-free survival in 244 patients with lymph node (LN) positive disease stratified by total number of lymph nodes involved with tumor (8 or fewer versus more than 8). (Reprinted from Stein et al[16] with permission from Elsevier.)

The number of positive nodes in context of number of nodes removed

While the number of lymph nodes involved with metastatic disease contains important prognostic information, simultaneous consideration of the extent of the lymphadenectomy performed appears to further enhance the prognostic significance. For example, consider two patients, both with four positive lymph nodes identified after

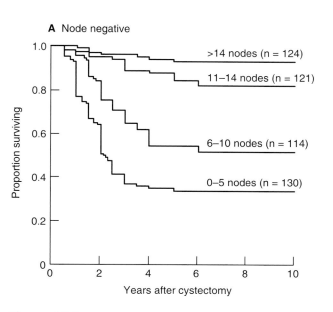

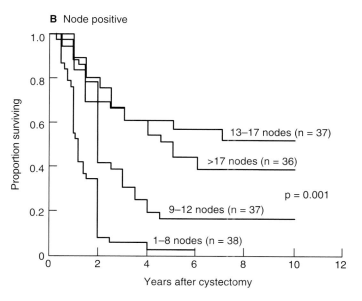

Figure 13.2
Data from Memorial Sloan Kettering Cancer Center indicating that the number of nodes removed impact survival in both node-negative and node-positive patients. (A) Disease-specific survival for node-negative patients by node-examined quartiles. (B) Disease-specific survival for node-positive patients by node-examined quartiles. (Reprinted from Herr et al17 with permission from Elsevier.)

cystectomy. The first patient had a total of 10 lymph nodes evaluated pathologically while the second patient had 40 lymph nodes analyzed. Should both patients be considered similarly staged? Would both patients have a similar anticipated outcome?

Data from both the University of Southern California and the Memorial Sloan-Kettering Cancer Center suggest that evaluation of the number of involved nodes in the context of the total number of lymph nodes removed provides a more accurate means to identify higher risk node-positive patients (Figure 13.3).[16,19] Using information obtained from the ratio of positive lymph nodes to the total number of lymph nodes evaluated (density of positive lymph nodes), both institutions have independently demonstrated an improved stratification of node-positive patients into differing risk groups. Using 20% as a cut-off for the percentage of involved lymph nodes, a 44% versus 17% 5-year recurrence-free survival probability was observed for patients with less than or more than 20% of their total nodes involved with disease, respectively.[16] An even greater difference in outcome was reported using a ratio-based analysis in a series of 162 node-positive patients that had undergone cystectomy and lymphadenectomy.[19] The 5-year disease-specific survival of patients with <20% of total nodes involved was approximately 65% compared to 5% for patients with >20% of evaluated lymph nodes involved with tumor. The ratio of positive nodes to total nodes removed and the number of nodes removed provided independent prognostic information, whereas pathologic stage was not significant in the multivariate analysis.[19] Furthermore, these variables were also associated with local pelvic recurrence.

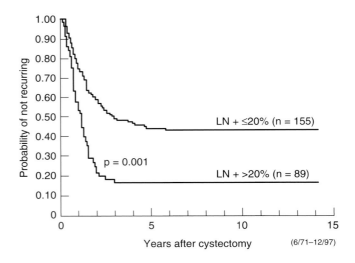

Figure 13.3
Recurrence-free survival in 244 patients with lymph node positive (LN+) disease stratified by lymph node density (20% or less versus more than 20%). Data from the University of Southern California. (Reprinted from Vieweg et al[15] with permission from Elsevier.)

Extent of lymphadenectomy

Importance

Given the importance of staging information provided by the lymphadenectomy, the question of the extent of the dissection required for adequate staging or therapeutic value remains to be clarified. An established set of necessary anatomic boundaries and extent (or number of lymph nodes) of the lymph node dissection that would provide optimal staging and therapeutic efficacy for bladder cancer is presently not available. The lack of prospectively validated studies has led to ongoing controversy regarding the necessary extent of dissection.

Wishnow et al attempted to determine the rate of involvement of the pelvic lymph nodes within the common iliac chain or more distally in the obturator, hypogastric, and external iliac nodes in bladder cancer patients undergoing radical cystectomy.[20] In a series of 130 patients with grossly negative lymph nodes at the time of cystectomy, 88% of whom had common iliac nodes resected, 18 (14%) patients were identified with microscopically involved nodes. Of these 18 patients, 17 had one or two positive nodes. None of the 17 patients had common iliac or lateral external iliac lymph nodes involved. Based on these findings, the authors recommended confining the proximal limit of the lymph node dissection to the bifurcation of the common iliac vessels for patients with no evidence of grossly positive lymph nodes.

More recently, at the Memorial Sloan-Kettering Cancer Center, a series of 144 bladder cancer patients undergoing radical cystectomy were prospectively evaluated to determine the site of regional lymph node involvement.[21] Eighteen patients (14%) were found to have microscopically involved regional lymph nodes including four with disease involving the common iliac nodes. In this series all but

one patient with common iliac nodes had simultaneous involvement of a more distal lymph node region (hypogastric, obturator, or external iliac), suggesting that excision of the common iliac nodes would benefit a subset of microscopically node-positive patients.

Additional information on the distribution of positive pelvic nodes is provided by a multicenter, prospective trial in which all patients underwent an extended PLND (proximal limits of dissection at or above the bifurcation of the aorta).[12] Of the 290 patients evaluated in this series, 81 (27.9%) demonstrated evidence of tumor involvement in 599 pelvic nodes. Involved nodes above the bifurcation of the common iliac vessels comprised 35% of all positive nodes. A total of 20 patients (6.9%) demonstrated involvement of the common iliac nodes without evidence of disease within the more distal nodal regions (obturator, hypogastric, or external iliac). While exact information on the nature of the nodes (gross or microscopically enlarged) was not available, in the 29 patients with only a single lymph node metastasis, 10% were located above the bifurcation of the common iliac vessels, providing further strong support for the need to extend the dissection to minimally include the common iliac chain. Indeed, if the obturator lymph nodal regions were the only sites excised, 74% of all positive nodes would have been inadequately eradicated.

Vazina and colleagues reported a retrospective node mapping study of 43 node-positive patients treated by a single surgeon with radical cystectomy and extended pelvic lymphadenectomy.[22] Positive nodes above the common iliac bifurcation were identified in 30% and 50% of patients with pT3 or pT4 disease, respectively. All but one patient with positive nodes at or above the common iliac bifurcation had positive nodes at more distal sites. This study also noted node metastases in the presacral region in 5% of patients. Importantly, 3 of 10 patients with pT2 tumors and positive nodes distal to the common iliac bifurcation had presacral node metastases. These data support inclusion of the presacral nodes as part of the standard node dissection template.

Outcome

The data describing the relationship between the extent of the node dissection and outcome are provided by single-institution, retrospective reviews. Poulsen et al reported a comparative analysis of two consecutive series of bladder cancer patients undergoing either a limited (proximal limit at the bifurcation of the common iliac vessels) or extended (including the nodes up to the level of the bifurcation of the aorta) lymphadenectomy performed at the time of radical cystectomy.[10] Previously untreated bladder cancer patients were included in the study in which 126 underwent an extended lymphadenectomy (between 1993 and 1997) and 68 received a limited lymph node dissection (between 1990 and 1993). The two groups were well matched demographically, with a slightly higher percentage of extravesical tumors in the extended lymphadenectomy group. As anticipated, the extended node dissection yielded a greater number of lymph nodes than the more limited excision (25 versus 14, $p<0.001$). Both groups had a similar proportion of node-positive patients, 27% in the extended and 24% in the limited lymph node groups. Despite the increased number of more advanced tumors in the extended dissection group, a similar 5-year recurrence-free survival, risk of local recurrence, and risk of distant metastasis were observed. In the subgroup of patients with organ-confined primary tumors, however, patients that underwent an extended dissection benefited with an improved 5-year recurrence (85% versus 64%, $p<0.02$).

Leissner and colleagues presented their analysis of 302 patients that received an extended lymph node dissection at the time of radical cystectomy for bladder cancer. They noted that patients with a greater number of lymph nodes identified in their pathology report had an improved disease-free and overall survival as well as improved local tumor control.[23] At 5 years, 51% of patients with ≤15 lymph nodes removed were alive and disease free compared to 65% for those with ≥16 lymph nodes evaluated. The improvement in local control was also significant, with pelvic recurrences identified in 27% compared to 17% of patients with ≤15 and ≥16 lymph nodes evaluated, respectively ($p<0.01$). Herr et al confirmed a similar improved outcome in 322 patients, in which those that underwent a more extensive node dissection, as represented by a greater number of lymph nodes identified in the pathology report, exhibited an improved overall survival.[24] All patients underwent cystectomy without preoperative radiation, or neoadjuvant or adjuvant chemotherapy. Of the 258 patients with negative nodes, the median number of nodes evaluated was 8, and for the 64 node-positive patients the median number of nodes was 11. The 5-year overall survival for node negative patients was 82% versus 41% for those patients with 9 or more nodes removed versus 8 or fewer nodes removed. For patients with node positive disease, approximately 44% versus 20% of patients with 11 or more versus fewer than 11 nodes removed, respectively. While these data provide additional evidence of the importance of a complete node dissection, the number of nodes removed in both node-negative and node-positive patients is lower than that reported by other institutions.

A recent analysis of 101 node-positive patients from Studer's group in Berne, Switzerland, emphasizes the importance of extranodal extension as an independent determinant of progression-free survival in patients with N1 or N2 disease.[25] In their series, the proximal limit of dissection was the common iliac artery at the level of the crossing of the ureter, and the median number of nodes removed was 21 (range 10–43). While number of nodes removed stratified as <5 or ≥5, node density of 20% and pathologic tumor stage were associated with outcome by univariate analysis, only extranodal extension was an independent predictor of progression by multivariate analysis. These data suggest that the number of lymph nodes reported may function mainly as a surrogate measure of the extent of dissection performed. If this is true then one would expect that if all patients received a similar PLND, outcomes would not be significantly affected by the number of lymph nodes reported by the pathologist. Variation in lymph node reporting and individual lymph node content, as well as other less well characterized variables, may all affect the number of lymph nodes reported despite similar anatomic dissections.

Additional supportive data obtained from a national cohort of patients are provided by a multivariate analysis of Surveillance, Epidemiology and End Results (SEER) registry data on 1923 radical cystectomy patients. This retrospective study found that the number of lymph nodes examined was positively associated with an improved survival, particularly in patients with higher stage disease. Patients with at least four lymph nodes evaluated demonstrated an improved outcome; however, patients with 10–14 nodes reported exhibited the greatest improvement in overall survival.[26]

A sobering statistic from this trial is that 40% of the patients had no nodes or fewer than four nodes removed with the cystectomy specimen, suggesting that a large number of patients may be undertreated surgically. This is an issue which should be addressed at each opportunity through continuing medical education programs, and the concept of the important contributions of pelvic lymphadenectomy should be incorporated into residency training programs as well.

Is laterality important?

The ability to limit the dissection to the ipsilateral side of the pelvis in patients with tumors located on one side of the bladder has also been proposed. Wishnow et al suggested that when there was clear laterality of the primary bladder tumor, lymph node metastases were confined to the ipsilateral side.[20] Contemporary data, however, clearly show that, despite a clear laterality of the primary bladder tumor, contralateral nodal involvement will frequently be identified. Leissner et al found that of 32 node positive patients with primary tumors located specifically to one side of the bladder, the risk of contralateral lymph node involvement was only slightly less than that found for the ipsilateral nodes.[12] Sentinel node studies have also confirmed that the initial node region involved with disease may be located in the contralateral side of the primary tumor.[27]

Surgical standard for bladder cancer and current practice

The establishment of the minimum number of lymph nodes needed for adequate staging, prognosis or improved outcome would provide a surgical standard that could be widely applied. Such standards have been established for the surgical management of colorectal, breast, and gastric cancers.[28–30] No such standard has been established to date for lymphadenectomy for bladder cancer. Major difficulties in establishing such a standard include the wide variation in reported node yields following either limited or extended dissections and the lack of prospective studies validating any such 'standard'. The variable extent of surgical dissection and differing techniques used for pathologic review contribute to the differences in reported median node number. Other variables include individual anatomic variation in the number of nodes present,[31] surgeon, patient age, and pretreatment. Our data indicate a range of 2–80 with a median of 26 nodes removed.[21] While increasing data confirm that surgeon experience is related to outcome following major surgical procedures,[32] Leissner et al demonstrated that node yield following radical cystectomy was not related to surgical experience.[23] In this series, some surgeons with the highest surgical volume reported the lowest node yields. In fact, in a single surgeon series from Baylor College of Medicine, the range of lymph nodes identified ranged from 2 to 80, despite consistent application of pelvic lymphadenectomy in 176 consecutive patients.[22] Recent data from Memorial Sloan-Kettering Cancer Center evaluating the factors associated with node yield variability in a series of 144 consecutive radical cystectomies demonstrated that only the extent of the dissection was associated with overall node yield within a group of four experienced surgeons.[21] Patient age, neoadjuvant systemic chemotherapy, the time from transurethral resection or prior use of bacillus Calmette–Guérin (BCG) did not exhibit a statistical association with node count. In contrast, others have found that increasing patient age is associated with lower node yields after an extended dissection.[12]

The way in which the nodes are submitted to pathology also affects the number of nodes reported. By sending separate nodal packets from the different anatomic node regions as opposed to an en bloc submission with the main specimen, Bochner et al reported a 3.5-fold increase in the number of reported nodes for a standard dissection and a 1.6-fold increase in node yield for an extended dissection.[33]

Conclusion

Anatomic and clinical experience with invasive bladder cancer has established the natural pathways of disease progression. Decades of experience with radical surgery for the management of muscle invasive bladder cancer clearly emphasizes the role that surgical quality may play in patient outcome. Future advances in establishing surgical standards for the treatment of bladder cancer will require well-controlled prospective trials that directly compare varying extents of surgery to their ability to provide local and distant disease control, as well as disease-specific survival. This will set the stage for clear benchmarks that can then be broadly applied to clinical practice. Technologic innovation in radiologic imaging will facilitate prospective identification of patients harboring occult pelvic lymph node metastases that will not only improve the accuracy of pretreatment staging but also facilitate appropriate surgical planning.

References

1. H.R. In Anatomy of the Human Lymphatic System. Ann Arbor, MI: Edwards Brothers, 1938, p 214.
2. Brunschwig A. Extended surgery in advanced cancer. Ann Surg 1951; 133(4): 574–6.
3. Whitmore WF Jr, Marshall VF. Radical surgery for carcinoma of the urinary bladder: one hundred consecutive cases four years later. Cancer 1956; 9(3): 596–608.
4. Leadbetter WF, Cooper JF. Regional gland dissection for carcinoma of the bladder; a technique for one-stage cystectomy, gland dissection, and bilateral uretero-enterostomy. J Urol 1950; 63(2): 242–60.
5. Skinner DG. Management of invasive bladder cancer: a meticulous pelvic node dissection can make a difference. J Urol 1982; 128(1): 34–36.
6. Mills RD, Turner WH, Fleischmann A, et al. Pelvic lymph node metastases from bladder cancer: outcome in 83 patients after radical cystectomy and pelvic lymphadenectomy. J Urol 2001; 166(1): 19–23.
7. Stein JP, Lieskovsky G, Cote R, et al. Radical cystectomy in the treatment of invasive bladder cancer: long-term results in 1,054 patients. J Clin Oncol 2001; 19(3): 666–75.
8. Vieweg J, Gschwend JE, Herr HW, et al. Pelvic lymph node dissection can be curative in patients with node positive bladder cancer. J Urol 1999; 161(2): 449–54.
9. Ghoneim MA, el-Mekresh MM, el-Baz MA, el-Attar IA, Ashamallah A. Radical cystectomy for carcinoma of the bladder: critical evaluation of the results in 1,026 cases. J Urol 1997; 158(2): 393–99.
10. Poulsen AL, Horn T, Steven K. Radical cystectomy: extending the limits of pelvic lymph node dissection improves survival for patients with bladder cancer confined to the bladder wall. J Urol 1998;160(6 Pt 1): 2015–19; discussion 2020.
11. Brossner C, Pycha A, Toth A, et al. Does extended lymphadenectomy increase the morbidity of radical cystectomy? BJU Int 2004; 93(1): 64–66.
12. Leissner J, Ghoneim MA, Abol-Enein H, et al. Extended radical lymphadenectomy in patients with urothelial bladder cancer: results of a prospective multicenter study. J Urol 2004; 171(1): 139–44.
13. Lerner S, Skinner D. Radical cystectomy for bladder cancer. In Vogelzang NJ, Scardino PT, Shipley WU, Coffey DS (eds): Comprehensive Textbook of Genitourinary Oncology, 2nd ed. Philadelphia: Lippincott Williams & Wilkins, 2000, pp 425–47.
14. Lerner SP, Skinner DG, Lieskovsky G, et al. The rationale for en bloc pelvic lymph node dissection for bladder cancer patients with nodal metastases: long-term results. J Urol 1993; 149(4): 758–64; discussion 764–65.
15. Vieweg J, Gschwend JE, Herr HW, et al. The impact of primary stage on survival in patients with lymph node positive bladder cancer. J Urol 1999; 161(1): 72–76.
16. Stein JP, Lieskovsky G, Cote R, et al. Risk factors for patients with pelvic lymph node metastases following radical cystectomy with en bloc pelvic lymphadenectomy: concept of lymph node density. J Urol 2003; 170(1): 35–41.
17. Herr HW. Extent of surgery and pathology evaluation has an impact on bladder cancer outcomes after radical cystectomy. Urology 2003; 61(1): 105–8.
18. Bella AJ, Stitt LW, Chin JL, Izawa JI. The prognostic significance of metastatic perivesical lymph nodes identified in radical cystectomy specimens for transitional cell carcinoma of the bladder. J Urol 2003; 170(6 Pt 1): 2253–7.
19. Herr HW. Superiority of ratio based lymph node staging for bladder cancer. J Urol 2003; 169(3): 943–45.
20. Wishnow KI, Johnson DE, Ro JY, et al. Incidence, extent and location of unsuspected pelvic lymph node metastasis in patients undergoing radical cystectomy for bladder cancer. J Urol 1987; 137(3): 408–10.
21. Bochner BH, Cho D, Herr HW, et al. Prospectively packaged lymph node dissections with radical cystectomy: evaluation of node count variability and node mapping. J Urol 2004; 172(4 Pt 1): 1286–90.
22. Vazina A, Dugi D, Shariat SF, et al. Stage specific lymph node metastasis mapping in radical cystectomy specimens. J Urol 2004; 171(5): 1830–34.
23. Leissner J, Hohenfellner R, Thuroff JW, et al. Lymphadenectomy in patients with transitional cell carcinoma of the urinary bladder; significance for staging and prognosis. BJU Int 2000; 85(7): 817–23.
24. Herr HW, Bochner BH, Dalbagni G, et al. Impact of the number of lymph nodes retrieved on outcome in patients with muscle invasive bladder cancer. J Urol 2002; 167(3): 1295–98.
25. Fleischmann A, Thalmann GN, Markwalder R, Studer UE. Extracapsular extension of pelvic lymph node metastases from urothelial carcinoma of the bladder is an independent prognostic factor. J Clin Oncol 2005; 23(10): 2358–65.
26. Konety BR, Joslyn SA, O'Donnell MA. Extent of pelvic lymphadenectomy and its impact on outcome in patients diagnosed with bladder cancer: analysis of data from the surveillance, epidemiology and end results program data base. J Urol 2003; 169(3): 946–50.

27. Sherif A, De La Torre M, Malmstrom PU, Thorn M. Lymphatic mapping and detection of sentinel nodes in patients with bladder cancer. J Urol 2001; 166(3): 812–15.

28. Siewert JR, Fink U, Sendler A, et al. Relevant prognostic factors in gastric cancer: ten-year results of the German Gastric Cancer Study. Ann Surg 1998; 228(4): 449–61.

29. Mathiesen O, Carl J, Bonderup O, Panduro J. Axillary sampling and the risk of erroneous staging of breast cancer. An analysis of 960 consecutive patients. Acta Oncol 1990; 29(6): 721–25.

30. Caplin S, Cerottini JP, Bosman FT. For patients with Dukes' B (TNM Stage II) colorectal carcinoma, examination of six or fewer lymph nodes is related to poor prognosis. Cancer 1998; 83(4): 666–72.

31. Weingartner K, Ramaswamy A, Bittinger A, et al. Anatomical basis for pelvic lymphadenectomy in prostate cancer: results of an autopsy study and implications for the clinic. J Urol 1996; 156(6): 1969–71.

32. Birkmeyer JD, Stukel TA, Siewers AE, et al. Surgeon volume and operative mortality in the United States. N Engl J Med 2003; 349(22): 2117–27.

33. Bochner BH, Herr HW, Reuter VE. Impact of separate versus en bloc pelvic lymph node dissection on the number of lymph nodes retrieved in cystectomy specimens. J Urol 2001; 166(6): 2295–6.

14

Management of the urethra in the cystectomy patient

Hendrik van Poppel

Introduction

Over the past 10 years, the indications for urethrectomy at the time of cystectomy have undergone substantial modification. While years ago a prophylactic urethrectomy was performed in many patients with cutaneous diversions, it has become clear that only patients with invasion from transitional cell carcinoma (TCC) at the level of the prostatic urethra or bladder neck have a substantial risk of developing subsequent urethral recurrence. Since the introduction of bladder replacement procedures, the indications for prophylactic urethrectomy have become more and more restricted. The pre- or intraoperative assessment of the prostatic urethra in males and of the bladder neck in females is the most important issue determining appropriate management of the urethra in patients with bladder cancer.

Historical perspective

Historically, there have been many reasons to advocate a prophylactic urethrectomy at the time of cystectomy for bladder cancer. Bladder replacement has now become a well-accepted procedure after cystectomy in both males and females and nowadays prophylactic urethrectomy is mandatory only in very unusual circumstances.[1]

The overall recurrence rate in the remnant urethra after cystectomy is about 10%.[2] Urethral recurrence may happen early or late after cystectomy and frequently is associated with advanced disease with distant metastases not found earlier because follow-up of the remnant urethra was not well established. At the time of symptomatic recurrence many patients have already developed metastatic disease. When a delayed urethrectomy has to be performed for urethral recurrence, the procedure is technically much more difficult, especially at the level of the urethral stump because of postoperative fibrotic changes.

The philosophy regarding prophylactic urethrectomy has changed dramatically, however, since the introduction of bladder replacement procedures using the native urethra. This has substantially reduced the patients' and urologists' reluctance to perform a cystectomy. The risk for urethral recurrence must, however, be weighed against the gain in quality of life, and recommendations for follow-up of the remnant urethra need to be established. Any patient that is a good candidate for cystectomy is a potential candidate for a bladder substitute connected to the urethra provided that the risk of recurrence, and subsequent tumor progression, is minimal.[3]

Etiology and risk factors for urethral invasion and recurrence

The origin of TCC in the prostate is not clearly understood. The tumor might extend in continuity from the bladder, starting at the bladder neck and the proximal prostatic urethra, growing along the urothelium into the prostatic ducts and the prostatic stroma. In this situation a urethral recurrence is nothing more than tumor persistence after cystoprostatectomy. Alternatively, TCC of the prostate can arise from implantation of cells shed from the primary tumor or de novo from urothelium affected by the same carcinogenic process that induced tumor growth in the bladder.[4]

Retrospective analyses of large cystectomy series have identified specific pathologic characteristics of primary bladder tumors that can help to predict a higher risk for urethral recurrence. These include high tumor stage and grade, multifocal recurrent tumors, upper tract involvement, carcinoma in situ (CIS), trigonal or bladder neck invasion, and involvement of the prostatic urethra, particularly invasion of the stroma of the prostate.[5–9] When all these situations would indicate prophylactic urethrectomy, the majority of bladder cancer patients would be in need of a cutaneous diversion because of the necessity to perform a prophylactic urethrectomy.[4]

The importance of prostatic urethral involvement was first recognized half a century ago when, in a cystectomy series, 71% of the urethral recurrences occurred in patients that had TCC in the prostatic urethra.[10] This association was later confirmed by other investigators that recognized different stages of prostatic urethral involvement.[5] There was a clear distinction between the presence of TCC limited to the urethral mucosa (TpU), invasion in the prostatic ducts (TpD), and invasion to the prostatic stroma (TpS) with, respectively, 0%, 25%, and 64% of urethral recurrence after cystectomy. Other groups have reported analogous figures of, respectively, 0%, 10%, and 30%.[11] These studies indicate that the invasion of the prostatic stroma is the single best prognostic indicator for development of urethral recurrence.

The association between the presence of CIS in the bladder and urethral recurrence is widely recognized. However, it has been shown in whole-mount step-sections that CIS of the bladder is not correlated with TCC of the prostatic urethra.[12] Conversely, CIS of the bladder neck and the trigone is clearly correlated with TCC of the prostate but not directly correlated with urethral recurrences.[12] Therefore, CIS at the bladder neck is a risk factor for TCC of the prostatic urethra and the latter is a risk factor for urethral recurrence.[9] The presence of CIS in the bladder or even at the bladder neck is not per se an absolute contraindication for urethral preservation.[6]

Investigation of the prostatic urethra before and during surgery

A rigorous pre- and intraoperative assessment of the prostatic urethra is mandatory since the invasion into the prostatic urethra is the most relevant prognosticator of urethral recurrence. For this purpose prostatic urethra cold-cup biopsies or transurethral resection biopsies were proposed.[13] In a prospective study of the prostatic involvement prior to cystectomy, a transurethral resection biopsy of the prostate accurately identified 9 out of 10 patients with prostatic involvement.[13] Core needle biopsies or needle aspirations were much less accurate. Consequently, 5 and 7 o'clock paracollicular biopsies have been advocated to identify involvement with TCC.[14,15] Recently, however, the value of this approach has been challenged. In a series of 371 consecutive patients that underwent cystectomy with negative preoperative paracollicular biopsies, urethral recurrence was diagnosed in 13 (3.5%) after a median time of 1 year.[16,17] The follow-up in these reports is, however, too short to definitively discourage the practice of transurethral resection (TUR) biopsying of the prostatic urethra.

At a time when even more bladder substitution procedures are performed, significantly more authors have chosen not to perform preoperative paramontanal biopsies and rather to rely on intraoperative frozen section analysis of the urethral resection margin at the prostatic apex.[6,18–22] This means that intraoperative assessment proved to be reliable for selection of patients that can have an orthotopic reconstruction, without subjecting the patients to unnecessary preoperative biopsies.[22] It is important, therefore, that all patients be counseled preoperatively about continent and incontinent diversion should intraoperative findings show that orthotopic bladder replacement is not feasible. The advantage of the preoperative assessment of the prostatic urethra with TUR biopsies is that patients can be counseled efficiently before surgery about what type of diversion probably will be performed.

Follow-up of the retained urethra after cystoprostatectomy

Urethral recurrence

One could presume that the introduction of the orthotopic neobladder and the increased frequency of conservation of the urethra would be associated with an increased recurrence rate in the retained urethra. The largest published series evaluating the recurrence rate of urethral TCC in patients with a cutaneous diversion and an intact defunctionalized urethra and in patients that had a neobladder and a functional urethra[6] reported an overall probability of urethral recurrence for all 436 male patients of 7.8% at 5 years. For patients with an ileal neobladder, this figure was 2.9% and in

those with a cutaneous diversion, 11.1%. The 5-year urethral recurrence rate was significantly higher in patients with prostatic involvement, but was only 5% in patients with a neobladder as compared with 24% in those with a Bricker diversion. The recently presented update of results in an even larger sample of 768 patients,[22] confirmed a urethral tumor recurrence rate of approximately 7% and clearly showed that patients undergoing orthotopic diversion and those without any prostate involvement with TCC had a significantly lower incidence of urethral recurrence. These results clearly indicate that a functional orthotopic neobladder may decrease the risk of developing recurrent TCC in the retained urethra.

The explanation of this finding remains incompletely elucidated. It is well known that primary malignancies are rare in the small bowel and even less common in the ileum,[23] and a number of intrinsic physiologic, biochemical, genetic, and immunologic characteristics of the ileum have been suggested.[6] On the other hand, the decreased risk of recurrent TCC in a urethra connected to an ileal neobladder might have nothing to do with its juxtaposition to ileum and exposure to ileal secretory products. The simple continued exposure to urine may be a responsible factor or there might be an unknown systemic cancer protective effect of the orthotopic reservoir.[4] Conversely, there may be a systemic effect of the non-orthotopic reservoir, which increases the risk of urethral recurrence in the defunctionalized urethra.[6]

These data have changed the management of the remnant urethra, the only absolute contraindications for bladder replacement being the presence of overt TCC in the anterior urethra and a positive frozen section of the urethral margin during cystectomy.[6,20–22]

Although reliable pre- or intraoperative tools are available to recognize patients at risk for urethral recurrence, there is always a (small) risk of tumor growth in the remnant urethra. This urethral recurrence should be detected while still curable by secondary urethrectomy or even by more conservative (endoscopic) treatment modalities. Follow-up of the retained urethra is mandatory, especially in those with cutaneous diversions, given their higher propensity to malignant change.[4]

Unfortunately, urethral recurrence can remain asymptomatic for a long time, and in many patients symptoms occur at the time of evolution to a metastatic stage. Clinically, carcinoma of the urethra is manifested as a bloody urethral discharge, penile or perineal pain, or a mass in the urethra or perineum. This is not the clinical picture that the urologist wants to face, but this type of recurrence has been reported to occur up to 20 years after cystectomy.[13] Once overt carcinoma becomes clinically manifest, the prognosis is indeed poor and nearly all patients will die within 5 years.[13,23] This poor outcome is related to the fact that the lamina propria is the only barrier between the urethral mucosa and the cavernous corpora.[14] If there were no reliable tests to detect urethral recurrence earlier, one would have to advocate prophylactic urethrectomy in many cases. This emphasizes the importance of careful routine follow-up with urethral cytology and/or urethroscopy.

Urethral wash cytology

Urethral wash cytology has been proposed for routine screening of patients with retained urethras.[24] Practically, a 14 Fr. catheter is introduced to the proximal blind end of the urethra. Normal saline (10–15 ml) is used to wash the urethra while the patient actively contracts the external urethral sphincter and pelvic floor.

The efflux is collected in an equal volume of a fixative and the specimen is then processed for cytologic examination.[4] In a review of urethral wash cytology performed every 6 months, lifelong, all recurrences were diagnosed while still confined to the urethra.[14] No patient developed a symptomatic urethral recurrence. No patient had false positive results or clinically obvious tumor in the absence of positive cytology. Therefore, urethral wash cytology of the remnant urethra, performed twice a year, was claimed to have a 100% sensitivity and specificity to detect urethral recurrence at a stage that was curable.[25] One might decrease the number of unnecessary urethral washings by selecting only those patients with CIS in the surgical specimen or in the precystectomy biopsies and thus reduce the frequency to a once yearly washing cytology. However, this approach has not been shown to be sufficiently safe until now, and every bladder cancer patient has a chance, though small in many of them, of developing a urethral recurrence.

The value of regular urethral cytology washings has recently been challenged. When the outcome was compared between patients that had routine urethral wash cytology and those that were not followed by urethral wash cytology but presented with bleeding or urethral discharge, there was no significant survival difference[26] or any statistically significant effect on disease progression.[27] Despite these data, this author does not discourage the continued use of urethral wash cytology since it is simple, well tolerated, and minimally invasive. In addition, symptoms such as urethral discharge may be overlooked by patients and, therefore, until prospective, preferably multi-institutional, evaluations are performed, the author continues to advocate close surveillance with routine urethral washing.[26] Monitoring the residual urethra with urethral washing cytology can spare patients a urethrectomy by allowing conservative endoscopic treatment and help to prevent the development of invasive carcinomas in this organ.[27,28]

In addition to urethral wash cytology, many urologists are performing routine urethroscopy. It has been proposed that urethrocystoscopies be performed twice a year for 3 years and then once yearly.[21]

Technique of simultaneous urethrectomy

When a patient cannot undergo a bladder substitution, the immediate urethrectomy can be performed en bloc with the cystoprostatectomy or after intraoperative decision making. While a delayed urethrectomy for urethral recurrence would most likely need to be performed through a perineal incision, a simultaneous urethrectomy could be done by a perineal or a prepubic approach.

Perineal approach

A urethrectomy performed through a perineal incision will add an hour to an already long and demanding operation.[14] A two-team approach by a perineal surgeon and an abdominal surgeon can somewhat shorten the procedure. The perineal urethrectomy will, however, also add to the morbidity and mortality. Indeed, an increased incidence of deep venous thrombosis was reported in patients undergoing a simultaneous perineal urethrectomy.[18] This outcome is probably related to the perineal pain and discomfort that is responsible for delayed mobilization of the patient after perineal urethrectomy.

Prepubic approach

The prepubic approach for simultaneous urethrectomy can avoid these problems. The technique was first described in 1989 by Van Poppel et al[29] and then further refined and detailed (Figures 14.1–14.8).[30,31] It was shown to be a safe technique without major complications. There is no need to place the patient in a lithotomy position, saving time and decreasing postoperative thromboembolic complications. The disadvantage of the classic perineal approach, hindering early postoperative mobilization, is thus

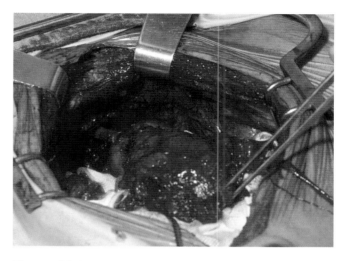

Figure 14.1
Dissection of the membranous urethra through the pelvic floor. Reproduced from Van Poppel & Baert.[31]

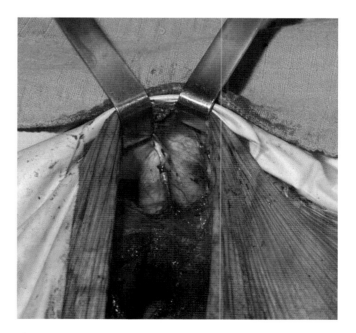

Figure 14.2
Prepubic exposure of the penile shaft. Reproduced from Van Poppel & Baert.[31]

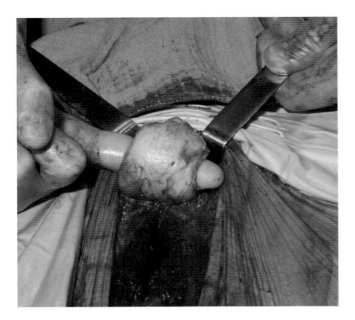

Figure 14.3
Inversion of the penis dissected upon Buck's fascia. Reproduced from Van Poppel & Baert.[31]

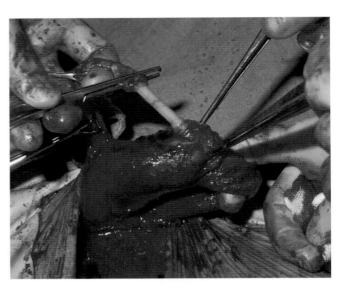

Figure 14.5
Transection of the glandular urethra. Reproduced from Van Poppel & Baert.[31]

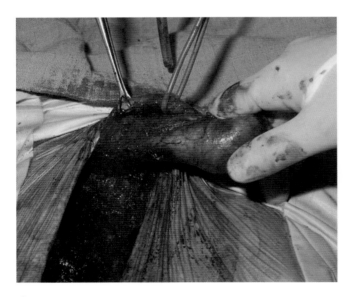

Figure 14.4
Separation of the corpus spongiosum from the corpora cavernosa. Reproduced from Van Poppel & Baert.[31]

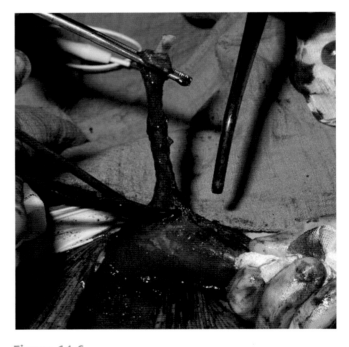

Figure 14.6
Dissection of the urethra towards the bladder. Reproduced from Van Poppel & Baert.[31]

avoided. The few complications are mainly due to hemorrhage and can be avoided by intraoperative hemostasis and adequate postoperative management.[32]

An interesting modification of the technique using urethral stripping was presented more recently.[33] It is clear that the entire urethra comprising the fossa navicularis and the urethral meatus needs to be excised since carcinoma can recur even at this distant level.[13]

Management of urethral recurrence in patients with a neobladder

Patients followed with routine urethral wash cytology that were noted to have positive cytology findings and subsequently underwent

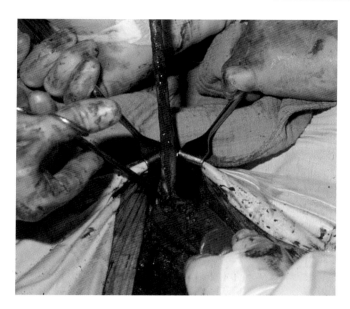

Figure 14.7
Blunt dissection of the bulbous urethra. Reproduced from Van Poppel & Baert.[31]

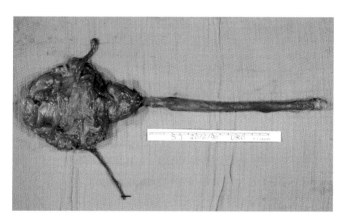

Figure 14.8
In continuity removed cystoprostatourethrectomy specimen. Reproduced from Van Poppel & Baert.[31]

therapeutic urethrectomy fared well.[14,25] Several reports have dealt with the therapeutic possibilities ranging from endoscopic treatments to formal urethrectomy and construction of an alternative continent/incontinent cutaneous or rectosigmoid diversion.[34,35] The median time to urethral recurrence is 24 months, and all diagnostic means should therefore be applied regularly during that time in order to detect superficial recurrences before any invasion has occurred that would necessitate urethrectomy.

The endoscopic approaches proposed for urethral recurrence are TUR,[20,34,36,37] instillation therapy with 5-fluorouracil,[2] and even bacillus Calmette–Guérin (BCG), which was indeed shown to be effective in urethral CIS.[34,38]

In the case of urethrectomy, pathologic evaluation has revealed a varied histology. About one-third of the specimens showed no evidence of disease (pT0) on pathologic examination. The authors explain this phenomenon by the occurrence of denudation of the urethral epithelium during urethral washing. It might be that vigorous saline irrigation during cytology specimen acquisition effectively washes away the neoplastic urothelium, particularly in cases of focal carcinoma in situ. Denudation of the mucosa during the operative procedure due to urethral manipulation is another possible explanation.[26]

Guidelines for the female urethra

Orthotopic bladder reconstruction has been much less widely applied in women, mainly because of more frequent voiding dysfunction in the female as well as a perceived increased risk for local recurrence. In the classic cystectomy with cutaneous diversion in women, urethrectomy is performed routinely. The female urethra, however, can also be preserved when invasive bladder cancer does not involve the trigone. It has been shown that the female continence mechanism may adequately function after cystectomy.[39–42] The key point is the preservation of the distal two-thirds of the urethra, and limiting the dissection above the endopelvic fascia in order to preserve the innervation of the sphincter by the pudendal nerve.

Urethral tumors occur only in female patients with TCC at the level of the bladder neck.[39] While some authors have recommended intraoperative frozen section at the urethral margin as the best method for determining patients' suitability for orthotopic reconstruction,[40] others have stated that a preoperative assessment is preferable because the quality of permanent imbedded sections is superior and because small tumor clusters and mucosal atypia can be missed by frozen section.[42]

Preservation of the female urethra is possible when the primary tumor does not involve the bladder neck. Before considering a bladder substitution in female patients, assessment of the sphincteric function is absolutely mandatory. When there is any doubt about continence before surgery, video-urodynamic studies are necessary. The successful functional outcome is not comparable with that in men because of the more frequent problems of incontinence and—even more common—hypercontinence. It is imperative that the radical nature of cancer surgery remains uncompromised.

Because follow-up of the remnant urethra in the female cannot be achieved with urethral wash cytology, and the value of sampling with a urethral swab has not been extensively studied, the physician must rely mainly on the voided urine specimen and on urethroscopy.

Conclusion

The indications for total urethrectomy at the time of cystectomy have undergone substantial modification. Historically, urethrectomy was performed in patients with multifocal tumors, diffuse CIS, and prostatic urethral involvement. Recent studies have shown that prostatic stromal invasion and diffuse CIS of the prostatic urethra are the primary risk factors. Routine preoperative prostatic urethral biopsies prior to cystectomy are not always performed but frozen section analysis of the urethral margin can be relied upon when deciding whether to proceed with neobladder construction. Suggested algorithms are described in Figures 14.9–14.11 to guide overall management and gender-specific management of the urethra.

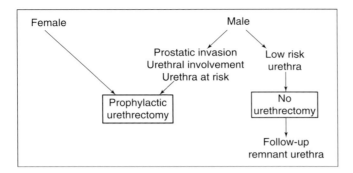

Figure 14.9
Management of the urethra in the cystectomy patient, candidate for cutaneous diversion.

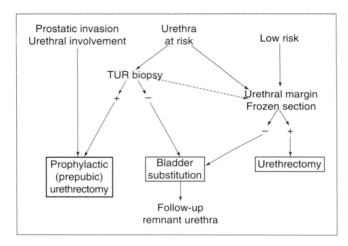

Figure 14.10
Management of the urethra in the male cystectomy patient, candidate for orthotopic bladder substitution. (TUR, transurethral resection.)

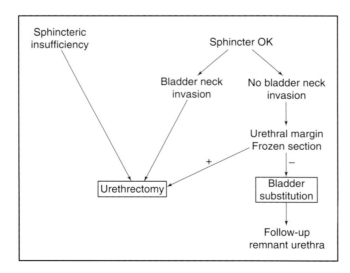

Figure 14.11
Management of the urethra in the female cystectomy patient, candidate for orthotopic bladder substitution.

In patients that are not candidates for a neobladder and have known prostatic stromal involvement by tumor, an en bloc urethrectomy is performed, preferably through a prepubic approach. In women, a classic radical cystectomy includes removal of the urethra and the anterior vaginal wall. In patients that are candidates for neobladders, a cystoscopy and preoperative bladder neck biopsies can be performed or, as in men, intraoperative frozen sections of the bladder neck are proposed to select those that could undergo bladder substitution. In women that are not candidates for neobladder, the urethra is routinely resected. When the urethra is not resected, early diagnosis of urethral recurrence remains important and urethral wash cytology and urethroscopy can help to detect recurrences at a stage when conservative measures can still provide a cure and avoid the need for a delayed urethrectomy.

References

1. Carrion R, Seigne J. Surgical management of bladder carcinoma. Cancer Control 2002; 9: 284–92.
2. Freeman JA, Ersig D, Stein JP, Skinner DG. Management of the patient with bladder cancer. Urethral recurrence. Urol Clin North Am 1994; 21: 645–51.
3. Hautman RE, de Petriconi R, Gottfried H-W, Kleinschmidt K, Mattes R, Pais T. The ileal neobladder: complications and functional results in 363 patients after 11 years follow-up. J Urol 1999; 161: 422–8.
4. Van Poppel H, Sorgeloose T. Radical cystectomy with or without urethrectomy? Crit Rev Oncol/Hematol 2003; 47: 141–5.
5. Hardeman SW, Soloway MS. Urethral recurrence following radical cystectomy. J Urol 1990; 144: 666–9.
6. Freeman JA, Tarter TA, Ersig D, et al. Urethral recurrence in patients with orthotopic ileal neobladders. J Urol 1996;156: 1615–9.
7. Tobisu KI, Tanaca Y, Mizutani T, Mizutane T, Kakizoe T. Transitional cell carcinoma of the urethra in men following cystectomy for bladder cancer: multivariate analysis for risk factors. J Urol 1991; 146: 1551–4.
8. Bell CR, Gujral S, Collins CM, Sibley GN, Persad RA. Review. The fate of the urethra after definitive treatment of invasive transitional cell carcinoma of the urinary bladder. BJU Int 1999; 83: 607–12.
9. Nixon RG, Chang SS, Lafleur BJ, Smith JA Jr, Cookson MS. Carcinoma in situ and tumor multifocality predict the risk of prostatic urethral involvement at radical cystectomy in men with transitional cell carcinoma of the bladder. J Urol 2002; 167: 502–5.
10. Ashworth A. Papillomatosis of the urethra. Br J Urol 1956; 28: 3.
11. Levinson AK, Johnson DE, Wishnow KI. Indications for urethrectomy in era of continent urinary diversion. J Urol 1990; 144: 73–5.
12. Wood DP, Montie JE, Pontes JE, Vanderberg Medendorp S, Levin HS. Transitional cell carcinoma of the prostate in cystoprostatectomy specimens removed for bladder cancer. J Urol 1989; 141: 346–9.
13. Schelhammer PF, Withmore FW. Transitional cell carcinoma of the urethra in men having cystectomy for bladder cancer. J Urol 1976; 115: 56–60.
14. Hickey DP, Soloway MS, Murphy WM. Selective urethrectomy following cystoprostatectomy for bladder cancer. J Urol 1986; 136: 828–30.
15. Wood DP, Montie JE, Pontes E, Levin HS. Identification of transitional cell carcinoma of the prostate in bladder cancer patients: a prospective study. J Urol 1989; 141: 83–5.
16. Donat SM, Wei DC, McGuire MS, Herr HW. The efficacy of transurethral biopsy for predicting the long-term clinical impact of prostatic invasive bladder cancer. J Urol 2001; 165: 1580.
17. Varol C, Burkhard F, Thalmann G, Studer UE. Urethral recurrence following cystectomy for bladder cancer: prevention and detection in patients with orthotopic bladder substitutes. J Urol 2003; 169(Suppl): 103; Abstr. 399.
18. Studer UE, Zingg EJ. Ileal orthotopic bladder substitutes. What have we learned from 12 years' experience with 200 patients? Urol Clin North Am 1997; 24: 781–93.

19. Elmajian AD. Indications for urethrectomy. Semin Urol Oncol 2001; 19: 37–44.
20. Iselin CE, Cary CN, Webster GD, Vieweg J, Paulson DF. Does prostate transitional cell carcinoma preclude orthotopic bladder reconstruction after radical cystoprostatectomy for bladder cancer? J Urol 1997; 158: 2123–6.
21. Lebret T, Hervé J-M, Barré P, et al. Urethral recurrence of transitional cell carcinoma of the bladder. Predictive value of preoperative lateromontanal biopsies and urethral frozen sections during prostatocystectomy. Eur Urol 1998; 33: 170–4.
22. Stein JP, Clark PE, Cai J, Groshen S, Miranda G, Skinner DG. Urethral tumor recurrence following cystectomy and urinary diversion: clinical and pathological characteristics in 768 patients. J Urol 2004; 171(Suppl): 80; Abstr. 306.
23. Taggart DP, Imrie WC. A new pattern in histologic predominance and distribution of malignant disease of the small intestine. Surg Gynec Obstet 1987; 165: 515–18.
24. Wolinska WH, Melamed MR, Schellhammer PF, Whitmore WF Jr. Urethral cytology following cystectomy for bladder carcinoma. Am J Surg Pathol 1977; 1: 225.
25. Tongaonkar HB, Dalal AV, Kulkarni JN, Kamat MR. Urethral recurrences following radical cystectomy for invasive transitional cell carcinoma of the bladder. Br J Urol 1993; 72: 910.
26. Lin DW, Herr H, Dalbagni G. Value of urethral wash cytology in the retained male urethra after radical cystoprostatectomy. J Urol 2003; 169: 961–3.
27. Knapik JA, Murphy WM. Urethral wash cytopathology for monitoring patients after cystoprostatectomy with urinary diversion. Cancer 2003; 99: 352–6.
28. Couts AG, Grigor MK, Fowler JW. Urethral dysplasia and bladder cancer in cystectomy specimens. Br J Urol 1985; 57: 535–41.
29. Van Poppel H, Strobbe E, Baert L. Prepubic urethrectomy. J Urol 1989; 1536–7.
30. Van Poppel H, Baert L. Prepubic urethrectomy. In Hohenfellner R, Novick A, Fichtner J (eds): Innovations in Urologic Surgery. Oxford: Isis Medical Media, 1997, pp 295–302.
31. Van Poppel H, Baert L. Prophylactic urethrectomy: When and how? In Petrovich Z, Baert L, Brady LW (eds): Carcinoma of the Bladder: Innovations in Management. Berlin: Springer-Verlag, 1998, pp 143–153.
32. Van Poppel H, Baert L. Innovative technique for urethrectomy. Prepubic technique and results in 41 patients. Progr Clin Biol Res 1991; 370: 147–50.
33. Hiebl R, Langen PH, Haben B, Polsky MS, Steffens J. Prepubic urethrectomy with urethral stripping. J Urol 1999; 162: 127–8.
34. Huguet J, Palou J, Serrallach M, Solé Balcells FJ, Salvador J, Villavicencio H. Management of urethral recurrence in patients with Studer ileal neobladder. Eur Urol 2003; 43: 495–8.
35. Bartoletti R, Natali A, Gacci M, Rizzo M, Selli C. Urethral carcinoma recurrence in ileal orthotopic neobladder: urethrectomy and conversion in a continent pouch with abdominal stoma. J Urol Int 1999; 62: 213–16.
36. Miller MI, Benson MC. Management of urethral recurrence after radical cystectomy and neobladder creation by urethroscopic resection and fulguration. J Urol 1996; 156: 1768.
37. Studer U, Danuser H, Hochreiter W. Summary of 10 years' experience with ileal low-pressure bladder substitute combined with an afferent tubular isoperistaltic segment. World J Urol 1996; 14(1): 29–39.
38. Witjes IA, Debruyne FM, Van Der Meijden AP. Treatment of carcinoma in situ of the urethra with intraurethra instillations of Bacillus Calmette–Guérin: case report and review of the literature. Eur Urol 1991; 20: 170–2.
39. Coloby PJ, Kakizoe T, Tobisu K, et al. Urethral involvement in female bladder cancer patients: mapping of 47 consecutive cysto-urethrectomy specimens. J Urol 1994; 152: 1438–42.
40. Stein JP, Cote RJ, Freeman JA, et al. Indications for lower urinary tract reconstruction in women after cystectomy for bladder cancer: a pathological review of female cystectomy specimens. J Urol 1995; 154: 1329–33.
41. Stenzl A, Draxl H, Posch B, et al. The risk of urethral tumors in female bladder cancer: can the urethra be used for orthotopic reconstruction of the lower urinary tract? J Urol 1995; 153: 950–5.
42. Mills RD, Studer UE. Female orthotopic bladder substitution: a good operation in the right circumstances. J Urol 2000; 163: 1501–4.

15

Role of radical cystectomy in patients with unresectable and/or locoregionally metastatic bladder cancer

S Machele Donat

Introduction

Approximately 19% of patients with bladder cancer will present with locally advanced disease, 3% with distant metastases, and about 25% with unsuspected positive regional nodes discovered at the time of cystectomy.[1-9] Although radical cystectomy with pelvic lymphadenectomy cures the majority of patients with invasive tumors confined to the bladder (stage pT1–2), and about half of those with microscopic extravesical tumor spread (stage pT3a), it cures only a minority of those with low-volume pelvic nodal (N1) or locally advanced disease (stage pT3b–4), and rarely cures those with extensive node-positive (N2–3) or metastatic (M+) bladder cancer.[2-9] The 5-year survival of non-organ-confined bladder cancer following cystectomy alone is reported in the vicinity of 43% for node-negative patients and 23% in node-positive patients, even in series in which an extended pelvic nodal dissection is standard practice (Table 15.1).[3-9] These findings indicate that the most important cause of surgical failure is the presence of occult metastasis outside the field of surgery, and, therefore, surgery alone in the treatment of locally advanced unresectable bladder cancer, gross regional nodal disease, and/or limited metastatic disease is destined to failure.[2-9,10]

Similarly, combination chemotherapy (methotrexate, vinblastine, adriamycin (doxorubicin), and cisplatin: MVAC) used alone will result in a major response in 39% to 72% of patients and a complete response in 20% to 36% of patients; however, the response is rarely durable, with the median survival approximately 1 year and only 4% to 9% of patients surviving more than 5 years.[11,12] These findings indicate that the use of either surgery or chemotherapy alone in advanced disease is unlikely to be curative. Therefore, both local tumor control and eradication of systemic disease are important treatment issues in terms of improved long-term survival and as a secondary goal in palliation of symptoms when cure is not possible.

Improvements in tumor response rates to combination chemotherapy, such as MVAC and more recent, less toxic cisplatin-based regimens, have given rise to the concept of multimodality therapy using surgery as an adjunct to chemotherapy to remove any previously unresectable and/or residual disease in an effort to improve survival.[11-13] The term 'postchemotherapy surgery' is often used interchangeably with the term 'salvage cystectomy' to describe radical cystectomy in patients that have failed a bladder-sparing approach or to describe a planned radical cystectomy following neoadjuvant chemotherapy in patients with surgically resectable muscle-invasive bladder cancer. For the purposes of this chapter, we will specifically discuss the concept of using surgery as an adjunct to combination chemotherapy in the treatment of patients that present with unresectable non-organ-confined or locally advanced bladder cancer, grossly positive regional nodal disease, and/or limited surgically resectable metastatic disease.

Clinical background

Radical cystectomy cures less than half of patients with measurable extravesical tumor spread, secondary to high-volume pelvic disease, positive lymph nodes in 40% or more, and preexisting distant metastases, increasing the risk for tumor relapse and surgical failure.[2-10] However, contemporary cystectomy series have reported higher survival among patients with resectable pelvic masses and negative lymph nodes, with 5-year survival rates in the range of 43% compared with 23% in those with grossly positive nodes (see Table 15.1).[3-9] Collectively, the data from these series suggest that few patients with bulky pelvic tumors and positive lymph nodes are cured with surgery alone and argue for combining multiagent chemotherapy with radical cystectomy.

The use of systemic chemotherapy has been explored in both the neoadjuvant (preoperative) and adjuvant (postoperative) settings,

Table 15.1 Survival rates following radical cystectomy alone for locally advanced (extravesical tumor) and regionally node-positive (gross) bladder cancer

Series (year)	Overall % node-positive patients	Stage pT3b–4, N0 % 5-year survival	Stage pT3b–4, N2–3 % 5-year survival
Stein (2001)[3]	23	47	24
Dalbagni (2001)[4]	36	26	13
Mills (2001)[6]	18	–	29
Herr (2001)[5]	23	–	24
Frank (2002)[8]	22	–	15
Maderbacher (2003)[7]	24	56	26
Herr (2003)[9]	23	42	28
Totals	**24**	**43**	**23**

with recent studies showing that neoadjuvant chemotherapy improves the survival of patients that are potentially curable by cystectomy.[14-16] A cooperative group-randomized study (SWOG 8710, Intergroup-0080) in patients with muscle-invasive bladder cancer found a clinically significant improvement (p=0.04) in survival with a median survival time 2.6 years longer among patients that received neoadjuvant chemotherapy than in those that received cystectomy alone.[14] The 5-year survival rate was 57% in the chemotherapy-plus-cystectomy group versus 43% in the cystectomy-alone group (p=0.06). A significantly higher proportion of deaths from bladder cancer occurred in the cystectomy-alone group than in the group receiving combination therapy (p=0.002), translating into a 14% reduction in absolute mortality and a 5% improvement in 5-year survival rate for the group receiving combination therapy. Furthermore, the survival benefit in the neoadjuvant MVAC group was strongly related to a significant improvement in tumor downstaging, with 38% having no evidence of cancer at cystectomy, compared with 15% of the patients in the cystectomy-alone group (p<0.001).

Of great interest for the treatment of locally advanced cancer patients was the observation that patients with locally advanced extravesical disease (stage T3 or T4) derived significant benefit (p=0.04) from neoadjuvant MVAC chemotherapy with a median survival time of 65 months in the MVAC-plus-cystectomy group compared with 24 months in the cystectomy-alone group. This translated into a 10% reduction in mortality in the combination-therapy group compared with the cystectomy-alone group in those with advanced disease (T3 or T4). For patients with clinical T2 tumors, the 5-year survival was improved by only 5%, whereas patients with stage T3B–4 tumors had a 20% improvement in 5-year survival (Figure 15.1).

Millikan et al also addressed combined chemotherapy and surgery in patients heavily weighted to have pathologic extravesical tumor extension and nodal involvement (94/140 or 67%), randomizing them to receive either two courses of neoadjuvant MVAC followed by cystectomy plus three additional cycles of chemotherapy, or, alternatively, to have initial cystectomy followed by five cycles of adjuvant chemotherapy.[17] Although there was no difference in outcome between the two groups, by intent-to-treat, 81 patients (58%) remained disease free, with a median follow-up of 6.8 years. Of particular relevance was the finding of a nearly 40% cure rate among patients with pathologically proven lymph node metastasis, better than any reported outcome with surgery alone in a similar cohort (see Table 15.1).[2-9] In addition, all patients in this study with pathologically extravesical extension also had nodal involvement, supporting an improved cure fraction among patients with locally advanced bladder cancer by a combination of multiagent chemotherapy and surgery. Collectively, these promising combination-therapy experiences suggest that therapeutic chemotherapy may improve survival after radical cystectomy, even for more advanced bladder cancer, and provide an impetus to explore further combined modality approaches in treatment of advanced bladder cancer.

Rationale for postChemotherapy surgery

Postchemotherapy surgery as an adjuvant treatment in locally advanced (≥pT3A) or limited metastatic (N+, M+) bladder cancer

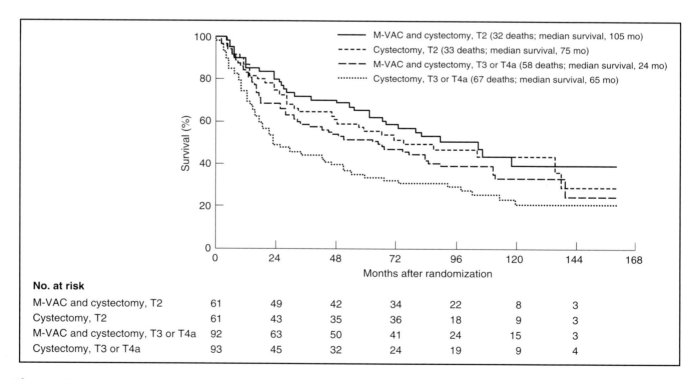

Figure 15.1

Survival analysis for neoadjuvant chemotherapy plus cystectomy versus cystectomy alone in locally advanced bladder cancer. Reproduced with permission from Grossman et al.[14] Copyright © 2003 Massachusetts Medical Society. All rights reserved.

has become a viable treatment option in select patients with the advent of more effective combination chemotherapy. The concept of combined modality therapy utilizing combination chemotherapy and radical surgery has evolved following several critical clinical observations over the past two decades.

- Available chemotherapy has limited curative potential in patients with locally advanced or metastatic urothelial tumors.[11,12,18]
- The majority of patients with nodal metastases tend to have recurrence at the initial sites of clinical disease following chemotherapy.[18]
- Extended lymph node dissection appears to contribute to long-term survival in a small subset of patients.[2–9]
- Incidence of both local recurrence and distant relapse following surgery increases with pathologic stage despite extended surgical dissection.[2–9,19]
- Improved modern combination chemotherapy can render disease surgically resectable in patients that initially might not have been surgical candidates.[20]

The challenge remains in the proper selection of patients that may benefit from postchemotherapy surgery, the optimal combination and dosing of systemic therapy, the optimal sequence for surgery and systemic therapy, and the extent of surgery to be performed.[11,13,21] There are compelling arguments for both neoadjuvant and adjuvant chemotherapy (Table 15.2). On one hand, upfront cystectomy may palliate symptoms such as clot retention, urinary incontinence, and ureteral obstruction, all of which would complicate the delivery of adequate and timely chemotherapy. On the other hand, perioperative complications may delay the timing of needed chemotherapy. Of note, in The University of Texas M.D. Anderson Cancer Center series reporting on cystectomy with adjuvant MVAC versus cystectomy with both pre- and postoperative MVAC, investigators found no difference in perioperative morbidity; however, patients were more likely to be able to receive at least two cycles of chemotherapy if given before surgery rather than after, even though there was no difference in the eventual outcome between the two groups.[17] The Memorial series evaluating postchemotherapy surgery in patients with unresectable or regionally metastatic disease also noted no increase in operative mortality or surgical morbidity although the surgery was more technically challenging.[22]

The role of surgery in patients with locally advanced bladder cancer and/or regionally metastatic disease in whom the timing of adjuvant chemotherapy may be critical is controversial and evolving. Inaccuracy in clinical staging remains a significant problem, with staging errors reported in the 35% to 65% range (Table 15.3).[17,23] Although computed tomography (CT) is routinely used for preoperative staging, it is relatively limited in its ability to distinguish extravesical spread of tumor and fails to detect positive lymph nodes in over half of cases.[24,25] These inaccuracies are accentuated in the postchemotherapy setting, where it can often be difficult to discern fibrosis/necrosis from viable tumor. This is especially important, particularly in light of the observations by Dimopoulos et al, who noted a higher incidence of relapse at earlier sites of disease in patients that had clinically responded to chemotherapy.[18]

Bladder-sparing procedures in locally advanced bladder cancer

Although radical cystectomy usually is advised after chemotherapy for invasive bladder cancers,[26] selected patients may be treated by partial cystectomy if they achieve a major reduction in tumor size and a complete endoscopic response to neoadjuvant chemotherapy.

Table 15.2 Advantages of neoadjuvant chemotherapy versus adjuvant chemotherapy

Neoadjuvant therapy	Adjuvant therapy
Measurable disease to assess response	Chemotherapy is limited to those that will benefit (based on pathologic staging)
Downstaging of the tumor allows better surgery	Local symptoms may be relieved, allowing easier delivery of chemotherapy
Surgical complications may delay needed therapy	No delay in definitive local therapy
Allows identification of candidates for bladder-sparing procedures	Avoids any increase in surgical morbidity secondary to chemotherapy side effects
Improves survival	May improve survival

Table 15.3 The inaccuracy of clinical staging*

Clinical T stage	No. pts	P0/Pa/Pis	P1	P2	P3A	P3B	Node-positive disease
		Pathologic stage[†]					
T1	113	17	73 (65%)	16	2	5 (4%)	10 (9%)
T2	181	22	23	65 (36%)	34	37 (20%)	33 (18%)
T3a	104	5	8	6	48 (46%)	37 (36%)	29 (28%)
T3b	56	3	1	6	13	33 (59%)	32 (57%)
Totals	**454**						**104 (22%)**

*Clinical stage matched pathologic stage in 48%.
[†]Reflects stages of the cystectomy specimen only.
Adapted from Herr.[23]

Herr and Scher reported a small series of 26 patients that underwent a partial cystectomy after MVAC, of which 17 (65%) survived beyond 5 years, including 14 (54%) with an intact functioning bladder.[27] The group with the best prognosis was patients found to have no tumor (pT0) in their surgical specimens, with a 5-year survival rate of 87% (14/16) compared with 30% (3/10) among patients with residual invasive cancer. Overall, 12 patients (46%) developed bladder recurrences, of which 5 (18%) were invasive and 7 (26%) were superficial. The experience indicates that neoadjuvant chemotherapy may permit bladder sparing in highly selected patients that have significant downsizing of their tumors located in sites favorable to partial cystectomy; however, they remain at risk for the development of new tumors in the bladder, the majority of which may be treated successfully by local therapy or salvage cystectomy.

Postchemotherapy surgery for unresectable and node-positive bladder cancer

After the MVAC regimen became established in 1983 as effective chemotherapy against metastatic bladder cancer,[28] it became reasonable to consider chemotherapy and surgery for patients with locally advanced but inoperable disease. Donat et al reported their initial experience with 41 consecutive patients that had stage pT4b, N2–3,M0 unresectable or extensive node-positive bladder cancer treated with MVAC followed by an attempt at postchemotherapy radical cystectomy.[20] Of the 41 patients, 34% achieved a complete clinical response, and 29 (71%) were deemed surgical candidates and underwent surgical exploration, with cystectomy being accomplished in 24. Cystectomy was not performed in 17 patients that had not responded to chemotherapy or refused the treatment. After a minimum follow-up of 4 years (range 4–7 years), nine patients (22%) survived and remained free of disease, including seven with a pathologic complete response in the bladder (complete response to chemotherapy) and two after resection of residual viable bladder cancer (complete response to MVAC plus surgery). There was an overall survival advantage for those that underwent chemotherapy with postchemotherapy surgery (p=0.009), with the authors concluding that chemotherapy allowed for potentially curative surgery to be performed as a combined modality strategy in patients whose disease was initially unresectable.

An update of the Memorial experience from 1984 to 1999 examining patients with unresectable and regionally metastatic bladder cancer treated with cisplatin-based chemotherapy regimens again showed patients responding to chemotherapy had a longer survival.[22] Of 207 patients, 92 (44%) responded sufficiently to undergo postchemotherapy surgery with the intent of removing all residual disease. Of these, 80 (39%) underwent surgery, and 12 refused surgery. Tumor progression while on chemotherapy or poor performance status accounted for the 115 patients that did not undergo cystectomy. Of the 80 patients that underwent surgery, 34 (42%) survived 9 months to 5 years, including 20 of 46 (41%) with complete resection of residual viable disease. Of 60 patients that received MVAC and had mature follow-up of 5 years or more, 10 of 34 (29%) survived after resection of persistent tumor. Postchemotherapy surgery did not benefit patients that failed to achieve a major clinical response to chemotherapy, and only one of 12 patients (8%) that refused surgery survived longer than 5 years.

The M.D. Anderson Cancer Center reported similar findings in a group of 11 patients that underwent postchemotherapy retroperitoneal lymph node dissection for nonvisceral metastasis restricted to the retroperitoneal nodes, 7 concurrently with cystectomy and 4 at the time of relapse in the retroperitoneum.[29] Although all 11 patients showed major clinical responses to chemotherapy, 9 had residual viable tumor in the retroperitoneal nodes. The 4-year disease-specific and recurrence-free survival rates were 36% and 27%, respectively. Of the 7 patients with a complete clinical response, only 1 had a true pathologic complete response, again emphasizing the inaccuracy of clinical staging in the postchemotherapy setting.

These two series demonstrate that postchemotherapy surgical resection of metastatic bladder cancer can be curative in selected patients. Further, the inaccuracy of clinical methods for assessing a complete response to chemotherapy alone and the high relapse rate at initial sites of disease suggest that surgical resection of prechemotherapy sites of local–regional disease may improve relapse-free survival.

Postchemotherapy surgery for metastatic bladder cancer

Although the role of surgical excision of viable residual cancer following chemotherapy to achieve complete response is well defined in other genitourinary tumors such as testis cancer, it is not yet established in urothelial cancer. However, in the original MVAC series,[28] 13 patients that underwent complete postchemotherapy resection of viable metastatic tumor achieved a median survival of 25 months, and several survived 5 years, indicating a possible benefit in selected patients. Following this initial experience, Dodd et al evaluated 203 patients with unresectable primary tumors and metastatic transitional cell carcinoma that received therapeutic MVAC chemotherapy.[30] Fifty responding patients underwent postchemotherapy surgery for suspected or known residual disease. In 17 patients, no viable tumor was found at surgery, pathologically confirming a complete response to chemotherapy, and in 30 patients residual viable bladder cancer was completely resected, and the patient had a complete response to chemotherapy plus surgery. Figure 15.2 shows that, of those 30 patients obtaining a complete response by the combination of surgery and chemotherapy, 7 (33%) remained alive at 5 years. Similarly, of 41% discovered at surgery to have a complete pathologic response to chemotherapy alone, those patients with unresectable primary tumors and metastases restricted to lymph node sites were most likely to survive 5 years. Of 7 patients that underwent postchemotherapy resection of visceral metastasis, 3 survived after thoracotomy to resect residual lung disease.

The most recent collective experience from the Memorial Sloan-Kettering Cancer Center includes a total of 276 patients, 89 (32%) of whom achieved major responses after cisplatin-based chemotherapy in nodal or distant metastatic sites and subsequently underwent postchemotherapy surgery.[13] Thirty of the 89 patients (34%) survived 5 years after postchemotherapy surgery, and 27 (30%) patients had no viable tumor in the resected specimen, confirming a complete response to chemotherapy. In 54 patients, residual, viable cancer was completely resected, resulting in a complete response utilizing chemotherapy plus surgery. Eighteen of these 54 patients (33%) remain alive at 5 years, a result similar to the results observed for patients that attained a complete response to chemotherapy alone (44%). Of the 14 responding patients that refused surgery,

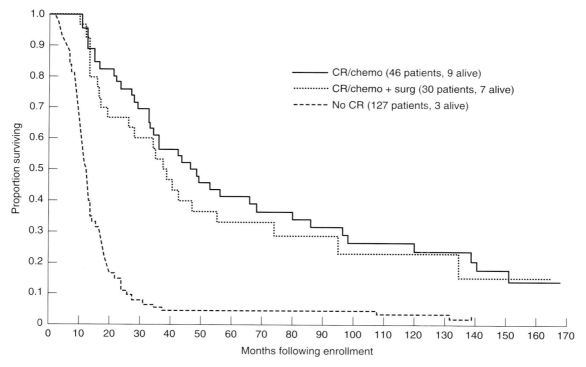

Figure 15.2
Outcomes of postchemotherapy surgery after treatment with MVAC in patients with unresectable or metastatic transitional cell carcinoma. From Dodd PM, McCaffrey JA, Herr HW, et al. Outcome of post-chemotherapy surgery after treatment with MVAC in patients with unresectable or metastatic transitional cell carcinoma. Journal of Clinical Oncology 1999;17:2546–2552. Reprinted with permission from the American Society of Oncology.

Table 15.4 Postchemotherapy surgery for unresectable primary and node-positive bladder cancer: MSKCC experience 1984–1999

Pathologic findings at surgery	No. pts clinically resectable postchemotherapy	% Complete clinical response to chemotherapy	% Alive (3–5 years)
Residual cancer	54	7 (13%)	18 (33%)
No residual cancer	27	14 (52%)	12 (44%)
Unresectable disease	8	0 (0%)	0 (0%)
Refused surgery	14	10 (71%)	1 (7%)
Overall	**103/276 (37%)**	**CR 30%, PR 57%, NR 13%**	**31/103 (30%)**

CR, complete response; NR, no response; PR, partial response.
Adapted from Herr et al.[13]

only 1 (7%) survived for 3 years. Table 15.4 summarizes survival outcome reported in the three Memorial series of patients after postchemotherapy resection of residual viable local or metastatic bladder cancer.[13,28,30] About a third of patients that undergo resection survive up to 5 years, and many have resection of both pelvic and distant metastatic sites of disease.

A recent M.D. Anderson Cancer Center experience specifically focused on 31 patients with metastatic bladder cancer that underwent metastasectomy performed with intent of rendering them free of disease.[31] All gross disease was completely resected in 30 patients (97%), including lung metastases in 24 cases (77%), distant lymph node metastases in 4 (13%), brain metastases in 2 (7%) and subcutaneous metastases in 1 (3%). The majority of patients (22 or 71%)

underwent resection in the postchemotherapy setting; 4 (13%) received chemotherapy adjuvantly, and 5 (16%) underwent surgical resection alone. The results in this highly selected cohort, with 33% alive at 5 years after metastasectomy, again suggest that resection of metastatic disease is feasible and may contribute to long-term disease control, especially when integrated with chemotherapy in patients that would otherwise succumb to disease. These experiences suggest that optimal candidates for surgery include patients whose postchemotherapy sites of disease are restricted to the bladder or pelvis, lymph nodes, or solitary visceral metastases and who have a major response to chemotherapy.

On the other hand, surgical resection of metastatic deposits unresponsive to chemotherapy is rarely reported or practiced, except to achieve palliation in selected cases. Otto et al reported their experience with resection of metastatic bladder cancer in 70 patients that failed to respond to MVAC chemotherapy.[32] Resected sites of disease included lymph nodes, peritoneum, skin, bone, lung, and liver. Seventy-six percent of the patients had multiple sites of disease, while 24% had a solitary site of disease. The median survival time was 7 months, with 30% and 19% surviving 1 and 2 years, respectively. Although the surgery did not appear to prolong survival, 42 of the 51 patients (83%) appeared to benefit from surgery in terms of tumor-related symptoms and improved performance scores. The WHO performance score changed from 3.3 to 2.1 (p=0.005). The authors reported no major adverse effects of surgery in such patients, although symptomatic patients felt worse after surgery.

Selection of patients for postchemotherapy surgery

Selection of patients that should undergo and are most likely to benefit from postchemotherapy surgery is evolving, but several generalizations can be made on the basis of previous experience.

1. A major clinical response (complete or partial) to chemotherapy portends the best chance for long-term survival with postchemotherapy surgery, based on the fact that there were no patients surviving 5 years in any of the reported series among patients that achieved less than a major response to chemotherapy despite postchemotherapy surgery.
2. Visceral metastasis, especially liver and bone, portends a poor outcome despite complete surgical resection of visible disease. This is in contrast to patients with locally advanced primary, pelvic soft tissue, and regional or distant nodal disease.
3. Limited nodal (one or two positive nodes) or a solitary (rather than multiple) visceral/lung lesion is most likely to benefit from surgical resection.
4. Long-term survival is greatest when disease is restricted to the bladder, pelvis, and regional nodes following chemotherapy. The majority of patients having residual tumor after chemotherapy in both distant sites and the bladder experience a rapid recurrence and death.
5. A complete clinical response to chemotherapy as measured by radiographic shrinkage of tumor, negative urine cytology, and negative transurethral or needle biopsy does not obviate the need for postchemotherapy surgical resection considering reports of less than 7% survival in this setting and a very high relapse rate at prior sites of disease, both locally and distantly. Unlike neoadjuvant chemotherapy given to patients with operable tumors confined to the bladder, TUR biopsies and CT images to evaluate advanced bladder cancer generally confirm absence of tumor progression, but not pathologic tumor response, rendering them of little use in selecting patients for postchemotherapy surgery.[24,25,29,33]

Conclusion

Platinum-based chemotherapy is the primary treatment for metastatic bladder cancer;[34] however, used alone it is rarely curative, with tumor relapse in the bladder, pelvic soft tissue, and lymph

nodes a common finding even after a complete clinical response to chemotherapy.[11,12,18] Current postchemotherapy clinical staging methods are imprecise, with minimal correlation between a clinical complete response to chemotherapy and the final pathologic specimen, limiting its usefulness in determining which patients may defer surgery.[13,20,22,29,30] The best correlation for survival after postchemotherapy surgery is the achievement of a major or complete clinical response to chemotherapy.[5,11,13,20,22] Current data show that many patients with advanced bladder cancer have residual viable cancer even after achieving a major response to chemotherapy. However, with complete resection of known or suspected sites of residual disease, up to 33% of these patients will survive up to 5 years. Furthermore, the need for postchemotherapy surgery in the setting of a complete clinical response is supported by the finding that over 90% of those that refused surgery died of recurrent metastatic bladder cancer.[13] Although a complete pathologic response promises the best prognosis, with 5-year survival of up to 58%, as many as 41% of patients achieve a complete response and 5-year survival with the combination of chemotherapy and surgery.[22] Conversely, patients that do not achieve a major response to chemotherapy, or that experience progression of disease while on chemotherapy, do not appear to benefit from postchemotherapy surgery with few, if any, surviving 5 years even with surgery,[13,17,20,22,30] although there may be a palliative benefit in selected patients.[32]

More effective chemotherapy regimens have made postchemotherapy surgery a viable option for selected patients with locally advanced or metastatic bladder cancer and suggest that a multidisciplinary approach to the treatment of these patients should be considered. Although the surgery is technically challenging, it may be done safely in experienced hands and provides improved survival in some and palliation in many more.

References

1. Jemal A, Tiwari RC, Murray T, et al. Cancer statistics 2004. CA Cancer J Clin 2004; 54(1): 8–29.
2. Vieweg J, Gschwend JE, Herr HW. Pelvic lymph node dissection can be curative in patients with node-positive bladder cancer. J Urol 1999; 161: 449–54.
3. Stein JP, Lieskovsky G, Skinner DG. Radical cystectomy in the treatment of invasive bladder cancer: long-term results in 1,054 patients. J Clin Oncol 2001; 19: 666–75.
4. Dalbagni G, Genega E, Herr HW, et al. Cystectomy for bladder cancer: a contemporary series. J Urol 2001; 165: 1111–16.
5. Herr HW, Donat SM. Outcome of patients with grossly node positive bladder cancer after pelvic lymph node dissection and radical cystectomy. J Urol 2001; 165: 62–64.
6. Mills RD, Turner WH, Fleishmann A, et al. Pelvic node metastases from bladder cancer: outcome in 83 patients after radical cystectomy and pelvic lymphadenectomy. J Urol 2001; 166: 19–23.
7. Maderbacher S, Hochreiter W, Studer UE. Radical cystectomy for bladder cancer today—homogeneous series without neoadjuvant therapy. J Clin Oncol 2003; 21: 690–6.
8. Frank I, Cheville JC, Zincke H. Transitional cell carcinoma of the urinary bladder with regional lymph node involvement treated by cystectomy. Cancer 2003; 97(10): 2425–31.
9. Herr HW. Superiority of ratio based lymph node staging for bladder cancer. J Urol 2003; 169: 943–945.
10. Quek ML, Stein JP, Clark PE, et al. Natural history of surgically treated bladder carcinoma with extravesical tumor extension. Cancer 2003; 98(5): 955–61.
11. Bajorin DF, Dodd PM, Mazumdar M, et al. Long-term survival in metastatic transitional cell carcinoma and prognostic factors predicting outcome of therapy. J Clin Oncol 1999; 17: 3173–81.

12. Saxman SB, Propert KJ, Einhorn LH, et al. Long-term followup of a phase III intergroup study of cisplatin alone or in combination with VAC in patients with metastatic urothelial carcinoma. J Clin Oncol 1997; 15: 2564–9.

13. Herr HW, Donat SM, Bajorin DF. Bladder cancer, the limits of surgical excision. When/how much? Urol Oncol 2001; 6: 221–4.

14. Grossman HB, Natale RB, Tangen CM, et al. Neoadjuvant chemotherapy plus cystectomy compared with cystectomy alone for locally advanced bladder cancer. N Engl J Med 2003; 349: 859–66.

15. Advanced Bladder Cancer (ABC) Meta-analysis Collaboration. Neoadjuvant chemotherapy in invasive bladder cancer: a systematic review and meta-analysis. Lancet 2003; 361: 1927–34.

16. Winquist E, Kirchner TS, Segal R, et al. Neoadjuvant chemotherapy for transitional cell carcinoma of the bladder: a systematic review and meta-analysis. J Urol 2004; 171: 561–9.

17. Millikan RE, Dinney CPN, Swanson D, et al. Integrated therapy for locally advanced bladder cancer: a final report of a randomized trial of cystectomy plus adjuvant MVAC versus cystectomy with both preoperative and postoperative MVAC. J Clin Oncol 2001; 19: 4005–13.

18. Dimopoulos MA, Finn L, Logothetis CJ. Pattern of failure and survival of patients with metastatic urothelial tumors relapsing after cisplatinum chemotherapy. J Urol 1994; 151: 598.

19. Stein JP, Skinner DG. Results with radical cystectomy for treating bladder cancer: a 'reference standard' for high-grade, invasive bladder cancer. BJU Int 2003; 92: 12–17.

20. Donat SM, Herr HW, Bajorin DF. MVAC chemotherapy and cystectomy for unresectable bladder cancer. J Urol 1996; 156: 368–71.

21. Millikan R, Siefker-Radtke A, Grossman HB. Neoadjuvant chemotherapy for bladder cancer. Urol Oncol: Semin Orig Investig 2003; 21: 464–7.

22. Herr HW, Donat SM, Bajorin DF. Post-chemotherapy surgery in patients with unresectable or regionally metastatic bladder cancer. J Urol 2001; 165: 811–14.

23. Herr HW. Uncertainty and outcome of invasive bladder tumors. Urol Oncol 1996; 2: 92–5.

24. See WA, Fuller JR. Staging of advanced bladder cancer: current concepts and pitfalls. Urol Clin North Am 1992; 19: 663–83.

25. Herr HW, Hilton SH. Routine CT scan in cystectomy patients: does it change management? Urology 1996; 47(3): 324–5.

26. Schultz PK, Herr HW, Zhang Z-F, et al. Neoadjuvant chemotherapy for invasive bladder cancer: prognostic factors for survival of patients treated with MVAC with 5-year follow-up. J Clin Oncol 1994; 12: 1394–401.

27. Herr HW, Scher HI. Neoadjuvant chemotherapy and partial cystectomy for invasive bladder cancer. J Clin Oncol 1994; 12: 975–980.

28. Sternberg CN, Yagoda A, Scher HI, et al. Preliminary results of MVAC for transitional cell carcinoma of the urothelium. J Urol 1985; 133: 403–7.

29. Sweeney P, Millikan R, Donat SM, et al. Is there a therapeutic role for post-chemotherapy retroperitoneal lymph node dissection in metastatic transitional cell carcinoma of the bladder? J Urol 2003; 169: 2113–17.

30. Dodd PM, McCaffrey JA, Herr HW, et al. Outcome of post-chemotherapy surgery after treatment with MVAC in patients with unresectable or metastatic transitional cell carcinoma. J Clin Oncol 1999; 17: 2546–52.

31. Siefker-Radtke AO, Walsh GL, Pisters LL, et al. Is there a role for surgery in the management of metastatic urothelial cancer? The M.D. Anderson experience. J Urol 2004; 171: 145–8.

32. Otto T, Krege S, Suhr J, et al. Impact of surgical resection of bladder cancer metastases refractory to systemic therapy on performance score: a Phase II trial. Urology 2001; 57: 55–9.

33. Schultz PK, Herr HW, Zhang Z-F, et al. Neoadjuvant chemotherapy for invasive bladder cancer: prognostic factors for survival of patients treated with MVAC with 5-year follow-up. J Clin Oncol 1994; 12: 1394–401.

34. Raghavan D. Progress in the chemotherapy of metastatic cancer of the urinary tract. Cancer 2002; 97: 2050–5.

Section 3

Primary bladder sparing therapy

16

Radical TURBT

Eduardo Solsona

Introduction

Radical cystectomy is the gold standard of therapy for patients with muscle-invasive bladder cancer. Although the quality of life of patients treated with radical cystectomy has improved substantially with the use of orthotopic, continent urinary diversions and preservation of sexual potency in selected cases, morbidity is high and there is no doubt that patients with their own bladders, even after undergoing one or more transurethral resections of the bladder (TURBs), have less morbidity and a better quality of life than patients treated with cystectomy. For this reason, bladder preservation programs have been developed for patients with muscle-invasive bladder cancer.[1-3] TURB is a fundamental procedure for the diagnosis and staging of bladder cancer. However, TURB alone is controversial as a therapeutic approach to invasive bladder cancer due to the different patterns of tumor spread (frontal, tentacular) and the presence of microfoci, both surrounding and at a distance from the primary tumor. This makes it difficult to achieve complete tumor resection. Nevertheless, retrospective studies of TURB alone have demonstrated the feasibility of this approach in patients with low invasive disease. In selected series, 5-year survival rates ranging from 31% to 53% have been reported.[4,5]

Rationale

In large series, the incidence of attaining P0 at cystectomy is approximately 12%.[6-9] The lack of residual cancer suggests that in some instances patients may be overtreated by cystectomy and that the tumor was completely controlled with TURB during the diagnostic work-up.

Cystectomy has little or no survival impact on patients with distant micrometastases, which are the main cause of failure. Consequently, many of these patients initially could have potentially been treated successfully with TURB alone. The incidence of P0, therefore, constitutes the main rationale for the use of radical TURB in selected patients with invasive bladder cancer. However, the absence of residual tumor in the cystectomy specimen does not necessarily mean that patients are cured with cystectomy, as the 5-year cause-specific survival rate in some series is around 80%.[8,10-13]

On the other hand, in univariate and multivariate analyses, a complete TURB is a good prognostic factor in patients included in bladder preservation programs with radiochemotherapy,[14,15] as well as in patients treated with cystectomy after preoperative radiotherapy[16] or with radical radiotherapy.[17] The prognostic value also suggests a potential therapeutic effect of complete TURB in patients with invasive bladder cancer.

Retrospective studies

In a retrospective study from Western Sweden, Holmäng et al[18] reported that cystectomy was superior to TURB and to radiotherapy in patients with clinical stages T2–3 bladder carcinoma when 5-year tumor-related mortality was evaluated, with rates of 56.6%, 75%, and 81.8%, respectively. In this study, patients unfit for cystectomy were treated with TURB or radiotherapy. Consequently, the survival rates with these approaches are not totally comparable. In another retrospective study of 114 patients with invasive bladder cancer, TURB resulted in a better 5-year overall survival rate than did cystectomy or radiotherapy or preoperative radiotherapy plus cystectomy.[19] However, combination therapy was slightly superior for patients with stage B2 (cT2b) disease. Both studies were retrospective and some important selection bias may have occurred.

A review of retrospective studies of patients with invasive bladder cancer initially treated with TURB revealed the results shown in Table 16.1.[4,5,19-23] Although some patients were salvaged with cystectomy after an invasive recurrence, 5-year survival rates ranged from 31% to 58.8%. This was particularly remarkable in patients with clinical stage B1 (cT2a) disease. However, this survival rate is inferior to that of patients treated with cystectomy—56% to 68% and 59% to 81% in P2a and P2b respectively.[6,9,24] Although cystectomy is superior to TURB in terms of survival, these results also demonstrated that a group of patients with invasive bladder cancer could be cured with TURB as monotherapy. The problem is how to identify clinically those patients in whom TURB can provide local control of the tumor. For this reason, it is important to analyze the prospective studies.

Prospective studies

Only two prospective studies dealing with TURB as a therapeutic approach in patients with invasive bladder cancer have been published. The basic aim of both series was to achieve a complete resection of invasive bladder tumor limited to the muscularis propria, T2a–b (2002 TNM classification). However, since the unreliability of the clinical staging assessment with respect to pathologic staging precludes its use as an inclusion criterion, Herr used the absence of invasive tumor on a repeat TURB performed 2–3 weeks after a complete TURB of the primary tumor as an inclusion criterion.[25]

Solsona et al systematically performed a fractionated TURB in large papillary tumors or small mixed or sessile tumors, including, first, resection of the exophytic part of the tumor, then removal of the endophytic part. Once the endophytic part was completely removed macroscopically, five or more biopsies were taken from the

Table 16.1 Survival in retrospective studies of patients treated with TURB alone

Lead author (reference)	No. pts	5-Year cancer-specific survival (%)		
		General	B1 (cT2a)	B2 (cT2b)
Flocks[21]	126	47.8	54.8	43
Milner[5]	190	53.8	57.8	23
Barnes[20]	114	40.8		
O'Flynn[23]	123	52.8	59.8	20
Barnes[4]	75	31.8		
Henry[19]	43	52.8	63.8	38
Kondas[22]	27	48.8	54.6	20
Total	698	45.8	58.8	31

Table 16.2 Prospective studies of patients treated with TURB alone

Series (year)	Herr 1987[25]	Solsona et al 1998[27]
No. patients	45	133
No recurrence (%)	9 (20)	61 (45.8)
Recurrence: cT1A (%)	21 (46.6)	35 (26.2)
Progression (%)	15 (33.3)	37 (27.7)
cT≥2M0	13 (28.8)	30 (22.4)
cT0M1	2 (4.4)	7 (5.3)
Cancer-specific survival (%)	37 (82.2)	107 (80.5)
Bladder preservation (%)	30 (67)	100 (75.2)
Median follow-up	5.1 (3–7 years)	83 (11–183 months)

healthy appearing muscularis propria of the tumor bed; cold-cup biopsies of the perivesical fat were then performed, if this structure had been reached during the TURB.[26,27] If all of these biopsies were negative, TURB was then considered radical and patients were included in a surveillance program. Although the inclusion criteria used by Herr[25] and Solsona et al[26,27] were not completely identical, initial results were comparable, with a progression rate of 33.3% and 27.7%, a cause-specific survival of 82.2% and 80.5%, and a bladder preservation rate of 67% and 75.2%, respectively (Table 16.2). More importantly, with a minimum follow-up of more than 10 years, the results continued to be comparable with slight modifications with respect to the initial evaluation (Table 16.3). Patients in both series were carefully selected, which is an important consideration that limits comparison of these results to survival of contemporary patients treated with radical cystectomy. Herr compared the survival of patients in his series with patients that fulfilled the same inclusion criteria but refused TURB and patients that preferred radical cystectomy.[28] The 10-year disease-specific survival was 76% in 99 patients that received TURB as definitive therapy (57% with bladder preserved) compared with 71% in 52 patients that had immediate cystectomy (p=0.3).

In Herr's series, of the 99 patients treated with TURB, 82% of 73 that had T0 on restaging TURB survived versus 57% of the 26 patients that had residual T1 tumor on restaging TURB (p=0.003).[28] Survival rates in patients that were P0 at cystectomy did not differ significantly between prospective studies of TURB (Table 16.4).

Of 133 patients in Solsona et al's series, 92 were followed for more than 15 years; 79 of these patients have died, 21 of tumor and 58

from intercurrent diseases.[27] The cause-specific survival was 77.2%, the progression rate was 31.5%, and the bladder preservation rate was 70.6% (Table 16.5). These figures strongly confirm the feasibility of TURB as monotherapy in a carefully selected group of patients with invasive bladder cancer. Although progression and recurrence occurred after 10 years, the negative impact on cause-specific survival was minimal.

Table 16.3 10-year outcome in prospective studies of TURB alone

Series (year)	Herr (2001)[28]	Solsona (2004)*
No. patients	99	133
Progression: T≥2- (%)	34 (34)	40 (30)
Cancer-specific survival (%)	75 (76)	106 (79.7)
Bladder preservation (%)	57 (57)	96 (72.1)
Cystectomy (%)	34 (34)	11 (8.9)

* Unpublished data, presented at the XXth Congress of the European Association of Urology 2005.

Table 16.4 Survival comparisons between patients with P0 at cystectomy and TURB alone (prospective studies)

Author (reference)	No. pts	5-year cancer-specific survival (%)
Radical cystectomy		
Mathur[11]	3	2 (67)
Brendler[10]	13	12 (92.3)
Pagano[8]	25	17 (67)
Thrasher[13]	66	50 (75)
Stein[9]	39	36 (92)
Total	146	117 (8.1)
Radical TURB		10-year cancer-specific survival (%)
Herr[28]	99	75 (76)
Solsona[27]	133	106 (79.7)
Total	232	181 (78.1)

Table 16.5 Prospective studies: 15-years' outcome

No. patients	92
Overall survival (%)	13 (14.1)
Cancer-specific survival (%)	71 (77.2)
Patients lost for follow-up (%)	9 (9.7)
Recurrence: T1A (%)	29 (31.5)
Progression: T≥2- (%)	29 (31.5)
Bladder preservation (%)	65 (70.6)
Patients alive with bladder (%)	12 (13)

Justification of the results in the prospective studies

These excellent results may have occurred for several reasons. The Spanish approach to bladder preservation in patients with invasive bladder cancer clearly relies heavily on patient selection. As previously mentioned, patients with negative biopsies of the muscularis propria after a macroscopically complete TURB were included in a surveillance program. However, patients with positive biopsies of the muscularis propria of the tumor bed were usually treated with radical cystectomy. Since 1989, these patients have been offered cystectomy or three courses of cisplatin-based systemic chemotherapy in order to preserve the bladder. Of these patients, 64 chose cystectomy and 61 chose TURB plus systemic chemotherapy. A significantly higher survival rate was achieved in patients treated with radical TURB alone as compared to patients treated with more aggressive procedures—TURB plus systemic chemotherapy or cystectomy (Figure 16.1). This clearly reflects patient selection. These patients met the same inclusion criteria used in both studies. The presence or absence of residual cancer on the biopsies of the muscularis propria of the tumor bed was the single most important variable in decision making regarding treatment selection. Univariate and multivariate analyses were performed in order to determine how this and other variables affected survival outcomes (Table 16.6). On univariate analysis, morphology, biopsies of the tumor bed, and treatment selection were all statistically significant factors. However, on multivariate analysis, biopsy of the tumor bed was the only independent prognostic variable. Thus, biopsy of the muscularis propria of the tumor bed which is macroscopically free of tumor is an important prognostic factor that differentiates between two groups: one with a good prognosis (negative biopsies of muscularis propria) and the other with a poor prognosis (positive biopsies of muscularis propria). This is despite the use of the most radical therapies in the latter group, including systemic chemotherapy.

The key to good results achieved by radical TURB alone in prospective studies is close follow-up and patient selection. The most important factor is biopsy of the tumor bed which, when negative, selects a group of patients with a good prognosis, and confirms the radicality of the endoscopic tumor resection. The prognostic value of radical TURB was also corroborated in a recent review by Dunst et al[15] in bladder preservation programs using multimodal approaches.

Concerns

Radical TURB in a very select group of patients with invasive bladder cancer can be a feasible alternative to cystectomy. All bladder preservation programs should provide long-term follow-up because patients remain at risk of disease progression throughout their lives. In series from Herr[28] and Solsona et al,[27] progression and recurrence developed after 5 and 10 years. With long-term follow-up many patients may die of causes that are not tumor related, and relapse percentages can be misleading. When at-risk patients were evaluated sequentially, the incidence rates of nonmuscle-invasive recurrence and progression were similar, with the highest proportion of events occurring during the first 3 years. Afterwards, the frequency dramatically decreased, but continued to occur up to 15 years. Patients developed distant metastases without local bladder tumor recurrence during the first 3 years. Thereafter, progression was due to invasive local recurrence (Table 16.7). This means that progression occurred primarily during the first 3 years, representing 67% of patients that progressed. Thereafter, the percentage was 17.5% in 3–5 years, 12.5% in 5–10 years, 2.5% in 10–15 years, and none after 15 years. According to these data, a strict follow-up schedule is proposed, including endoscopic evaluation every 3 months during the first 3 years due to the risk of recurrence during this period. Subsequent follow-up every 6 months is recommended up to the fifth year and then annually up to the tenth year. On the first endoscopic evaluations at 3 months, as well as in the second evaluation at 6 months, a new TURB of the scar tissue where the tumor was initially located is strongly recommended, along with routine urinary cytology, random biopsies, and bimanual examination in order to identify residual tumors. When these initial follow-up evaluations are negative, cystoscopy and cytology can be performed in the outpatient clinic and biopsies performed if needed in response to abnormal results. In order to evaluate locoregional progression, CT scans and chest x-rays should be performed every 6 months for 3 years.

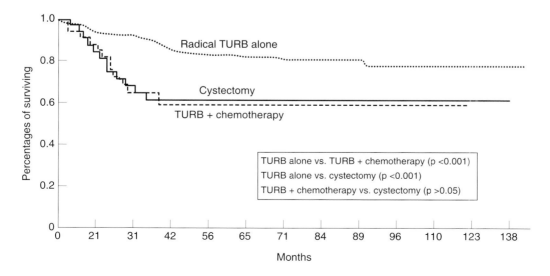

Figure 16.1
Survival comparison between the three series of the bladder preservation programs.

Table 16.6 Prognostic factors for cancer-specific survival including 133 patients with negative biopsies of tumor bed treated with radical TURB alone and 125 patients with positive biopsies of the tumor bed, 61 treated with TURB plus chemotherapy and 64 with radical cystectomy

Univariate analysis Variables incuded	Percentages	p value
Recurrent tumor (yes vs. no)	26.3 vs. 24.1	0.6903
Biopsies of tumor bed (positive vs. negative)	33.6 vs. 20.3	0.0004
Age (continuous)	25.4 vs. 27.2	0.9716
Grade (2 vs. 3)	20 vs. 28.9	0.097
Tumor morphology (papillary vs. sessile)	21.2 vs. 29.5	0.0452
Number of tumors (unique vs. multiple)	25.1 vs. 34.3	0.4284
Sex (women vs. men)	43.1 vs. 25	0.1381
Tumor size ($\geq$3 cm vs. >3 cm)	26.6 vs. 26.1	0.7421
Bladder Tis associated (yes vs. no)	31.9 vs. 25.6	0.3955
Treatment: TURB alone vs.	20.3 vs.	
TURB + chemotherapy vs.	36	0.0007
Radical cystectomy	31.2	0.0015
Multivariate analysis Variables	p value	Exp (B)
Biopsies of muscularis propria (tumor bed)	0.0007	2.6423

Table 16.7 Final outcome: sequential assessment

	Minimum months of follow-up						
	Initial (%)	$\geq$12 (%)	$\geq$24 (%)	$\geq$36 (%)	$\geq$60 (%)	$\geq$120 (%)	$\geq$180 (%)
Pts at risk	130	132	128	118	98	50	17
Progression	40 (30)	25 (18.9)	22 (17.2)	12 (10.1)	6 (6.1)	2 (4)	0
T$\geq$2,M0	33 (24.8)	19 (14.4)	19 (14.8)	12 (10.1)	6 (6.1)	2 (4)	0
T0,M1	7 (5.2)	6 (4.5)	3 (2.3)	0	0	0	0
Recurrence: T1A	40 (30)	26 (19.7)	18 (12.7)	15 (12.7)	8 (8.1)	8 (6)	0

The greatest concern associated with this approach is the progression rate: 34% in Herr's series[28] and 32% in Solsona et al's series.[27] It is important to clarify that some patients were understaged (invasive recurrence at the 3-month evaluation) and other patients developed true progression (after a disease-free interval).

Attempting to address both problems, Solsona et al carried out univariate and multivariate analyses including clinical–pathologic variables (Table 16.8).[22] Regarding true progression, the presence of carcinoma in situ (CIS) was the only significant variable in the multivariate analysis. However, this variable was clinically irrelevant since the biologic behavior of CIS in these patients was similar to that in patients with nonmuscle-invasive bladder tumors associated with CIS. In consequence, the initial presence of CIS is not an exclusion criterion for patients with muscle-invasive bladder tumors included in a bladder preservation program of radical TURB, but these patients do need intravesical bacillus Calmette–Guérin (BCG) as adjuvant therapy. The recurrence rate of nonmuscle-invasive bladder cancer was not very high in Solsona et al's and Herr's series and did not affect prognosis.[27,28] Therefore, intravesical therapy should be used only in patients with bladder-associated CIS and for patients that develop nonmuscle-invasive recurrences.

With respect to understaging, no single variable was statistically significant, but a relationship between tumor size and morphology was noted. Stratifying variables, such as tumor size of more than 3 cm and solid morphology had a close relationship to understaging, reaching statistical significance (p = 0.0236). When the primary tumor had a papillary morphology, size had no prognostic value (p = 0.647) following radical transurethral resection of bladder tumor (TURBT).[27] However, given the relationship with understaging, one must be very cautious about using radical TURB alone for patients with solid tumors of more than 3 cm.

In a separate analysis, p53 overexpression was tested in a pilot study of 60 patients in Solsona et al's series.[27] Among these patients, 10/18 (55.5%) with p53 overexpression and 16/42 (38%) with negative p53 developed progression. This difference was not statistically significant. Recently, Herr[28] observed a significantly superior local progression-free rate of 68% and survival of 82% in patients with no residual tumor (T0) upon repeat TURB versus 28% and 57%, respectively, in those with nonmuscle-invasive residual tumors (T1A). In summary, patients with invasive bladder cancer that are the best candidates for TURB as monotherapy are those patients with negative biopsies of the muscularis propria of the tumor bed or no residual tumor at repeat TURB after a macroscopically initial complete resection, regardless of size if the primary tumor is papillary, and less than 3 cm if the primary tumor is sessile.

Another concern is that some tumors might have been overstaged pathologically because of confusion between muscularis mucosae and muscularis propria. The histologic structures of muscularis mucosae and propria are different: smooth muscle fibers are associated with blood vessels in muscularis mucosae and thick muscle fibers in muscularis propria. However, in fragmented biopsies it is difficult to determine whether the smooth muscle present represents

Table 16.8 Predictive factors for progression differentiating between understaging (progression at 3-months' evaluation in the scar) and true progression (after a progression-free interval): univariate analysis

Univariate analysis Variables	True progression percentages (p value)	Understanding percentages (p value)
Tumor size (≤3 cm vs. >3 cm)	23.1 vs. 24.5 (0.813)	1.9 vs. 8.5 (0.057)
Age (≤65 vs. >65 years)	25 vs. 20.7 (0.791)	7.5 vs. 3.7 (0.652)
Grade (2 vs. 3)	20.3 vs. 26 (0.445)	1.5 vs. 10.1 (0.117)
Tumor morphology (papillary vs. sessile)	22.1 vs. 25 (0.517)	3.9 vs. 9.6 (0.135)
No. tumors (unique vs. multiples)	22.8 vs. 26.3 (0.968)	6.1 vs. 5.5 (0.532)
Primary vs. recurrent tumors	23.1 vs. 25 (0.698)	6.8 vs. 0 (0.250)
Sex (women vs. men)	13.9 vs. 18.7 (0.686)	12.5 vs. 5.1 (0.072)
Bladder Tis (yes vs. no)	17 vs. 42.4 (0.013)	6.9 vs. 3.1 (0.346)

Multivariate analysis: True progression Variable		
Bladder Tis	p value	Exp (B)
	0.026	2.27

muscularis mucosae or muscularis propria. The necessary presence of muscularis propria with no tumor invasion in the third sample from the fractionated TURB as an inclusion criterion is crucial in the differentiation between both muscular structures. Pathologists can compare the histologic structure of the muscle fibers from the third sample clearly as muscularis propria and the second sample which should include muscle fibers infiltrated by tumor.

Comments

The importance of these prospective studies is that they have been able to identify a group of patients with muscle-invasive bladder tumors whose survival rates are approximately equivalent to those of patients with P0 in cystectomy specimens. This select group of patients represents 21% and 19%, respectively, of patients with invasive bladder tumors treated at the Memorial Sloan-Kettering Cancer Center and the Instituto Valenciano de Oncología.

Whether radiochemotherapy associated with radical TURB might improve the outcome of radical TURB is not entirely clear. One of the most important aims of radiochemotherapy in combination with TURB is to eliminate residual tumor after TURB. The incidence of negative biopsies indicating persistent muscle-invasive cancer at the initial 3-month follow-up in Solsona et al's series was 6.7%.[26] Therefore, only a modest number of patients may have benefited from additional radiation and chemotherapy, while all of these patients would have suffered the toxicity and long-term side effects of these radiochemotherapy programs. In fact, radiochemotherapy programs have never been prospectively compared to radical TURB alone or to cystectomy.

In a recent meta-analysis the survival benefit of neoadjuvant chemotherapy programs was small but significant, i.e. 5%.[29]

The role of pelvic lymphadenectomy in this group of patients is also controversial. The incidence of lymph node metastases in patients with P2 ranges from 9.9% to 20%,[29,30–33] 12.6% in P2A tumors,[33] and from 0% to 5% in P0 tumors.[30,31] Because our patients are potentially those with P0 in the cystectomy specimen, the incidence of micrometastases in lymph nodes should be very low. This incidence could be included in the 5.2% of patients that develop distant metastases with no bladder-invasive recurrence and those with synchronous bladder tumors. Taking into account the low incidence of occult positive lymph nodes and that the 5-year survival rate ranges from 14% to 40% in cases of positive lymph nodes in patients treated with cystectomy and lymphadenectomy, in this selected group of invasive bladder cancer patients the potential survival benefit should be minimal, adding unnecessary morbidity in most of the patients.

Conclusion

The key to success of radical TURB is careful patient selection according to very strict inclusion criteria based upon fractionated TURB performed in patients suspected of having invasive bladder tumors including those with large papillary tumors, tumors with thick papillae, or sessile tumors less than 3 cm, or using a second TURB after a complete initial TURB as selection criteria. A second TURB with no tumor in chips, or with negative biopsies on muscular layer and perivesical fat of tumor bed, supports the use of radical TURB as initial monotherapy.

Regardless of these very careful patient selections, with long-term follow-up the progression rate is high. Consequently, a strict follow-up schedule is mandatory, particularly during the first 3 years. At the first endoscopic evaluation, a TURB of the scar tissue where the initial tumor was located is essential in order to preclude understaging. This approach achieves similar cause-specific survival for patients with P0 on cystectomy specimen.

In summary, a small and select group of patients with invasive bladder cancer, identified by a second TURB with no tumor in chips or with negative biopsies of the muscular layer and perivesical fat of the tumor bed, can be treated with TURB as an initial monotherapy.

References

1. Kachnic LA, Kaufmann DS, Griffin FF, et al. Bladder preservation by combined modality therapy for invasive bladder cancer. J Clin Oncol 1997; 15: 1022–9.
2. Rödel C, Grabenbauer GG, Kühn R, et al. Combined-modality treatment and selective organ preservation in invasive bladder cancer: long-term results. J Clin Oncol 2002; 20: 3061–71.

3. Sternberg CN, Pansadoro V, Calabro F, et al. Can patient selection for bladder preservation be based on response to chemotherapy? Cancer 2003; 97: 1644–52.

4. Barnes RW, Dick AL, Hadley HL, Johnston OL. Survival following transurethral resection of bladder carcinoma. Cancer Res 1977; 37: 2895–7.

5. Milner WA. The role of conservative surgery in the treatment of bladder tumours. Br J Urol 1954; 26: 375.

6. Dalbagni G, Genega E, Hashibe M, et al. Cystectomy for bladder cancer: a contemporary series. J Urol 2001; 165: 1111–16.

7. Frazier HA, Robertson JE, Dodge RK, Paulson DF. The value of pathological factors in predicting cancer-specific survival among patients treated with radical cystectomy for transitional cell carcinoma of the bladder and prostate. Cancer 1993; 71: 3993–4001.

8. Pagano F, Bassi P, Galetti TP, et al. Results of contemporary radical cystectomy for invasive bladder cancer: a clinicopathological study with an emphasis on the inadequacy of the tumor, nodes, and metastasis classification. J Urol 1991; 145: 45–50.

9. Stein JP, Lieskosvsky G, Cote R, et al. Radical cystectomy in the treatment of invasive bladder cancer: long-term results in 1054 patients. J Clin Oncol 2001; 19: 666–75.

10. Brendler C, Steinberg GD, Marshall FF, Mostwin JL, Walsh PC. Local recurrence and survival following nerve-sparing radical cystoprostatectomy. J Urol 1990; 144: 1137–40.

11. Mathur VK, Krahn HP, Ramsey EW. Total cystectomy for bladder cancer. J Urol 1981; 125: 784–86.

12. Stein JP, Freeman JA, Boyd SD, et al. Radical cystectomy in the treatment of invasive bladder cancer: long-term results in a large group of patients. J Urol 1998; 159: 213.

13. Thrasher JB, Frazier HA, Robertson JE, Paulson DF. Does stage pT0 cystectomy specimen confer a survival advantage in patients with minimally invasive bladder cancer? J Urol 1994; 152: 393–96.

14. Fung CY, Shipley WU, Young RH, et al. Prognostic factors in invasive bladder carcinoma in a prospective trial of preoperative adjuvant chemotherapy and radiotherapy. J Clin Oncol 1991; 9: 1533–42.

15. Dunst J, Rodel C, Zietman A, Schrott KM, Sauer R, Shipley WU. Bladder preservation in muscle-invasive bladder cancer by conservative surgery and radiochemotherapy. Semin Surg Oncol 2001; 20: 24–32.

16. Fossa SD, Waehre H, Aass N, Jacobsen AB, Olsen DR, Ous S. Bladder cancer definitive radiation therapy of muscle-invasive bladder cancer. A retrospective analysis of 317 patients. Cancer 1993; 72: 3036–43.

17. Gospodarowicz MK, Hawkins NV, Rawlings GA, et al. Radical radiotherapy for muscle invasive transitional cell carcinoma of the bladder: failure analysis. J Urol 1989; 142: 1488–1453.

18. Holmäng S, Hedelin H, Anderstrom C, Johansson SL. Long-term followup of all patients with muscle invasive (stages T2, T3 and T4) bladder carcinoma in a geographical region. J Urol 1997; 158: 389–92.

19. Henry K, Miller J, Mori M, Loening S, Fallon B. Comparison of transurethral resection to radical therapies for stage B bladder tumors. J Urol 1988; 140: 964–67.

20. Barnes RW, Bergman RT, Hadley HL, Love D. Control of bladder tumors by endoscopic surgery. J Urol 1967; 97: 864.

21. Flocks RH. Treatment of patients with carcinoma of the bladder. JAMA 1951; 145: 295–301.

22. Kondas J, Vaczi L, Scecso L, Konder G. Transurethral resection for muscle-invasive bladder cancer. Int Urol Nephrol 1993; 25: 557–567.

23. O'Flynn JD, Smith JD, Hanson JS. Transurethral resection for the assessment and treatment of vesical neoplasms. A review of 800 consecutive cases. Eur Urol 1975; 1: 38.

24. Marderbacher S, Hochreiter W, Bukhard F, Thalmenn GN, Danuse H, Studer U. Radical cystectomy for bladder cancer today—a homogeneous series without neo-adjuvant therapy. J Clin Oncol 2003; 21: 690–96.

25. Herr HW. Conservative treatment of muscle-infiltrating bladder cancer prospective experience. J Urol 1987; 138: 1162–63.

26. Solsona E, Iborra I, Ricós JV, Monrós JL, Dumont R. Feasibility of transurethral resection for muscle-infiltrating carcinoma of the bladder: prospective study. J Urol 1992; 147: 1513.

27. Solsona E, Iborra I, Ricós JV, Monrós JL, Casanova J, Calabuig C. Feasibility of transurethral resection for muscle infiltrating carcinoma of the bladder: long-term followup of a prospective study. J Urol 1998; 159: 95–98; discussion 98–99.

28. Herr HW. Transurethral resection of muscle-invasive bladder cancer: 10-year outcome. J Clin Oncol 2001; 19: 89–93.

29. (No authors) Neoadjuvant chemotherapy in invasive bladder cancer: a systematic review and meta-analysis. Lancet 2003; 361: 1927–34.

30. Lerner SP, Skinner DG, Lieskovsky G, et al. The rationale for en bloc pelvic lymph node dissection for bladder cancer patients with nodal metastases: long-term results. J Urol 1993; 149: 758–64; discussion 764–65.

31. Poulsen AL, Horn T, Steven K. Radical cystectomy extending the limits of pelvic lymph node dissection improves survival for patients with bladder confined to the bladder wall. J Urol 1998; 160: 2015–20.

32. Vieweg J, Gschwend JE, Herr HW, Fair WR. Pelvic lymph node dissection can be curative in patients with node positive bladder cancer. J Urol 1999; 161: 449–54.

33. Leissner J, Hohenfellner R, Thuroff JW, Wolf HK. Lymphadenectomy in patients with transitional cell carcinoma of the urinary bladder; significance for staging and prognosis. BJU Int 2000; 85: 817–23.

17

Partial cystectomy

Yair Lotan, David A Swanson, Arthur I Sagalowsky

Introduction

Bladder cancer is the fourth most common cancer in men (6%) and the tenth most common cancer in women (2%), accounting in men for 3% of cancer deaths in the year 2004 in the US.[1] On average, 15% to 30% of all patients with bladder cancer are diagnosed with muscle-invasive tumors and radical cystectomy represents the gold standard therapy.[2] In an effort to reduce the morbidity of radical cystectomy, attempts have been made to utilize bladder-preserving therapy such as aggressive transurethral resection (TUR) followed by combined chemotherapy/radiotherapy or partial cystectomy. The advantage of partial cystectomy over TUR is that it allows for complete pathologic staging of the tumor and pelvic lymph nodes with preservation of normal bladder and sexual function. The popularity of this procedure peaked in the 1950s and 1960s, but reports in the 1970s emphasized the problems, particularly high recurrence rates. Unfortunately, partial cystectomy virtually disappeared thereafter, despite the fact that good results are possible, even with T2 and T3 tumors. Many of the recurrences were due, not to incomplete removal of tumor, but to the appearance of new tumors, suggesting that patient selection is critically important to the potential for success of partial cystectomy.[3–7]

Although partial cystectomy can be performed when adequate transurethral biopsy cannot be confidently performed because of location or other considerations, and it may be appropriate as palliative therapy in highly selected patients instead of radical cystectomy, our discussion in this chapter will focus on its potential to provide definitive therapy for transitional carcinoma of the bladder.

Indications

As stated, the most important factor in performing a successful partial cystectomy is proper patient selection. Bladder cancer is an aggressive disease that places the entire urothelium at risk. Once it metastasizes, treatment options such as radical cystectomy, radiotherapy, and systemic chemotherapy do not significantly change the overall survival rates.[8,9] Accordingly, the best opportunity to cure patients of their disease is offering the appropriate treatment at the start of therapy. In fact, a review of the literature concluded that only 5.8% to 18.9% of patients with muscle-invasive bladder cancer were suited for partial cystectomy, and that would be considered too permissive by many.[10] Another study evaluating initial management of all stages of bladder cancer in Canada found that only 3.5% of cases underwent partial cystectomy or open excision as their initial treatment.[11] At The University of Texas M.D. Anderson Cancer Center, 842 radical cystectomies were performed between January 1982 and

January 1993. In that same period, 36 patients (4.1% of all patients requiring extirpative surgery) underwent partial cystectomy as a planned procedure, selected with intent to cure, because radical cystectomy was deemed unnecessary to remove all tumor.

In well-selected patients, partial cystectomy offers outcomes equivalent to those of radical cystectomy. Early recurrences are due to incomplete tumor excision, either because of unrecognized tumor or inadequate surgical margins. Conceptually, radical cystectomy is simply a partial cystectomy with the widest possible margins! New tumors in the remnant bladder, obviously an argument for removing the entire bladder, can be minimized by selecting patients with a solitary tumor and no antecedent history of prior transitional carcinoma of the bladder. Candidates for partial cystectomy should have a solitary lesion in the mobile portion of the bladder (particularly the dome and posterior wall) where it is possible to resect the tumor with a margin of at least 2 cm. As such, larger lesions increase the difficulty of complete resection with negative margins and there is a practical limit to the size of lesion that will allow for a partial cystectomy. While the need for ureteral reimplantation can increase the difficulty of the procedure, it is not an absolute contraindication.[12] Although there is no intrinsic reason for not permitting ureteral reimplantation, it is a strong relative contraindication because it provides an added check that the tumor is located in an appropriate position to ensure success. The surgeon will not be tempted to offer it to patients whose tumor is on the bladder base (where the results have been historically poorer), and will not be tempted to 'cheat' and take <2 cm margin of normal mucosa around the tumor to avoid reimplanting the ureter. Evaluation should be performed either cystoscopically or with random bladder biopsies to confirm that all other areas in the bladder have normal mucosa. Furthermore, patients should have a good bladder capacity with a normally functioning bladder.

Those patients with urachal adenocarcinomas, or tumors in bladder diverticula, represent special categories of patients that may specifically benefit from partial cystectomy. Some previous reports also recommended partial cystectomy for tumors that are inaccessible to TUR or large enough to make TUR technically difficult.[12] However, as stated earlier, if partial cystectomy is being offered to such patients, they should fulfill the other criteria of first tumor, solitary tumor, and tumor located where it is possible to achieve a 2 cm margin. Sternberg et al recommended using response to chemotherapy as the basis for selecting patients for partial cystectomy.[13] Only those patients that attained a complete or partial response to combination chemotherapy (methotrexate, vinblastine, adriamycin (doxorubicin), and cisplatin: MVAC) with solitary lesions in favorable anatomic locations were eligible for partial cystectomy but the results were reasonably good. Similarly, Herr and Scher recommended somewhat expanding the indications for performing partial cystectomy in patients that responded well to neoadjuvant chemotherapy.[14]

The main contraindications to partial cystectomy include the presence of carcinoma in situ (CIS) and multifocal disease, as well as a history of prior tumors. The risk of developing recurrence increases with the presence of multicentric disease (p < 0.03) and when neoplasm is found at the margin of resection (p < 0.05).[3,15]

Cancer in bladder diverticulum

Because of the absence of a muscular layer, resection of cancer in a bladder diverticulum is difficult and carries a high risk of perforation. These cancers are also prone to early metastases.[16–18] Partial cystectomy offers a good treatment option for patients with isolated tumors in a diverticulum or those difficult to resect. It is important that they fulfill the other criteria for a partial cystectomy including a solitary lesion with negative random biopsies, no prior history of bladder tumors, and the ability to achieve a 2 cm negative margin. Furthermore, partial cystectomy is not ideal for large high-grade or invasive tumor, as the most important predictor of outcome is the stage of the tumor.[19] In order to improve outcomes, Garzotto et al recommended combining partial cystectomy with chemotherapy or radiation therapy.[20] Unfortunately, there are no randomized trials comparing combination therapies with partial cystectomy due to the infrequent nature of cancers in bladder diverticula.

Non-transitional cell carcinoma

Partial cystectomy has been utilized successfully for management of nontransitional cell carcinoma of the bladder. A multitude of case reports describe the use of partial cystectomy for benign lesions such as leiomyoma,[21] inflammatory pseudotumor,[22] neurofibroma,[23] pheochromocytoma,[24] and paragangliomas.[25] While partial cystectomy has been used for treatment of bladder sarcomas, recurrences have been reported, and these tumors should be widely excised.[26,27]

Partial cystectomy can also be necessary[27] in cases with non-urologic malignancies such as locally advanced colorectal carcinoma. If clear margins are achievable then those patients can have good local control without sacrificing survival.[28,29]

Adenocarcinoma and urachal tumors

Adenocarcinomas of the bladder are rare and often aggressive cancers. They can be primary or urachal in origin.[30] In one of the largest series of adenocarcinoma of the bladder (n=185), el-Mekresh and colleagues found an overall 5-year disease-free survival of 55%.[31] Only three factors had a significant impact on survival: the tumor pathologic stage, grade of the tumor, and lymph node involvement. They recommended radical cystectomy over partial cystectomy in managing these tumors. While partial cystectomy was appropriate for some patients, Xiaoxu et al also found poor 3-year survival rates (33%) after partial cystectomy for primary adenocarcinoma of the bladder.[32]

There is generally less controversy about performing partial cystectomy for urachal tumors, in large part because they commonly appear in a location where the procedure is technically possible. In evaluating the surgical management of urachal tumors at the Mayo Clinic, Henly et al found that these cancers comprised only 0.22% of bladder cancers diagnosed at their institution over a 35-year period.[33] They found no difference in 5-year survival of patients with partial and those with radical cystectomy (43% and 50%, respectively). They attributed the low survival to the aggressiveness of the disease. Herr recommended performing an extended partial cystectomy, including complete excision of the umbilicus, overlying peritoneum, and posterior rectus fascia lateral to the medial obliterated umbilical ligaments.[34] He found that 10 of 12 patients were free of disease at 1–13 years with no recurrences in bladder or pelvis. Santucci and coauthors also found that 88% of patients (n=16) with well-differentiated colonic-type adenocarcinomas of the urachus were cured by partial cystectomy.[35]

Preoperative considerations

The main objective of preoperative evaluation is proper staging of the bladder tumor. Cystoscopy with random bladder biopsy can help exclude patients with multifocal disease or CIS. Bimanual examination under anesthesia allows for evaluation of the extent of tumor involvement and bladder mobility. When there is a concern regarding bladder function, an evaluation of bladder capacity is in order. Preoperative testing should include a computed tomography (CT) scan and chest radiograph to look for evidence of metastatic disease. The overall health of the patient should also be assessed in determining appropriateness of surgical intervention.

Surgical technique

The surgical technique has been well described elsewhere.[10,36,37] The main objectives include:

1. bilateral pelvic lymphadenectomy
2. full mobilization of the bladder with ligation of the superior vesical artery on the affected side or the vas deferens, if necessary
3. identification of the tumor either cystoscopically or through a small vertical cystotomy in order to avoid cutting across tumor
4. excision of the tumor with a clear 2 cm margin of normal bladder
5. watertight closure of the bladder and pelvic drain. A Foley catheter is preferred over a suprapubic tube due to the risk of spilling tumor cells into the pelvis or along the suprapubic tube tract.

One of us (DAS) believes strongly that the procedure should be done extraperitoneally.

After mobilizing the anterior and lateral aspects of the bladder, the surgeon should peel the parietal peritoneum from the bladder with blunt and sharp dissection, leaving the peritoneum attached only over the area adjacent to the tumor (Figure 17.1). Next, the peritoneum is cut so that a patch is left adherent to the bladder overlying the tumor. The peritoneal defect is closed, and the peritoneum and contents are packed out of the way, converting the remainder of the operation to an extravesical one before the cystotomy is performed.

Of concern during partial cystectomy is recurrence of disease in the wound or pelvis secondary to spillage of tumor cells during surgery. Recurrence rates range from 0% to 40% and can lead to significant morbidity and mortality (Table 17.1). While most authors recommend only carefully packing the pelvis to prevent tumor spill from the bladder, that approach protects the pelvis better than the wound, and several other techniques have been advocated. In one

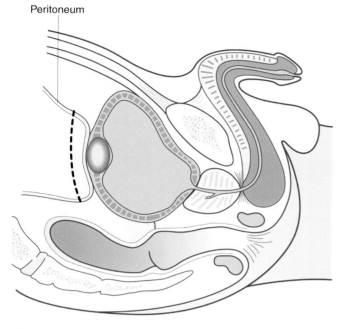

Peritoneum

Figure 17.1
The appearance after dissecting the peritoneum off the bladder except for that portion overlying the tumor. The peritoneum is then opened (dashed line), a peritoneal patch left attached to the bladder over the tumor, and the peritoneal defect closed.

approach, the area of tumor is identified endoscopically, and clamps (e.g. Pean or Satinsky) are used to isolate the area of bladder that is to be excised. The tumor is removed and the cut edge is oversewn without opening the bladder.[38] During this maneuver, one surgeon identifies the tumor cystoscopically while the other places clamps that exclude the tumor with a 2 cm margin. Two sets of clamps are used with one closing the normal bladder and the other closing the tumor side. This prevents spillage of cancer cells as the tumor is excised. Other recommendations include the instillation of intravesical chemotherapy such as mitomycin C into the bladder prior to beginning the procedure to reduce the number of viable cancer cells.[38] While the evidence for benefit of such an approach is sparse, mitomycin C has been shown to prevent bladder tumor cell implantation and reduce recurrence of superficial bladder cancers.[39-41] One caveat, however, is that it is important to irrigate the bladder carefully before opening it to prevent systemic absorption of the intravesical agent.

Postoperative Complications

Complications after partial cystectomy can be divided into those that occur perioperatively (<30 days) and those that appear long term (>30 days). Operative mortality is less than 5% in most large series but has been reported as high as 20% (see Table 17.1). These series are not contemporary, however, and there is no reason to believe the mortality should be any higher than for radical cystectomy, and is probably lower.

Urinary leakage from the bladder closure is not infrequent and can usually be managed conservatively.[36,42] Other complications include wound infection, which rarely can lead to sepsis. Cases of bladder wall necrosis leading to vesicocutaneous fistulas and peritonitis have also been reported, but not recently.[12] When the ureter

Table 17.1 Partial cystectomy series with operative mortality and recurrence rates

Authors	Years of accrual	No. pts	Operative mortality (%)	Overall recurrence (%)	Wound recurrence (%)	Bladder recurrence (%)
Dandekar et al[42]	1984–1993	32	3.1	43.8	0	43.8% (n=14/32); Bladder (n=12/32); Superficial (n=5); Invasive (n=7); Distant (n=2)
Kaneti[15]	25 years	62	1.6	38.0	NA	41 patients received postoperative XRT, only 1 needed cystectomy
Lindahl et al[12]	1958–1978	55	7.3	58.0	NA	NA
Schoborg et al[44]	1955–1975	45	4.4	70.0	NA	NA
Faysal & Freiha[7]	1962–1977	117	0.0	78.0	3.4	54 patients received XRT; 14 patients had cystectomy and 9 had salvage cystectomy
Merrell et al[47]	1958–1973	54	NA	29.0	NA	10 had XRT and 2 had cystectomy
Brannan et al[48]	1950–1974	49	2.0	NA	0	12 patients received XRT with 5 receiving salvage cystectomy
Cummings et al[4]	1945–1971	101	0.0	49.0	NA	NA
Novick & Stewart[3]	1960–1972	50	0.0	50 (n=25)	NA	15 patients had pelvic recurrence or metastases
Evans & Texter[49]	25 years	47	0.0	NA	NA	10 patients with repeat partial cystectomy and 8 patients requiring cystectomy
Utz et al[5]	1945–1965	153	3.0	NA	2	50
Resnick & O'Conor[6]	1955–1965	102	NA	75.6	7.8	Overall (75.6%); resection margin recurrence (29.4%)
Long et al[50]	1940–1971	27	20.0	NA	40	NA
Magri[43]	1952–1959	104	9.6	32.7	11.5	21.2

NA, not applicable; XRT, radiotherapy.

has been reimplanted, ureteric fistulae and ureteral anastomotic strictures have occurred.[15]

Decreased bladder capacity can cause problems with bladder function. Cummings et al found that 18% (19/101) of their patients experienced compromised bladder function with significant irritative symptoms, with five patients requiring palliative diversion.[4]

Follow-up and outcomes

The use of perioperative radiation therapy as an adjuvant to partial cystectomy has been shown to improve survival in some series[43] but to have no benefit in others.[5,6] It should be emphasized, however, that most of the papers discussing preoperative radiation therapy were written in an era when this approach was common, if not standard, for patients undergoing extirpative surgery for bladder cancer—including radical cystectomy. One difficulty in assessing benefits of adjuvant radiation therapy is the significant selection bias in treating those patients more likely to have recurrence[4,5,44] as well as treating patients only after they show evidence of local recurrence.[6] The important fact to remember is that it is possible to

perform partial cystectomy safely after preoperative doses up to 5000 cGy, and possibly higher, as long as the bladder volume is sufficient. Even after 5000 cGy, the bladder will usually expand with time to approach normal volumes, although this is less likely after higher preoperative doses.

Patients with bladder cancer undergoing partial cystectomy require close monitoring. Overall recurrence rates have been reported from 29% to 78% (see Table 17.1). Most recurrences are new tumors and occur in the bladder secondary to the multifocal nature of bladder cancer. Consequently, cystoscopy and cytology should be continued at 3-month intervals for at least 2 years, and then at appropriate intervals thereafter on a schedule similar to that for tumors managed endoscopically.[36] Unfortunately, patients may experience distant metastases, especially with high-grade and high-stage tumors, and regular CT scans of the abdomen and pelvis, plus chest x-rays, are recommended.

Survival for patients with bladder cancer who undergo partial cystectomy depends on the grade and stage of the tumor (Table 17.2). Overall, 5-year survival ranging from 40% to 80% has been reported in various series and depends on the stage distribution of bladder cancer in the study cohort. Patients with low-grade and low-stage tumors have the best overall survival.[12] It should be emphasized,

Table 17.2 Partial cystectomy series with 5- and 10-year survival rates

Authors	No. pts	5-year survival (overall %)	A	B1	B2	C	D	10-year survival
Dandekar et al[42]	32	80.1		T2=100% (n=5)	T3a=88.5% (n=18)	T3b=45.7% (n=9)		NA
Kaneti15	62	50.0	0–A=68% (n=15/23)	B=40% (n=8/20)		33% (n=26)	0% (n=0/3)	22
Lindahl et al[12]	55	47.1						35.4
Schoborg et al[44]	45	NA	0–A=69% (n=9/13)	29% (n=2/7)	50% (n=3/6)	12% (n=2/17)	100% (n=1/1)	0–A=37% (n=3/8); B1=0% (n=0/5); B2=20% (n=1/5); C=0% (n=0/15); D=0% (n=0/1)
Faysal & Freiha[7]	117	40.0	58% (n=7/12)	29% (n=4/14)	32% (n=8/25)	7% (n=1/15)	0% (n=0/2)	NA
Merrell et al[47]	54	48.0		67% (n=21)	37% (n=16)	25% (n=8)	0% (n=5)	Overall=30%; B1=33% (n=18); B2=25% (n=12); C=0% (n=2); D=0% (n=3)
Brannan et al[48]	49	57.7	68.8% (n=11/16)	54.5% (n=6/11)	62.5% (n=5/8)	33% (n=3/9)		Overall=32.4%; A=45.5% (n=5/11); B1=44.4% (n=4/9); B2=20% (n=1/5); C=11% (n=1/9)
Cummings et al[4]	101	60.0	79% (n=23/29)	80% (n=17/21)	45% (n=10/22)	6% (n=1/17)		NA
Novick & Stewart[3]	50	NA	67% (n=10/15)	B=53% (n=8/15)		17% (n=1/6)	25% (n=1/4)	A=67% (n=4/6); B=44% (n=4/9); C=0% (n=0/3); D=0% (n=0/4)
Evans & Texter[49]	47	46.7	68% (n=17/26)	42% (n=3/7)	14% (n=1/7)	0% (n=0/7)		NA
Utz et al[5]	153	43.3	68% (n=17/26)	47% (n=18/38)	40% (n=14/35)	29% (n=11/38)	0% (n=0/19)	NA
Resnick & O'Conor[6]	102	41.9	70.7% (n=17/24)	76.9% (n=10/13)	18.3% (n=3/16)	13% (n=2/7)	20% (n=1/5)	NA
Long et al[50]	27	NA	75% (n=6)	48% (n=7)	23% (n=5)	11% (n=11)		NA
Magri[43]	104	41.8	Ta=80% (8/10)	T2=38.4% (10/26)		T3=26.3% (5/19)		NA

NA, not applicable.

however, that even T2 and T3 tumors can be controlled with partial cystectomy if all tumor is excised. For adverse prognostic features such as extensive invasion of the perivesical fat or nodal metastases, adjuvant chemotherapy is appropriate, as it would be if the patient had undergone a radical cystectomy.

The experience at the M.D. Anderson Cancer Center illustrates the potential efficacy of partial cystectomy for muscle-invasive tumors. From January 1982 through July 1996, 24 patients with muscle-invasive tumors (transitional cell carcinoma 23, squamous cell carcinoma 1) underwent partial cystectomy as definitive therapy with intent to cure. There were 13 patients with T2, four with T3a, and seven with T3b tumors. With a median follow-up of 36 months (range 6–165), of 17 patients with no bladder recurrences, four died of intercurrent disease, and two of metastatic bladder cancer. Eleven patients were alive, although, in truth, three patients were at risk for recurrence for <12 months. Seven patients had recurrent tumors in their bladder remnants:

- two were treated with TUR-BT ± Bacillus Calmette–Guérin (BCG) and remain clinically free of disease (NED)
- two were NED after delayed radical cystectomy
- one received MVAC adjuvant chemotherapy for N1 disease with good response
- two patients, however, died of metastatic disease after late recurrence.

Patient P.L.M. received five courses of adjuvant MVAC after partial cystectomy for pT3b tumor with vascular invasion. He had a grade 2 Ta solitary recurrence 33 months after partial cystectomy, and a grade 3 T1 recurrence 8 months after that. Evaluation soon afterwards revealed metastases to lungs, bones, adrenal gland, and retroperitoneal lymph nodes, and he died 43 months after his original surgery.

Patient J.E.H. underwent partial cystectomy for T3b tumor, followed by five courses of CISCA (cisplatin, cyclophosphamide (Cytoxan), adriamycin). He did well until 89 months later at which time he had a grade 3 T1 recurrence, which was treated with TUR-BT and BCG. Fifty months later, his cytology became positive, and he was found to have transitional cell carcinoma in the prostatic ducts and stroma, with positive pelvic lymph nodes found on CT scan. He underwent salvage chemotherapy and became clinically NED; TUR biopsy of the prostate revealed only a single focus of transitional cell carcinoma in the prostatic ducts. However, salvage surgery was delayed for medical reasons and he developed bony metastases 156 months after his partial cystectomy. He died of disease shortly thereafter.

Conclusion

Considering the relatively poor survival outcomes for patients with partial cystectomy historically, it can be concluded that patient selection is critical in determining the best treatment course for patients with invasive bladder cancer. Bladder preservation with partial cystectomy and combined therapy, either neoadjuvant or adjuvant chemotherapy, or possibly combined trimodality surgery–chemotherapy–radiation therapy, may improve survival outcomes in selected patients.[13,14,45,46] It is apparent that some patients, even with T2 or T3 tumors if solitary and without prior history of bladder cancer, can be treated successfully with partial cystectomy with or without adjuvant therapy, but they are still at risk of developing

recurrent bladder cancer. Although many of the recurrences will be superficial and potentially manageable endoscopically, some will be invasive and some patients may develop metastatic disease. It is *critically* important that all patients treated for T2 or T3 disease with partial cystectomy be followed with regular cystoscopies and urinary cytologies for their *lifetimes*. If invasive disease occurs, delayed radical cystectomy is the most conservative approach. Nonetheless, with the appropriate caveats, partial cystectomy can be effective therapy for 3% to 4% of patients that need extirpative surgery for bladder cancer, and many patients are very grateful for the opportunity to preserve normal bladder and sexual function.

References

1. Jemal A, Tiwari RC, Murray T, et al. Cancer statistics, 2004. CA Cancer J Clin 2004; 54: 8–29.
2. Lerner SP, Skinner E, Skinner DG. Radical cystectomy in regionally advanced bladder cancer. Urol Clin North Am 1992; 19: 713–23.
3. Novick AC, Stewart BH. Partial cystectomy in the treatment of primary and secondary carcinoma of the bladder. J Urol 1976; 116: 570–74.
4. Cummings KB, Mason JT, Correa RJ Jr, Gibbons RP. Segmental resection in the management of bladder carcinoma. J Urol 1978; 119: 56–58.
5. Utz DC, Schmitz SE, Fugelso PD, Farrow GM. Proceedings: a clinicopathologic evaluation of partial cystectomy for carcinoma of the urinary bladder. Cancer 1973; 32: 1075–77.
6. Resnick MI, O'Conor VJ Jr. Segmental resection for carcinoma of the bladder: review of 102 patients. J Urol 1973; 109: 1007–10.
7. Faysal MH, Freiha FS. Evaluation of partial cystectomy for carcinoma of bladder. Urology 1979;14: 352–356.
8. Borden LS Jr, Clark PE, Hall MC. Bladder cancer. Curr Opin Oncol 2003; 15: 227–233.
9. Pashos CL, Botteman MF, Laskin BL, Redaelli A. Bladder cancer: epidemiology, diagnosis, and management. Cancer Pract 2002; 10: 311–22.
10. Sweeney P, Kursh ED, Resnick MI. Partial cystectomy. Urol Clin North Am 1992; 19: 701–11.
11. Hayter CR, Paszat LF, Groome PA, Schulze K, Mackillop WJ. The management and outcome of bladder carcinoma in Ontario, 1982–1994. Cancer 2000; 89: 142–51.
12. Lindahl F, Jorgensen D, Egvad K. Partial cystectomy for transitional cell carcinoma of the bladder. Scand J Urol Nephrol 1984; 18: 125–29.
13. Sternberg CN, Pansadoro V, Calabro F, et al. Can patient selection for bladder preservation be based on response to chemotherapy? Cancer 2003; 97: 1644–52.
14. Herr HW, Scher HI. Neoadjuvant chemotherapy and partial cystectomy for invasive bladder cancer. J Clin Oncol 1994; 12: 975–80.
15. Kaneti J. Partial cystectomy in the management of bladder carcinoma. Eur Urol 1986; 12: 249–52.
16. Das S, Amar A D. Vesical diverticulum associated with bladder carcinoma: therapeutic implications. J Urol 1986; 136: 1013–4.
17. Yu CC, Huang JK, Lee YH, Chen KK, Chen MT, Chang LS. Intradiverticular tumors of the bladder: surgical implications—an eleven-year review. Eur Urol 1993; 24: 190–96.
18. Melekos MD, Asbach HW, Barbalias GA. Vesical diverticula: etiology, diagnosis, tumorigenesis, and treatment. Analysis of 74 cases. Urology 1987; 30: 453–7.
19. Golijanin D, Yossepowitch O, Beck SD, Sogani P, Dalbagni G. Carcinoma in a bladder diverticulum: presentation and treatment outcome. J Urol 2003; 170: 1761–4.
20. Garzotto MG, Tewari A, Wajsman Z. Multimodal therapy for neoplasms arising from a vesical diverticulum. J Surg Oncol 1996; 62: 46.
21. Sakellariou P, Protopapas A, Kyritsis N, Voulgaris Z, Papaspirou E, Diakomanolis E. Intramural leiomyoma of the bladder. Eur Radiol 2000; 10: 906–8.

22. Poon KS, Moreira O, Jones EC, Treissman S, Gleave ME. Inflammatory pseudotumor of the urinary bladder: a report of five cases and review of the literature. Can J Urol 2001; 8: 1409–15.

23. Cheng L, Scheithauer BW, Leibovich BC, et al. Neurofibroma of the urinary bladder. Cancer 1999; 86: 505–13.

24. Kozlowski PM, Mihm F, Winfield HN. Laparoscopic management of bladder pheochromocytoma. Urology 2001; 57: 365.

25. Cheng L, Leibovich BC, Cheville JC, et al. Paraganglioma of the urinary bladder: can biologic potential be predicted? Cancer 2000; 88: 844–52.

26. Iczkowski KA, Shanks JH, Gadaleanu V, et al. Inflammatory pseudotumor and sarcoma of urinary bladder: differential diagnosis and outcome in thirty-eight spindle cell neoplasms. Mod Pathol 2001; 14: 1043–51.

27. Martin SA, Sears DL, Sebo TJ, Lohse CM, Cheville JC. Smooth muscle neoplasms of the urinary bladder: a clinicopathologic comparison of leiomyoma and leiomyosarcoma. Am J Surg Pathol 2002; 26: 292–300.

28. Balbay MD, Slaton JW, Trane N, Skibber J, Dinney CP. Rationale for bladder-sparing surgery in patients with locally advanced colorectal carcinoma. Cancer 1999; 86: 2212–16.

29. Weinstein RP, Grob BM, Pachter EM, Soloway S, Fair WR. Partial cystectomy during radical surgery for nonurological malignancy. J Urol 2001; 166: 79–81.

30. Burnett AL, Epstein JI, Marshall FF. Adenocarcinoma of urinary bladder: classification and management. Urology 1991; 37: 315–21.

31. el-Mekresh MM, el-Baz MA, Abol-Enein H, Ghoneim MA. Primary adenocarcinoma of the urinary bladder: a report of 185 cases. Br J Urol 1998; 82: 206–16.

32. Xiaoxu L, Jianhong L, Jinfeng W, Klotz LH. Bladder adenocarcinoma: 31 reported cases. Can J Urol 2001; 8(5): 1380–3.

33. Henly DR, Farrow GM, Zincke H. Urachal cancer: role of conservative surgery. Urology 1993; 42: 635–9.

34. Herr HW. Urachal carcinoma: the case for extended partial cystectomy. J Urol 1994; 151: 365–6.

35. Santucci RA, True LD, Lange PH. Is partial cystectomy the treatment of choice for mucinous adenocarcinoma of the urachus? Urology 1997; 49: 536–40.

36. Jiminez VK, Marshall FF. Surgery of bladder cancer. In Walsh PC, Retik AB, Stamey TA, Vaughan (eds): Campbell's Urology. Philadelphia: Saunders, 2002, p 2841.

37. Boileau MA. Segmental or partial cystectomy. In Johnson DE, Boileau MA (eds): Genitourinary Tumors: Fundamental Principles and Surgical Techniques. New York: Grune & Stratton, 1982, p 457.

38. Haddad FS. Partial cystectomy for bladder cancer. A new technique. Urology 1991; 38: 458–9.

39. Pode D, Horowitz AT, Vlodavsky I, Shapiro A, Biran S. Prevention of human bladder tumor cell implantation in an in vitro assay. J Urol 1987; 137: 777–81.

40. Zincke H, Benson RC Jr, Hilton JF, Taylor WF. Intravesical thiotepa and mitomycin C treatment immediately after transurethral resection and later for superficial (stages Ta and Tis) bladder cancer: a prospective, randomized, stratified study with crossover design. J Urol 1985; 134: 1110–14.

41. Solsona E, Iborra I, Ricos JV, Monros JL, Casanova J, Dumont R. Effectiveness of a single immediate mitomycin C instillation in patients with low risk superficial bladder cancer: short and long-term followup. J Urol 1999; 161: 1120–3.

42. Dandekar NP, Tongaonkar HB, Dalal AV, Kulkarni JN, Kamat MR. Partial cystectomy for invasive bladder cancer. J Surg Oncol 1995; 60: 24–9.

43. Magri J. Partial cystectomy: a review of 104 cases. Br J Urol 1962; 34: 74–87.

44. Schoborg TW, Sapolsky JL, Lewis CW Jr. Carcinoma of the bladder treated by segmental resection. J Urol 1979; 122: 473–5.

45. Angulo JC, Sanchez-Chapado M, Lopez JI, Flores N. Primary cisplatin, methotrexate and vinblastine aiming at bladder preservation in invasive bladder cancer: multivariate analysis on prognostic factors. J Urol 1996; 155: 1897–902.

46. Sternberg CN, Arena MG, Calabresi F, et al. Neoadjuvant M-VAC (methotrexate, vinblastine, doxorubicin, and cisplatin) for infiltrating transitional cell carcinoma of the bladder. Cancer 1993; 72: 1975–82.

47. Merrell RW, Brown HE, Rose JF. Bladder carcinoma treated by partial cystectomy: a review of 54 cases. J Urol 1979; 122: 471–2.

48. Brannan W, Ochsner MG, Fuselier HA Jr, Landry GR. Partial cystectomy in the treatment of transitional cell carcinoma of the bladder. J Urol 1978; 119: 213–15.

49. Evans RA, Texter JH Jr. Partial cystectomy in the treatment of bladder cancer. J Urol 1975; 114: 391–93.

50. Long RT, Grummon RA, Spratt JS Jr, Perez-Mesa C. Carcinoma of the urinary bladder. Comparison with radical, simple, and partial cystectomy and intravesical formalin. Cancer 1972; 29: 98–105.

18

Optimal radiotherapy for bladder cancer

Michael F Milosevic, Robert Bristow, Mary K Gospodarowicz

Introduction

There is extensive experience using radiation, either alone or in combination with surgery or chemotherapy to treat muscle-invasive bladder cancer. The goal of radiation treatment is to eradicate the tumor while preserving the structure and function of the bladder and other surrounding normal tissues. The utility of radiation in treating cancer arises because of differences in the radiation response of tumors and normal tissues. In general, tumor cells are less able than normal cells to repair DNA damage produced by radiation. DNA and other intracellular damage from radiation induce downstream molecular events leading to cell death. Differences in the molecular and cellular radiation responses of malignant and normal tissues result in a favorable therapeutic ratio. The tumoricidal effects of carefully planned and delivered radiation treatment should outweigh the potential for serious toxicity to normal surrounding tissues. Advances in high-precision, image-guided radiotherapy, coupled with an improved understanding of bladder cancer radiobiology and specific targeting of molecular pathways that contribute to radiation resistance, have the potential to dramatically improve tumor control in bladder cancer patients while maintaining normal bladder function.

This chapter will review the current literature concerning the use of radiation to treat muscle-invasive bladder cancer, including patient selection, treatment planning and delivery, and the results of radiation alone or in combination with neoadjuvant or concurrent chemotherapy. Much of the evidence for radiotherapy is based on large series of unselected patients treated at single institutions over many years. Many of these patients received radiotherapy instead of cystectomy because of advanced age, concurrent medical problems, or extensive disease at the time of diagnosis. Most were treated before the introduction of modern, high-precision, image-guided radiation planning and delivery techniques. Therefore, the current literature reflects the worst possible results of radiotherapy rather than the optimal outcomes that might be achieved in patients that are carefully selected using clinical, radiographic, and novel molecular markers of response, and treated with biologically targeted, high-precision techniques. This chapter will emphasize possible approaches to improving the outcome of patients with bladder cancer through the integrated application of emerging radiobiologic and technologic concepts. In particular, the radiobiology of bladder cancer will be discussed with a focus on molecular markers of radiation response that might be used in the future to select optimal patients for radiotherapy or stratify patients in clinical studies. These biomarkers of tumor response are also potential targets for novel molecular-based agents that can be used in combination with radiation to improve the therapeutic outcome.

Patient selection for radiotherapy

Radiotherapy for muscle-invasive bladder cancer, administered with the aim of permanently controlling the tumor and preserving normal bladder function, is most appropriate in situations in which the prior probability of achieving this goal is high. Numerous factors may influence the success of radiotherapy in patients with bladder cancer, and they can be broadly classified as those relating to the characteristics of the tumor, the bladder, and the patient. Table 18.1[6–9,22] summarizes the results of multivariate analyses of local control and survival in several large contemporary series.

In general, there is limited evidence to support the use of radiotherapy to treat superficial bladder cancer. Given the effectiveness and convenience of other management strategies, radiation should be reserved for circumstances in which these other options have either been exhausted or are otherwise inappropriate for patient-specific reasons.

Tumor factors for local control

Sustained local control of muscle-invasive bladder cancer treated with radiotherapy is strongly influenced by the bulk of local disease at the time of treatment, and the propensity for new tumors to develop in the bladder after treatment. Advanced T category, large tumor size, the presence of an extravesical mass, and hydronephrosis have all been associated with either incomplete response to radiation or local disease recurrence.[1–10] Overall, approximately 50% of patients treated with external beam radiotherapy have complete regression of disease: 50% to 70% of those with T2 or T3a disease and 40% to 50% with T3 or T4a tumors.[1,2,4,5,11–13] Sustained local control can be expected in 30% to 50% and 20% to 30% of patients with T2 and T3 disease, respectively.[2,6,14] A gross complete transurethral resection of the bladder tumor before radiotherapy has been associated with improved local control,[7,15] although this has not been observed consistently.[4,13,16]

Treatment of bladder cancer with radiotherapy is associated with long-term risk of new tumor development in the preserved bladder. For example, Gospodarowicz et al[6] reported a continuous decline in local relapse-free rate and cause-specific cystectomy-free survival to beyond 10 years in 355 patients treated with radiotherapy alone. Patients at greatest risk of new tumor development are those with multifocal superficial disease at the time of initial diagnosis.[6–9,17] Extensive carcinoma in situ (CIS), when present in association with

Table 18.1 Prognostic factors by multivariate analysis for local control and survival following treatment with radiotherapy, with or without chemotherapy

Lead author (year)	No. pts	Local control	Survival
Gospodarowicz (1991)[6]*	355	T stage	Grade T stage Tumor bulk Hydronephrosis
Fossa (1993)[22]	308		Age Year of treatment† T category Serum creatinine
Mameghan (1995)[8]	342	Multifocal disease Hydronephrosis T stage	
Moonen (1998)[9]	379	Multifocal disease Radiation dose	Age T category
Rodel (2002)[7]	415	Multifocal disease	Age Extent of TURBT T category Lymphatic invasion Treatment‡

*Cause-specific survival.
†1980–1985 versus 1986–1990.
‡Radiotherapy alone, versus radiotherapy + carboplatin, versus radiotherapy + cisplatin, versus radiotherapy + 5-fluorouracil/cisplatin; p=0.06.
TURBT, transurethral resection of bladder tumor prior to radiotherapy.

muscle-invasive bladder cancer, is a particularly strong adverse prognostic factor for sustained local control with radiotherapy.[1,18,19] Wolf et al[19] reported the development of new bladder cancers after radiotherapy in 58% of patients with dysplasia or CIS at initial presentation, but in none of the patients without concomitant CIS. Zietman et al[20] described the Massachusetts General Hospital experience with superficial disease recurrence in 121 patients who presented initially with muscle-invasive cancer and were treated with a combination of surgery, radiation, and chemotherapy. Superficial disease recurrence was seen at 57 sites in 32 patients (26%), at a median interval of 2.1 years from the completion of initial treatment. CIS associated with the original muscle-invasive tumor was a strong predictor of subsequent superficial recurrence. Conservative treatment with transurethral resection and intravesical therapy was undertaken in 27 patients, 10 of whom eventually required cystectomy because of further superficial recurrence or progression to invasive cancer. There was no difference in survival among patients who remained permanently free of disease following initial treatment and those who developed a superficial recurrence. These results indicate that, while CIS is associated with reduced long-term disease control in the bladder, it is not an absolute contraindication to the use of radiotherapy in patients with muscle-invasive disease, and should be considered in the context of other tumor- and patient-related factors when treatment options are evaluated.

the completion of transurethral resection of the bladder prior to radiotherapy have all been associated with reduced survival.[1,6,7,9,22]

Several surgical series have demonstrated pelvic lymph node metastases at diagnosis in 10% to 50% of patients with muscle-invasive bladder cancer depending on primary tumor extent.[26–29] Nodal metastases imply a high risk of occult distant metastases, a high risk of recurrence outside of the pelvis following local treatment alone, and significantly lower survival relative to node-negative patients. Nevertheless, the impact of nodal metastases on the outcome of bladder cancer patients treated with radiotherapy has not been extensively studied. This in part reflects the difficulty of reliably identifying subclinical nodal disease in the absence of surgical dissection. Very few of the modern radiotherapy series have described the prognostic impact of nodal status at diagnosis. Rodel et al[7] showed that lymph node involvement was predictive of inferior local control by univariate analysis, but not by multivariate analysis. However, patients with positive nodes were more likely to develop distant metastases independent of other tumor-, patient-, and treatment-related factors. The potential for radiotherapy, with or without concurrent chemotherapy to control bulky nodal disease, is limited by normal tissue toxicity and the relatively modest doses that can be delivered safely.[30] In addition, these patients are at particularly high risk of having occult distant metastases. Patients in this situation desiring bladder conservation should be managed by multimodality strategies that incorporate initial chemotherapy followed by consolidative pelvic radiotherapy for complete responders.

Tumor factors for survival

The prognostic factors for survival are similar to those for local control, and generally reflect primary tumor bulk. Patients with T2 tumors have an expected survival of 30% to 50%, and those with T3 disease a survival of 15% to 35%.[1–6,9,11–14,21–25] In addition, advanced age at diagnosis, high histologic grade, and gross residual disease at

Patient factors

Radiotherapy is generally tolerated well in elderly patients[31] and in those with concurrent medical problems, and this has contributed to an imbalance in the underlying likelihood of long-term survival between patients who undergo cystectomy and those treated with radiotherapy. However, the benefit of definitive radiotherapy with bladder conservation is likely to be limited in situations in which pretreatment bladder function is compromised and in patients at high risk of developing intolerable acute or long-term treatment complications. Those with severe irritable bladder symptoms due to factors such as longstanding outflow obstruction, chronic infection, multiple prior transurethral resections, or prior intravesical chemotherapy may have permanent impairment of bladder function after radiotherapy that diminishes the benefit of organ preservation. Anatomic and technical factors that limit the accuracy and reproducibility of radiation delivery, and increase the likelihood of missing the target—such as atonic bladders and large bladder diverticula—may contribute to a higher risk of local tumor recurrence and treatment complications. New image-guided radiation delivery systems may help to overcome these challenges.

Overall, the ideal candidate for definitive radiotherapy with bladder preservation has a small, solitary tumor less than 5 cm in size with no associated CIS, no evidence of lymph node or distant metastases, and a normal (or normally functioning) bladder. The patient must be highly motivated to preserve the bladder, committed to frequent invasive follow-up examinations, and willing to accept the uncertainty that accompanies life-long bladder surveillance and the possibility of requiring treatment of new, superficial, invasive, or metastatic disease.

Radiotherapy treatment planning and delivery

The goal of radiotherapy is to eradicate all gross and microscopic tumor in the bladder and often also in the pelvic lymph nodes, while minimizing patient toxicity. Therefore, the success of radiotherapy depends not only on the selection of appropriate patients, but also on knowledge of tumor patterns of spread, accurate localization of the primary tumor and lymph node metastases, selection of appropriate treatment volumes to encompass all tumor and exclude as much normal tissue as possible, and careful tracking of tumor movement. The bladder is not a fixed structure but rather varies in size and position as a function of urine volume and rectal contents. Compensation for frequent variations in bladder positioning and tumor movement during a fractionated course of treatment is an important component of the radiotherapy treatment plan.

Radiotherapy for the primary bladder tumor

Radiotherapy for bladder cancer implies the need for accurate and reproducible delivery of multiple radiation fractions to the gross tumor and regions of subclinical disease extension. Microscopic infiltrative tumor is likely to be present in the lamina propria, muscularis propria, and lymphovascular spaces adjacent to the primary tumor, although the degree of extension beyond gross disease has not been studied and is likely to be highly variable. Disease may also extend into paravesical tissues. The location and extent of gross tumor determined from diagnostic and staging tests—including cystoscopy, pelvic computed tomography (CT), and pelvic magnetic resonance imaging (MRI)—should be integrated with results of CT imaging of the patient in the treatment position to develop a three-dimensional radiotherapy plan. CT-based treatment planning has been shown to be more accurate than conventional planning techniques that rely on cystogram alone.[32–35] However, there probably is significant interobserver variability in the definition of gross tumor using CT, particularly in the region of the trigone and bladder neck.[36,37] This may be improved in the future with the use of planning MRI and registration of the CT and MR images. MRI provides greater soft tissue resolution than CT, and valuable information about the extent of local disease. Figure 18.1 shows axial, sagittal and coronal images of a tumor extensively involving the dome and posterior wall of the bladder and causing ureteric obstruction and hydronephrosis.

The clinical target volume (CTV) for treatment of the primary bladder tumor is often considered to be the entire bladder. However, lateralized solitary tumors that can be accurately localized are probably safely treated with a reduced CTV that encompasses the gross tumor and a surrounding margin to account for microscopic disease extension. Cowan et al[38] reported the results of a three-arm phase III study in which patients with bladder cancer were

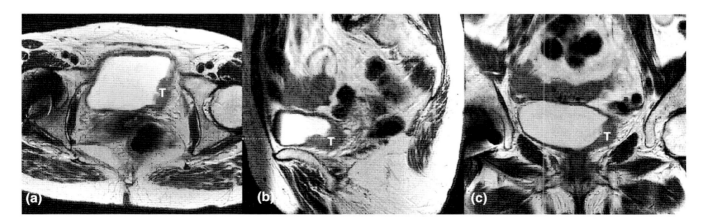

Figure 18.1
(a) Axial, (b) sagittal, and (c) coronal T$_2$-weighted MR images of a muscle-invasive bladder tumor (T) involving the left posterolateral wall. MR provides high-resolution images of bladder cancer that can be used to accurately determine radiation treatment volumes.

randomized to either whole-bladder treatment, or escalated dose partial-bladder treatment with two different dose regimens. The median irradiated pelvic volume was 61% lower in the partial-volume arms of the study than in the whole-bladder arm. While statistically significant, there were no differences in complete response, sustained local control, long-term survival, or toxicity; the trial was closed early due to slow accrual and only 72 patients of a planned 123 reached the clinical endpoint of failure of local control.

Variability in the position of the bladder tumor from day to day during a course of fractionated radiotherapy theoretically may be minimized by asking patients to completely empty their bladders immediately prior to imaging for treatment planning, and prior to receiving each radiation fraction. However, the efficacy of this maneuver has not been rigorously evaluated, and there still may be significant changes in bladder volume depending on factors such as the interval between voiding and treatment delivery, the state of hydration of the patient, and the use of diuretic medications or beverages. Movement may also be influenced by extrinsic pressure, such as might arise from differences in rectal filling,[39] and by the characteristics of the tumor, including size and degree of extravesical extension. Turner et al[39] demonstrated interfraction bladder wall movement of at least 1.5 cm in 18 of 30 patients, with the greatest movement being seen in those with large initial bladder volumes. Bladder movement resulted in inadequate coverage of the CTV in 10 patients. An isotropic planning target volume (PTV) of 2 cm around the CTV was recommended to account for random internal movement.[39] Muren et al[40] studied 20 patients with bladder cancer

using weekly CT scans. In 89% of the repeat scans during treatment, the bladder wall extended beyond the bladder contour as outlined using the original planning CT. The greatest displacements during treatment occurred along the superior, left, anterior, and posterior aspects of the bladder and measured up to 3.6 cm. Anisotropic margins (CTV–PTV) of 1.1–2.3 cm were necessary to encompass all bladder displacements simultaneously except in the most extreme cases. Similarly, Meijer et al[37] advocated anisotropic margins (CTV–PTV) of 2.3 cm superiorly and 1 cm inferiorly (behind the symphysis) and laterally.

The choice of radiation treatment margin around the gross bladder tumor is likely to influence not only local control, but also toxicity. In a recent analysis, conformal three- or four-field treatment plans for 15 patients were developed using either isotropic margins of 1 cm around the bladder wall CTV, or wider anisotropic margins of 1.2 cm laterally and 2 cm elsewhere. The wider margins were associated with a 1.5- to 2.4-fold increase in the volume of small bowel and rectum receiving greater than 50% of the prescribed dose. The fractional rectal volume receiving greater than 75% of the prescribed dose was 3.6- to 5-fold higher. The higher doses to critical normal structures correlated with model predictions of higher complication rates.[41] In the future, image-guided radiotherapy that allows day-to-day optimization of the treatment volumes should further reduce the possibility of accidentally underdosing mobile tumors while at the same time minimizing the dose to critical adjacent normal tissues. Figure 18.2 is an axial image through the bladder acquired using cone-beam CT[42] that is integrated with the

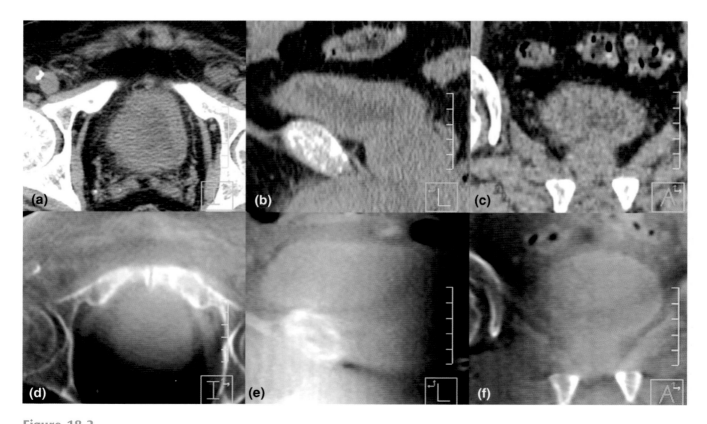

Figure 18.2
(a) Axial and reconstructed (b) sagittal and (c) coronal planning CT images in a patient with bladder cancer. (d) Axial, (e) sagittal, and (f) coronal cone-beam CT images in the same patient acquired during treatment. The cone-beam CT imager is incorporated into the radiation treatment unit. Daily imaging prior to radiation and correction for patient positioning errors and internal organ movement have the potential to greatly improve the accuracy of bladder cancer radiotherapy.

radiation treatment unit. Anatomic imaging prior to each daily fraction and correction of errors would greatly improve the accuracy of bladder cancer radiotherapy.

Radiotherapy for pelvic lymph node metastases

Pelvic lymph node metastases occur in 10% to 50% of patients with muscle-invasive bladder cancer. Radiotherapy treatment volumes historically have encompassed pelvic lymph nodes, whether or not there is radiographic evidence of gross nodal metastases. However, the benefit of nodal irradiation in bladder cancer has not been extensively studied. Several surgical series have suggested long-term survival of 15% to 30% in patients with nodal metastases who undergo thorough lymph node dissection at the time of cystectomy.[27,28,43–49] By extrapolation, there may also be a benefit of aggressive nodal treatment in patients who are managed primarily with radiotherapy. Pelvic lymph node radiation typically is delivered using a four-field technique, which encompasses a large volume of small bowel and rectum. Therefore, the dose of radiation that can be prescribed safely is limited by the radiation tolerance of these critical normal tissues, and is probably inadequate to control gross or, in some cases, even 'bulky' subclinical nodal disease that is near the threshold of radiographic detection. Intensity modulated radiotherapy (IMRT), which allows the radiation dose to be 'sculpted' in three dimensions to a predefined lymph node volume while excluding surrounding normal tissue, may facilitate higher lymph node doses.[30] Figure 18.3 shows an optimized radiation treatment plan in which the whole bladder and pelvic lymph nodes are treated with IMRT to facilitate dose escalation with relative sparing of the surrounding normal tissues.

Conventional radiation fractionation

Using current radiation techniques, the dose that can be delivered safely to pelvic lymph nodes is limited by the radiation tolerance of the surrounding normal tissues, and is typically 40–50 Gy in 1.8–2.0 Gy daily fractions. The future implementation of precision IMRT techniques may allow escalation of the lymph node dose, with the expectation of improved nodal control.[30]

Radiation doses of 50–70 Gy in 1.8–2.5 Gy fractions over 4–7 weeks are commonly used to treat the primary bladder tumor. The clinical dose–response relationship for bladder cancer is poorly defined, and it remains unclear to what extent differences in total dose in this range influence local tumor control and patient survival. In practice, the prescribed dose is usually determined by the radiation tolerance of the surrounding normal tissues on the assumption that a higher bladder cancer dose will always be desirable and produce improved local control. Therefore, phase III randomized studies comparing different conventionally fractionated dosage schedules have never been undertaken. At least four case series have suggested improved local tumor control with doses greater than 55–60 Gy,[2,13,17,50] although others have found no evidence to support such a relationship.[3,10] The dose–response relationship in these and other retrospective studies may have been obscured to some extent by differences among the dose strata

in the distribution of other important tumor-, patient-, and treatment-related factors.

Side effects of radiotherapy

Conventionally fractionated radiotherapy to total doses of less than 70 Gy is typically well tolerated by patients with bladder cancer. Most experience acute gastrointestinal and lower urinary tract side effects during treatment that usually are easily controlled with dietary modification and medications. Late complications primarily affect the bowel and normal bladder, and typically arise from 1 to 4 years after treatment is completed. Approximately 75% of late complications are present by 3 years.[5,14] Late bladder side effects, which include urinary frequency, dysuria, and hematuria, have been reported in 7% to 15% of patients,[2,5,6,14,51] and in some circumstances necessitate cystectomy. Severe gastrointestinal toxicity is seen in 6% to 17% of patients.[5,6,14] Doses above 70 Gy are likely to be associated with an unacceptably high rate of serious complications if delivered using standard radiation techniques,[3] but may be feasible in the future with image-guided intensity-modulated radiotherapy.

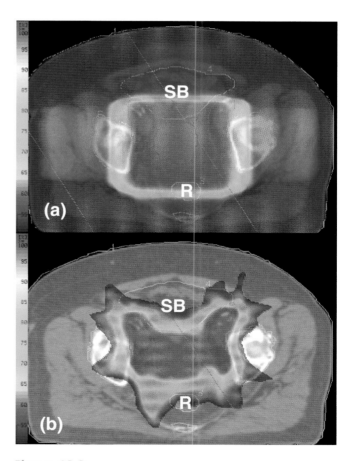

Figure 18.3
Radiation treatment plans for bladder cancer (including the pelvic lymph nodes) using (a) a standard four-field approach, and (b) intensity-modulated radiotherapy (IMRT). The IMRT plan results in relative dose sparing of the small bowel (SB) and rectum (R).

Follow-up after radiotherapy

Patients with muscle-invasive bladder cancer are at risk of developing progressive tumor both in the bladder and at metastatic sites after completing radiation treatment. This underscores the importance of life-long bladder surveillance and prompt treatment of bladder recurrences.[20] Several studies have demonstrated that new superficial disease in the bladder following radiotherapy, including new CIS, can often be managed effectively with transurethral resection and intravesical bacillus Calmette–Guérin (BCG).[20,52,53] However, persistent or new muscle-invasive cancer usually implies the need for salvage cystectomy. Most modern radiotherapy series have reported salvage cystectomy rates of only 20% to 30% of patients.[2,6,7,22,51,54,55] Many patients referred for radiotherapy have bulky unresectable tumors and a high risk of occult micrometastases, or concurrent medical problems, making them unsuitable for initial surgery. For the same reasons, these patients often are not considered for salvage cystectomy in the event of radiation failure. However, cystectomy frequently is the only remaining option for patients with recurrent localized muscle-invasive bladder cancer. In general, all patients with residual or recurrent bladder cancer following radiotherapy should be evaluated for cystectomy.

The rate of bladder cancer regression following radiotherapy influences both the optimal timing of cystoscopy to evaluate response and the optimal timing of salvage cystectomy. Several reports have identified disease status at the completion of radiotherapy (with or without concurrent chemotherapy) as an important prognostic factor for overall patient outcome.[6,7] In most radiotherapy series, response has been evaluated 1–3 months after completion of treatment.[6,7] However, the Massachusetts General Hospital has adopted a policy of earlier evaluation.[56] After initial thorough transurethral resection, patients receive induction radiotherapy to a dose of approximately 40 Gy with concurrent cisplatin chemotherapy. Cystoscopy is performed 2–4 weeks later to assess disease regression. Patients that have had complete regression receive consolidative radiotherapy, while those with residual bladder cancer proceed to immediate cystectomy. The advantage is early cystectomy after only a modest dose of radiotherapy, which should maximize the curative potential of cystectomy and minimize toxicity. However, early response assessment before completion of full-course radical radiotherapy theoretically may decrease the likelihood of bladder preservation if slow responders, who would have achieved complete regression of disease given sufficient time, are evaluated prematurely. Although there has not been a randomized comparison of early versus delayed response assessment and cystectomy, the results from several series suggest comparable results with respect to local control, patient survival, the proportion of patients undergoing cystectomy, and treatment complications.[6,7,9,56] At the Princess Margaret Hospital, it is our practice to assess response no later than 6 weeks after completing radiotherapy.

Patient outcome following radiotherapy for bladder cancer

There is substantial evidence that radiotherapy is effective treatment for bladder cancer. However, many patients with muscle-invasive disease have bulky tumors at presentation and are at high risk of harboring occult lymph node or distant metastases. Radiotherapy and chemotherapy are therefore frequently used in combination with the aim of enhancing local tumor control, reducing metastasis development, and improving patient survival.

Radiotherapy alone

Table 18.2[2–6,9,11–14,21–25,32] summarizes the published experience with external beam radiotherapy alone as treatment for bladder cancer.

Table 18.2 External beam radiotherapy alone for muscle-invasive bladder cancer

Lead author (year)	No. Pts	5-year survival by T category (%)			
		T2	T3 (T3a/T3b)	T4	Overall
Goffinet (1975)[23]	384	35–42	20		
Yu (1985)[24]	356	42	(35/23)		
Goodman (1981)[25]	470				38
Duncan (1986)[5]	963	40	26	12	30
Blandy (1988)[11]	614	27	38	9	
Jenkins (1988)[12]*	182	46	35		40
Gospodarowicz (1991)[6]*	355	50	(38/28)		46
Jahnson (1991)[14]*	319	31	16	6	28
Davidson (1990)[21]*	709	49	28	2	25
Greven (1990)[2]	116	59	10	0	
Smaaland (1991)[13]	146	26	10†		
Fossa (1993)[22]	308	38‡	14§		24
Vale (1993)[4]	60	38	12		
Pollack (1994)[3]	135	42	20	0	26
Moonen (1998)[9]	379	25	17		22
Borgaonkar (2002)[32]*	163	48	26		45

*Cause-specific survival.
†T3/T4.
‡T2/T3a.
§T3b/T4.

Most are retrospective descriptions of the experience at a single institution over several decades, and often do not consider changes with time in patient assessment, imaging, stage classification, radiotherapy technique, and supportive treatment. Management strategies vary from institution to institution, including the criteria for salvage cystectomy, making detailed comparisons of results problematic. Nevertheless, there are consistent patterns among the studies with respect to both short- and long-term response to radiation. Together, they provide strong evidence that a substantial proportion of patients, particularly those with small tumors at presentation, are cured with radiotherapy and maintain normal bladder function.

Radical external beam radiotherapy produces complete regression of muscle-invasive bladder cancer in approximately 70% of patients,[1,2,4,5,11–13] and 30% to 50% have sustained local control (complete tumor regression without subsequent recurrence in the bladder).[2,6,14] Nevertheless, distant metastases develop in more than 50% of patients,[1] and long-term overall survival is in the range of only 25% to 30%.[1,3,5,9,22] Salvage cystectomy for progressive or recurrent disease after radiotherapy, which is an important part of the integrated management plan, has historically been undertaken in less than 30% of patients.[1,2,22,54] This, at least in part, reflects the poor general health, age, and prognosis of patients treated with radiation, who often have concomitant medical contraindications to surgery. Overall, approximately 80% of patients that survive long-term following external beam radiotherapy have intact, well-functioning bladders.[7]

Radiotherapy and concurrent chemotherapy

Rodel et al[7] recently updated their large accumulated experience in 415 patients with T1–4 bladder cancer. More than 50% of patients had T3 or T4 disease. All were treated with transurethral resection followed by pelvic radiotherapy. Chemotherapy with cisplatin, carboplatin, and/or 5-fluorouracil (5-FU) was used concurrently with radiation in 289 patients. Complete tumor regression occurred in 72% of patients, as assessed by cystoscopy and biopsy 6 weeks after completing treatment. Among patients that achieved a complete response, 50% remained free of any relapse in the bladder at

10 years, and 64% had no recurrence of muscle-invasive disease. Overall, 20% of patients underwent salvage cystectomy. Distant metastases developed in 35% of patients. The 10-year cause-specific survival was 42%.

In other studies, the Massachusetts General Hospital has pursued an aggressive program of bladder conservation with conservative surgery, radiation, and chemotherapy in selected patients since 1986. Patients initially underwent a thorough transurethral resection, followed by induction treatment with radiotherapy to 40 Gy, and concurrent cisplatin chemotherapy. Those with complete regression of disease proceeded to consolidative radiotherapy (a further 24–25 Gy with chemotherapy), while those with residual disease underwent cystectomy. Among 190 patients, 82% completed treatment according to protocol. Sixty percent of patients treated with chemoradiation alone remained free of bladder cancer long term. Superficial disease recurred in the bladder in 24 patients, and in the majority of cases was managed conservatively with further resection and intravesical chemotherapy. A muscle-invasive recurrence developed in 16%. The 10-year cause-specific survival rates were 60% overall, and 45% with an intact bladder. Bladder function was normal by urodynamic assessment in 75% of these patients.[56,57]

The only phase III trial of radiotherapy and concurrent chemotherapy was conducted by the National Cancer Institute of Canada[58] and is summarized in Table 18.3 along with other neoadjuvant and concurrent chemoradiation studies.[59–63] Patients with T2–4b urothelial carcinoma of the bladder received local regional therapy alone (full-dose radiotherapy or preoperative radiotherapy and cystectomy), with or without concurrent cisplatin. There was no difference in overall survival or distant relapse-free survival. However, patients that received concurrent chemotherapy had a significantly lower rate of pelvic recurrence than those treated with radiation alone. There was no difference in the risk of serious side effects.

Neoadjuvant chemotherapy and radiotherapy

Initial phase II studies of neoadjuvant chemotherapy suggested improved local control and prolonged survival.[64–66] However, phase

Table 18.3 Randomized studies of combination radiation and chemotherapy

Lead author (year)	No. pts	Stage	Experimental arm	Control arm	3–5 year survival*
Shearer (1988)[59]	423	T3	± Neo and Adj MTX	RT alone 64 Gy or preRT 44 Gy + cyst	39% vs. 37%, NS
Wallace (1991)[60]	255	T2–4	± Neo Cis	RT alone	NS
Coppin (1996)[58†]	99	T2–4	± Con Cis ×3 with induction RT	Induction RT 40 Gy RT boost 20 Gy or Cyst	47% vs. 33%, NS
Shipley (1998)[61] (RTOG 89-03)	123	T2–4	± Neo CMV ×2 after TURBT	TURBT RT 39.6 Gy + Con Cis RT boost 25.2 Gy + Cis if CR Cyst if no CR	48% vs. 49%, NS
Ghersi (1999)[63]	976	T2–4	± Neo CMV ×3	RT or Cyst	55% vs. 50%, NS
Senglov (2002)[62]	153	T2–4	± Neo Cis and MTX ×3	RT or Cyst	29% vs. 29%, NS

*Experimental versus control arm.
†Improved pelvic control.
Adj, adjuvant; Cis, cisplatin; CMV, cisplatin, methotrexate, vinblastine; Con, concurrent; CR, complete response; Cyst, cystectomy; MTX, methotrexate; Neo, neoadjuvant; NS, not significant; preRT, planned preoperative RT; RT, radiotherapy; TURBT, transurethral resection of bladder tumor.

III studies have, in general, failed to confirm these results. The largest phase III neoadjuvant study comprised 976 patients with T2–4 bladder cancer randomized to receive three cycles of chemotherapy with cisplatin, methotrexate and vinblastine (CMV) followed by cystectomy or radiotherapy, versus the same treatment without chemotherapy.[63] A total of 485 patients underwent cystectomy; 415 were treated with radiotherapy and 76 received preoperative radiation followed by cystectomy. There was no difference in overall survival between the chemotherapy and no-chemotherapy arms (55% versus 50%, respectively). Locoregional control was not affected by chemotherapy, although there was a suggestion that the development of metastasis was delayed.

Although the results of individual phase III randomized studies of neoadjuvant chemotherapy have been disappointing, a recent meta-analysis that combined individual data from 2688 patients in 10 studies has shown a survival advantage with combination platinum-based chemotherapy.[67] There was a 13% relative reduction in the risk of death and an improvement in survival at 5 years from 45% to 50%. Local disease-free survival and metastasis-free survival were also improved (relative risk reductions of 13% and 18%, respectively).

High Precision Radiation Treatment for Bladder Cancer

The potential of radiotherapy to eradicate bladder cancer has been limited over the years by technologic factors that prevented the accurate and reproducible delivery of sufficient radiation dose to the primary tumor and pelvic lymph nodes while at the same time sparing important adjacent normal tissues and minimizing toxicity. Little appreciation of the potential for the bladder and tumor to move between and during radiation fractions, coupled with inadequate treatment planning and delivery, has probably contributed to inadvertent underdosing of tumor and an excess number of local treatment failures. In addition, the radiation dose that can be delivered safely to pelvic lymph nodes is limited because of normal tissue tolerance to between 45 and 50 Gy, which is insufficient for reliable control of gross nodal disease or even 'bulky' subclinical metastases that are just below the threshold of radiographic detection. Therefore, it is likely that the pelvic lymph nodes have historically been inadequately treated with conventional radiotherapy in a large proportion of patients.

Recent advances in radiation treatment technology have the potential to overcome the limitations of previous techniques, thereby dramatically improving the likelihood of permanently eradicating bladder cancer and at the same time minimizing the risk of complications and preserving normal bladder function. IMRT allows dose escalation to the primary bladder tumor and pelvic lymph nodes (see Figure 18.3) with the expectation of improved tumor and equal or reduced toxicity.[30] Tighter radiation treatment margins around the tumor imply the need for greater accuracy in tumor delineation at the time of treatment planning using high-definition imaging modalities such as MRI (see Figure 18.1), and an enhanced capacity to ensure that the radiotherapy is actually delivered as planned each day during a course of fractionated treatment. This can be accomplished through daily imaging of patients prior to treatment, with correction of individual radiation beams to account for variation in patient positioning and tumor movement. Radiation treatment units that incorporate volumetric imaging, such as cone-beam CT[42] (see Figure 18.2), coupled with fast and accurate software

to automatically calculate beam corrections, are well suited to this application.

Overall, image-guided IMRT, coupled with advances in our understanding of tumor and normal tissue radiobiology, has the potential to revolutionize the treatment of bladder cancer. However, further development is necessary to assure its safe implementation in routine clinical practice. The success of IMRT in this setting will depend on the combined efforts of radiation oncologists, physicists, radiation therapists, and nurses. Coordination and communication among these professional groups is essential to ensure that important technical and patient-related issues are adequately addressed.

Modern Concepts in Bladder Cancer Radiobiology

Although radiation has proven efficacy in the treatment of muscle-invasive bladder cancer, there is the potential to significantly enhance the therapeutic effect by better understanding the molecular events that lead to radiation-induced cell death in tumors and normal tissues, and modulating the radiosensitivity of these tissues using molecularly targeted treatments.

The aim of clinical radiotherapy is to sterilize all malignant clonogenic cells that are capable of regrowing the tumor. Ionizing radiation leads to the rapid generation of reactive free radicals that randomly interact with the DNA, RNA, and proteins within the cell membrane and nucleus. Clustering of ionizations close to DNA leads to multiply damaged DNA sites consisting of DNA single- and double-strand breaks (DNA-ssb, DNA-dsb), DNA base damage, and DNA–DNA or DNA–protein crosslinks. The most lethal of these lesions is a non-repaired DNA-dsb.[68] Within seconds following irradiation, a cascade of signaling pathways is activated, which together control cell proliferation, DNA repair, and initiation of cell death. Many of these signaling pathways, which are associated with activated oncogenes (H-ras, raf or EGFR mutations) or inactivated tumor suppressor proteins (mutated p53 or pRb-retinoblastoma), are abnormal in bladder cancer cells.[69–71]

Following a lethal dose of ionizing radiation, cells may: 1) undergo apoptosis; 2) proceed through up to four abortive mitotic cycles, and then undergo mitotic catastrophe and cell lysis; or 3) undergo permanent growth arrest such as that observed for irradiated fibroblasts.[72] Complex, inter-related molecular mechanisms that regulate the cell cycle and DNA repair determine whether or not cell death occurs following exposure to ionizing radiation, and which of these morphologic patterns dominates in a particular tumor. Figure 18.4 illustrates the molecular pathways involved in the cellular response to radiation, and Table 18.4 summarizes the molecular targets that might be used to radiosensitize bladder cancer.

Altered cell cycle dynamics

Human cells respond to radiotherapy through altered cell cycle dynamics. Delayed progression through the G1, S, and G2 phases of the cell cycle (the G1, S, and G2 cell cycle checkpoints) potentially allows repair of DNA and cellular damage to occur, thereby preventing cell death.[73] Central to these checkpoints is the activation of the ATM (ataxia telangiectasia mutated) protein kinase, which initiates the G1 checkpoint by stabilizing the p53 tumor suppressor protein.

This in turn leads to an upregulation of the cyclin-kinase inhibitor, p21^{WAF}, hypophosphorylation of the RB protein, and inhibition of DNA replication.[74] The radiation-induced G1 arrest is lost in cells without functional p53 or RB proteins, and this may

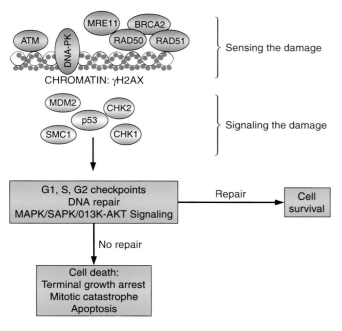

CHROMATIN: γH2AX

Sensing the damage

Signaling the damage

G1, S, G2 checkpoints
DNA repair
MAPK/SAPK/013K-AKT Signaling

Repair → Cell survival

No repair

Cell death:
Terminal growth arrest
Mitotic catastrophe
Apoptosis

Figure 18.4
Radiation-induced DNA breaks are sensed by a series of chromatin-binding kinases that mediate intracellular signaling within the cell. This activates a variety of downstream signaling pathways that ultimately result in either cell survival or cell death. Cell death occurs as a result of apoptosis, mitotic catastrophe or terminal growth arrest, the last two being the dominant mechanisms in the majority of human solid tumors.

influence local tumor control and survival of patients with bladder cancer.[75,76]

The S-phase checkpoint following DNA damage is controlled though an ATM-mediated phosphorylation of the BRCA1, NBS1, and SMC1 proteins, which modify transcription factors and other proteins (RPA, PCNA) required during DNA replication.[77] The G2 delay occurs as a result of decreased expression, reduced stability, or nuclear accumulation of cyclin B complexes, which prevent the formation of active nuclear cyclin B-CDC2 complexes required for the transition from G2 to mitosis.[78] Radiosensitization theoretically may be achieved with drugs that abrogate the G2 checkpoint (caffeine, methylxanthines, UCN-01) leading to increased mitotic catastrophe. These agents are currently being tested, together with radiation in phase I–II clinical trials.[79–81]

DNA repair

Repair of DNA damage is an important determinant of malignant and normal tissue cellular response to ionizing radiation. Clinical radiotherapy endeavors to maximize the therapeutic ratio, so that maximal tumor cell killing occurs with minimal normal tissue toxicity. The utopian goal, therefore, is to completely inhibit DNA repair in malignant cells, while at the same time maximizing repair in normal tissue cells. The repair of DNA-dsb breaks has been correlated with bladder cancer cell survival following irradiation in vitro.[82–86]

Radiation-induced DNA breaks are initially sensed by the ATM, DNA-PK$_{CS}$ and RAD50 proteins, which in turn recruit other proteins involved in DNA repair and cell cycle control.[87] Two main pathways for DNA-dsb repair exist in human cells. The homologous recombination (HR) pathway includes the concerted actions of the RAD51, RAD50-57, RPA, and BRCA2 proteins, and dominates in the S and G2 phases of the cell cycle. In contrast, the nonhomologous end-joining (NHEJ) pathway includes the DNA-PK$_{CS}$, Ku70/Ku80, DNA ligase IV, and XRCC4 proteins, and is the preferred pathway

Table 18.4 Biomarkers of bladder cancer radioresistance

Biomarker	Detection technique	Affected pathway	Treatment strategy
Mutant p53	IHC DNA sequencing	Defective checkpoints and apoptosis Increased cell proliferation and metastasis	Increase radiation dose and radioprotect normal tissues Utilize pro-p53 gene therapy Convert abnormal p53 expression using pharmacologic manipulation
Decreased BAX:BCL2 ratio	IHC	Defective apoptotic response	Anti-BCL2 gene therapy or pro-BAX gene therapy
EGFR overexpression	IHC ELISA, FISH	Defective EGFR signaling and increased tumor cell proliferation, survival and angiogenesis	Target EGFR receptor (C225-Cetuximab) or abnormal tyrosine kinase activity (ZD1389-Iressa)
Mutation in RAS or PI3K/AKT pathway	IHC ELISA	Increased tumor cell survival and proliferation	Farnesyl transferase inhibitors or PI3K inhibitors ARCON radiotherapy
High expression of CAIX, HIF1α, GLUT1, or VEGF	IHC	Increased acute and chronic hypoxia and angiogenesis, leading to tumor cell resistance and increased metastases	Selective hypoxic cell toxins (tirapazamine) Antiangiogenesis (COX2 inhibitors)
Overexpression of Ki67, cyclins A and D Short tumor doubling time (Tpot or labeling index)	IHC Flow cytometry	Increased cell proliferation and tumor cell repopulation	Accelerated fractionation

ARCON, accelerated radiotherapy and carbogen and nicotinamide; FISH, fluorescent in situ hybridization; IHC, immunohistochemistry.

for cells in the G1 phase of the cell cycle.[78,88] In addition, the HR and NHEJ repair pathways have recently been shown to influence the repair of platinum- and gemcitabine-induced DNA crosslinks and DNA-dsbs in bladder cancer cells.[89–92] This supported previous work in which the interaction of ionizing radiation and cisplatin was shown to be secondary to increased fixation of chemotherapy-induced DNA adducts by ionizing radiation.[92,93] This may in part explain the efficacy of combining radiation with cisplatin chemotherapy that has been demonstrated in randomized clinical studies of patients with bladder cancer.[58,94]

Taken together, the biologic responses outlined above interact to control the extent of cell death in malignant or normal tissues by recognizing whether the damage is sublethal or lethal, and whether sublethal damage can be effectively repaired. For each different type of tissue within the radiation volume, different mechanisms of cell death and cellular repair may be involved. In the context of clinical practice with fractionated radiotherapy, the factors that most prominently influence the response of a particular tissue may be summarized as the five Rs of radiotherapy:

- intrinsic *radiosensitivity*
- *redistribution* of cells within the cell cycle
- *reoxygenation* of cells during the course of radiotherapy
- *repopulation* of cells during radiotherapy
- cellular repair of tumor relative to normal tissue cells.[68]

Intrinsic radiosensitivity

In many bladder cancer radiobiology studies, survival has been determined using a clonogenic assay that represents the total or cumulative cell death within an irradiated cell population as a result of all types of cell death.[82] The surviving fraction of cells following a dose of 2 Gy (SF2), which is in the clinically relevant range for fractionated radiotherapy, varies between 0.3 and 0.8 for most bladder cancer cell lines. The SF2 value of primary explanted patient biopsies has been shown to correlate with outcome following radiotherapy in cervical cancer, supporting the concept that intrinsic radiosensitivity is an important determinant of clinical response.[78,95] Unfortunately, human ex vivo clonogenic assays are unlikely to be clinically valuable as an indicator of bladder cancer radiocurability in individual patients because the results take 5–9 weeks to generate and the growth of bladder cancer biopsies ex vivo is poor. Surrogate tests of intrinsic radiosensitivity such as the relative repair of DNA breaks or DNA crosslinks in irradiated or chemotherapy-treated bladder biopsies show promise, but require further confirmatory studies.[84–86]

There have been reports of a correlation between increased pretreatment apoptosis and improved local control following radiotherapy in patients with bladder cancer.[96] This relationship between pretreatment apoptotic index and radioresponse relates to activation of the extrinsic, receptor-based (TNF or TRAIL family members) and intrinsic, mitochondrial-based (BAX, BCL2 family members) pathways.[97] The threshold for activation of apoptosis is controlled by p53 protein function and by the relative levels of the BAX and BCL2 proteins. Mutations of the p53 gene and decreased BAX:BCL2 ratio have been associated with increased radioresistance in vitro and decreased bladder cancer clinical radioresponse.[96,98–110] This has led to a series of preclinical experiments pro-p53 or anti-BCL2 gene therapy to augment radiation-induced apoptosis.[74,111–113]

Although apoptosis is an important pathway leading to radiation-induced cell death, it is insufficient to account for the total therapeutic effect of anticancer agents in solid epithelial tumors.

In fact, the level of radiation-induced apoptosis rarely correlates with eventual clonogenic cell survival as measured by colony-forming assays.[72,114] Other antiproliferative responses that directly impact on radiation clonogenic survival include mitotic catastrophe and terminal growth arrest.

Mitotic catastrophe is the failure of human tumor cells to undergo mitosis after DNA damage because of defective cell cycle checkpoint control and DNA repair. This leads to chromosomal abnormalities (tetraploidy or aneuploidy), which have been observed in bladder cancer cells.[115,116] Survivin is a member of the inhibitors of the apoptosis (IAP) protein family, and controls both apoptosis and mitosis. Increased levels of survivin have been observed in malignant relative to normal bladder.[117] Survivin may also be a powerful new biomarker of prognosis and local recurrence following radical cystectomy.[118,119] Ionizing radiation can activate transcriptional downregulation of survivin mRNA in a p53-dependent and PI3K/AKT-dependent manner. Early preclinical studies have shown that reduction in survivin expression using antisense or silencing RNA (siRNA) in bladder cancer cells leads to radiosensitization in vitro.[72,120,121]

Cellular senescence was originally linked to the observation that human diploid cells can undergo only a finite number of divisions before their growth is terminally arrested because of critical shortening of chromosome telomeres. The fact that tumor cell lines may also undergo accelerated senescence after irradiation in vitro explains the correlation between pretreatment or post-treatment expression of terminal growth arrest biomarkers (p53, p21[WAF], p16[INK4a], senescence-associated β-galactosidase) and clinical outcome following radiotherapy.[72,101,102,104,108,122] Agents that differentially increase terminal arrest in bladder cancer cells, such as retinoids or histone deacetylase (HDAC) inhibitors, might therefore be useful as radiosensitizers in patients with bladder cancer.[123,124]

Redistribution, reoxygenation, repopulation and repair

The remaining four Rs of radiotherapy also modify bladder radioresponse. During the typical 24-hour interval between daily radiotherapy treatments, tumor cells can reoxygenate and also redistribute to more radiosensitive phases of the cell cycle. Radioresistant S-phase cells that survive a single radiation fraction will eventually cycle into the more radiosensitive G2, M, and G1 phases of the cell cycle by the time the next radiation treatment is administered. Fractionation also allows normal cells to undergo cellular repair and to repopulate in order to maintain organ function. Fractionation, therefore, results in relatively greater cell killing in tumor cells with tolerable normal tissue toxicity. An improved therapeutic ratio might be achieved in patients with bladder cancer by targeting radioresistant hypoxic subpopulations or using altered radiation fractionation schemes.

Most solid malignant tumors, including bladder cancer, have regions of hypoxia that arise largely because of abnormal vascular anatomy, distribution, organization, and functional dynamics.[125] Hypoxic cells are more resistant to the effects of radiation, are genetically unstable, and are more likely to metastasize.[126,127] High pretreatment levels of tumor hypoxia have been associated with decreased local control, disease-free survival, and overall survival following radiotherapy in a number of tumor types.[125] Hoskin et al[128] evaluated tumor hypoxia in 64 patients with bladder cancer using the intrinsic hypoxic markers carbonic anhydrase IX (CAIX) and glucose transporter-1 protein (GLUT1). There was no association between hypoxia and control of the primary bladder tumor following treatment with radiotherapy, carbogen, and nicotinamide. However, hypoxia was strongly predictive of both cause-specific and overall survival independent of clinical prognostic factors. This is consistent with the results in cervical cancer and other tumors, where hypoxia has been shown to have only a minimal effect on local control with radiotherapy, perhaps in part because of the effect of reoxygenation between radiation fractions, but a profound effect on the development of lymph node and distant metastases.[129,130] The combination of accelerated radiotherapy and the hypoxia-modifying agents carbogen and nicotinamide (ARCON) has shown promise in clinical studies of patients with bladder cancer.[131] Other agents that specifically target hypoxic cells or the abnormal tumor vasculature may be useful additions to bladder cancer radiotherapy.[126,132–134]

Laboratory and clinical studies have shown that tumor growth kinetics can increase during a course of fractionated radiotherapy relative to the pretreatment state as a result of changes in the balance between cellular proliferation and cell loss.[135] This may offset the beneficial effects of radiation, and decrease the probability of tumor eradication. Poorly differentiated urothelial carcinoma has been reported to have a high labeling index and short potential doubling time,[136–138] both indicators of rapid tumor growth and repopulation. In addition, high levels of the proliferative markers Ki67 and cyclins A and D have been correlated with decreased clinical radioresponse.[99,110,139] It has been estimated that prolongation of bladder cancer radiotherapy by 20% or more will decrease local control by a factor of 5 to 10.[140]

Accelerated radiotherapy regimens are designed to deliver the same total dose of radiation in a shorter interval of time relative to conventionally fractionated regimens to offset tumor cell repopulation. At least six phase II studies of accelerated radiotherapy have reported encouraging locoregional control rates and acceptable toxicity.[141–146] Horwich et al[147] reported the results of a prospective study in which 229 patients with bladder cancer were randomly assigned to receive accelerated radiation consisting of 60.8 Gy in 32 fractions over 26 days or conventional radiation with 64 Gy in 32 fractions over 45 days. There was no difference in local control, time to metastases, or overall survival between the groups, and patients in the accelerated arm had a significantly higher rate of bowel injury.

Finally, the therapeutic ratio theoretically can be enhanced in patients with bladder cancer by exploiting differences in the intrinsic DNA repair capacity between tumor and normal tissue cells. Hyperfractionated regimens, defined as the delivery of a larger number of smaller fractions (usually 1.5 Gy or less) with no increase in overall treatment time, should allow an increase in radiation dose leading to a greater likelihood of tumor control with no increase in the risk of late bowel or bladder complications. There have been at least two phase III randomized studies of hyperfractionated versus conventional radiotherapy in patients with bladder cancer.[148,149] Clinical complete response and long-term local control were improved in the hyperfractionated arms relative to conventional fractionation. A meta-analysis based on the pooled data from these studies indicated a significant improvement in overall survival with hyperfractionated treatment.[150]

Future directions in bladder cancer radiobiology

Both tumors and patients are heterogeneous. Multiple genetic and microenvironmental factors must be assessed to accurately predict the response of the bladder cancer, normal bladder, and adjacent normal tissues to radiation. Genomic and proteomic analyses have

shown that radiation-induced gene expression can be cell-type specific, dose dependent, and vary under in vitro versus in vivo conditions. This observation supports the concept that, in the future, 'molecular profiling' of an individual patient may predict the relevant radiation-associated stress responses within that patient.[151–153] Biopsies taken during radiotherapy may be required to optimize the patient profile, as they will better reflect radiation-associated stress responses than will the pretreatment state. These data will be required to fully utilize molecular-targeted agents in combination with radiotherapy and/or alternative radiotherapy fractionation protocols.

Noninvasive, molecular, and microenvironmental imaging has the potential to track changes in tumor and normal tissue biology over time during a course of fractionated radiotherapy, thereby allowing adaptation of treatment to optimize outcome. Imaging of cell death (apoptosis or necrosis), hypoxia, or the induction of radiation-induced signaling pathways (increased expression of p21^{WAF} or cell proliferation genes) will become increasingly important as bladder-specific molecular biology is incorporated into clinic practice.[154–156]

In summary, future developments in our understanding of radiobiology will allow patients to be selected more accurately for either radical cystectomy or radiation at initial presentation. They will also greatly facilitate the use of modifiers of radiation response to increase tumor cell killing and yet protect normal tissues. Together with developments in anatomic imaging of bladder cancer and image-guided precision radiation treatment planning and delivery, the use of novel biomarkers and molecularly targeted agents has the potential to dramatically improve tumor control, organ preservation, and quality of life for patients with bladder cancer.

References

1. Gospodarowicz MK, Hawkins NV, Rawlings GA, et al. Radical radiotherapy for the muscle invasive transitional cell carcinoma of the bladder: failure analysis. J Urol 1989; 142: 1448–54.
2. Greven KM, Solin LJ, Hanks GE. Prognostic factors in patients with bladder carcinoma treated with definitive irradiation. Cancer 1990; 65: 908–12.
3. Pollack A, Zagars GK, Swanson DA. Muscle-invasive bladder cancer treated with external beam radiotherapy: prognostic factors. Int J Radiat Oncol Biol Phys 1994; 30: 267–77.
4. Vale JA, A'Hern RP, Liu K, et al. Predicting the outcome of radical radiotherapy for invasive bladder cancer. Eur Urol 1993; 24: 48–51.
5. Duncan W, Quilty PM. The results of a series of 963 patients with transitional cell carcinoma of the urinary bladder primarily treated by radical megavoltage x-ray therapy. Radiother Oncol 1986; 7: 299–310.
6. Gospodarowicz MK, Rider WD, Keen CW, et al. Bladder cancer: long term follow-up results of patients treated with radical radiation. Clin Oncol 1991; 3: 155–61.
7. Rodel C, Grabenbauer G, Kuhn R, et al. Combined-modality treatment and selective organ preservation in invasive bladder cancer: long-term results. J Clin Oncol 2002; 20: 3061–71.
8. Mameghan H, Fisher R, Mameghan J, Brook S. Analysis of failure following definitive radiotherapy for invasive transitional cell carcinoma of the bladder. Int J Radiat Oncol Biol Phys 1995; 31: 247–54.
9. Moonen L, vd Voet H, de Nijs R, Hart AA, Horenblas S, Bartelink H. Muscle-invasive bladder cancer treated with external beam radiotherapy: pretreatment prognostic factors and the predictive value of cystoscopic re-evaluation during treatment. Radiother Oncol 1998; 49: 149–55.
10. Shipley WU, Rose MA, Perrone TL, Mannix CM, Heney NM, Prout GR. Full-dose irradiation for patients with invasive bladder carcinoma: clinical and histologic factors prognostic of improved survival. J Urol 1985; 134: 679–83.

11. Blandy JP, Jenkins BJ, Fowler CG, et al. Radical radiotherapy and salvage cystectomy for T2/3 cancer of the bladder. Progr Clin Biol Res 1988; 260: 447–51.

12. Jenkins BJ, Caulfield MJ, Fowler, et al. Reappraisal of the role of radical radiotherapy and salvage cystectomy in the treatment of invasive (T2/T3) bladder cancer. Br J Urol 1988; 62: 342–6.

13. Smaaland R, Akslen L, Tonder B, Mehus A, Lote K, Albrektsen G. Radical radiation treatment of invasive and locally advanced bladder cancer in elderly patients. Br J Urol 1991; 67: 61–9.

14. Jahnson S, Pedersen J, Westman G. Bladder carcinoma—a 20-year review of radical irradiation therapy. Radiother Oncol 1991; 22: 111–17.

15. Shipley WU, Prout GR, Kaufman SD, Perrone TL. Invasive bladder carcinoma. The importance of initial transurethral surgery and other significant prognostic factors for improved survival with full-dose irradiation. Cancer 1987; 60: 514–20.

16. Timmer PR, Harlief HA, Hooijkaas JA. Bladder cancer: pattern of recurrence in 142 patients. Int J Radiat Oncol Biol Phys 1985; 11: 899–905.

17. Moonen L, vd Voet H, de Nijs R, Horenblas S, Hart AA, Bartelink. H. Muscle-invasive bladder cancer treated with external beam radiation: influence of total dose, overall treatment time, and treatment interruption on local control. Int J Radiat Oncol Biol Phys 1998; 42: 525–30.

18. Fung CY, Shipley WU, Young RH, et al. Prognostic factors in invasive bladder carcinoma in a prospective trial of preoperative adjuvant chemotherapy and radiotherapy. J Clin Oncol 1991; 9: 1533–42.

19. Wolf H, Olsen PR, Hojgaard K. Urothelial dysplasia concomitant with bladder tumours: a determinant for future new occurrences in patients treated by full-course radiotherapy. Lancet 1985; 1: 1005–8.

20. Zietman A, Grocela J, Zehr E, et al. Selective bladder conservation using transurethral resection, chemotherapy, and radiation: management and consequences of Ta, T1, and Tis recurrence within the retained bladder. Urology 2001; 58: 380–5.

21. Davidson SE, Symonds RP, Snee MP, Upadhyay S, Habeshaw T, Robertson AG. Assessment of factors influencing the outcome of radiotherapy for bladder cancer. Br J Urol 1990; 66: 288–93.

22. Fossa SD, Waehre H, Aass N, Jacobsen AB, Olsen DR, Ous S. Bladder cancer definitive radiation therapy of muscle-invasive bladder cancer. A retrospective analysis of 317 patients. Cancer 1993; 72: 3036–43.

23. Goffinet DR, Schneider MJ, Glatstein EJ, et al. Bladder cancer: results of radiation therapy in 384 patients. Radiology 1975; 117: 149–53.

24. Yu WS, Sagerman RH, Chung CT, Dalal PS, King GA. Bladder carcinoma. Experience with radical and preoperative radiotherapy in 421 patients. Cancer 1985; 56: 1293–9.

25. Goodman GB, Hislop TG, Elwood JM, Balfour J. Conservation of bladder function in patients with invasive bladder cancer treated by definitive irradiation and selective cystectomy. Int J Radiat Oncol Biol Phys 1981; 7: 569–73.

26. Lerner SP, Skinner DG, Lieskovsky G, et al. The rationale for en bloc pelvic lymph node dissection for bladder cancer patients with nodal metastases: long-term results. J Urol 1993; 149: 758–64.

27. Frazier HA, Robertson JE, Dodge RK, Paulson DF. The value of pathologic factors in predicting cancer-specific survival among patients treated with radical cystectomy for transitional cell carcinoma of the bladder and prostate. Cancer 1993; 71: 3993–4001.

28. Bassi P, Ferrante GD, Piazza N, et al. Prognostic factors of outcome after radical cystectomy for bladder cancer: a retrospective study of a homogeneous patient cohort. J Urol 1999; 161: 1494–7.

29. Skinner DG, Tift JP, Kaufman JJ. High dose, short course preoperative radiation therapy and immediate single stage radical cystectomy with pelvic node dissection in the management of bladder cancer. J Urol 1982; 127: 671–4.

30. Milosevic M, Gospodarowicz M, Jewett M, Bristow R, Haycocks T. Intensity-modulated radiation therapy (IMRT) for lymph node metastases in bladder cancer. In Gregoire V, Scalliet P, Ang K (eds): Clinical Target Volumes in Conformal and Intensity Modulated Radiation Therapy. New York: Springer-Verlag, 2003, pp 157–69.

31. Agranovich A, Czaykowski P, Hui D, Pickles T, Kwan W. Radiotherapy for muscle-invasive urinary bladder cancer in elderly patients. Can J Urol 2003; 10: 2056–61.

32. Borgaonkar S, Jain A, Bollina P, et al. Radical radiotherapy and salvage cystectomy as the primary management of transitional cell carcinoma of the bladder. Results following the introduction of a CT planning technique. Clin Oncol 2002; 14: 141–7.

33. Larsen LE, Engelholm SA. The value of three-dimensional radiotherapy planning in advanced carcinoma of the urinary bladder based on computed tomography. Acta Oncol 1994; 33: 655–9.

34. Bentzen SM, Jessen KA, Jorgensen J, Sell A. Impact of CT-based treatment planning on radiation therapy of carcinoma of the bladder. Acta Radiol Oncol 1984; 23: 199–203.

35. Rothwell RI, Ash DV, Jones WG. Radiation treatment planning for bladder cancer: a comparison of cystogram localisation with computed tomography. Clin Radiol 1983; 34: 103–11.

36. Logue JP, Sharrock CL, Cowan RA, Read G, Marrs J, Mott D. Clinical variability of target volume description in conformal radiotherapy planning. Int J Radiat Oncol Biol Phys 1998; 41: 929–31.

37. Meijer G, Rasch C, Remeijer P, Lebesque J. Three-dimensional analysis of delineation errors, setup errors, and organ motion during radiotherapy of bladder cancer. Int J Radiat Oncol Biol Phys 2003; 55: 1277–87.

38. Cowan R, McBain C, Ryder W, et al. Radiotherapy for muscle-invasive carcinoma of the bladder: results of a randomized trial comparing conventional whole bladder with dose-escalated partial bladder radiotherapy. Int J Radiat Oncol Biol Phys 2004; 59: 197–207.

39. Turner SL, Swindell SL, Bowl N, et al. Bladder movement during radiation therapy for bladder cancer: implications for treatment planning. Int J Radiat Oncol Biol Phys 1997; 39: 355–60.

40. Muren L, Smaaland R, Dahl O. Organ motion, set-up variation and treatment margins in radical radiotherapy of urinary bladder cancer. Radiother Oncol 2003; 69: 291–304.

41. Muren L, Redpath A, McLaren D. Treatment margins and treatment fractionation in conformal radiotherapy of muscle-invading urinary bladder cancer. Radiother Oncol 2004; 71: 65–71.

42. Jaffray DA, Siewerdsen JH, Wong JW, Martinez AA. Flat-panel cone-beam computed tomography for image-guided radiation therapy. Int J Radiat Oncol Biol Phys 2002; 53: 1337–49.

43. Turner WH, Markwalder R, Perrig S, Studer UE. Meticulous pelvic lymphadenectomy in surgical treatment of the invasive bladder cancer: an option or a must? Eur Urol 1998; 33(Suppl 4): 21–2.

44. Vieweg J, Gschwend JE, Herr HW, Fair WR. Pelvic lymph node dissection can be curative in patients with node positive bladder cancer. J Urol 1999; 161: 449–54.

45. Stein JP, Lieskovsky G, Cote R, et al. Radical cystectomy in the treatment of invasive bladder cancer: long-term results in 1,054 patients. J Clin Oncol 2001; 19: 666–75.

46. Smith JA, Whitmore WF. Regional lymph node metastases from bladder cancer. J Urol 1981; 126: 591–3.

47. Zincke H, Patterson DE, Utz DC, Benson RC. Pelvic lymphadenectomy and radical cystectomy for transitional cell carcinoma of the bladder with pelvic lymph node disease. Br J Urol 1985; 57: 156–9.

48. Poulson AL, Horn T, Steven K. Radical cystectomy: extending the limits of pelvic lymph node dissection improves survival for patients with bladder cancer confined to the bladder wall. J Urol 1998; 160: 2015–21.

49. Bretheau D, Ponthieu A. Results of radical cystectomy and pelvic lymphadenectomy for bladder cancer with pelvic node metastases. Urol Int 1996; 57: 27–31.

50. Quilty PM, Kerr GR, Duncan W. Prognostic indices for bladder cancer: an analysis of patients with transitional cell carcinoma of the bladder primarily treated by radical megavoltage x-ray therapy. Radiother Oncol 1986; 7: 311–21.

51. Sell A, Jakobsen A, Nerstrom B, Sorensen B, Steven K, Barlebo H. Treatment of advanced bladder cancer category T2, T3 and T4a. Scand J Urol Nephrol 1991; 138: 193–201.

52. Pisters LL, Tykochinsky G, Wajsman Z. Intravesical bacillus Calmette–Guérin or mitomycin C in the treatment of carcinoma in situ of the bladder following prior pelvic radiation therapy. J Urol 1991; 146: 1514–17.

53. Palou J, Sanchez-Martin FM, Rosales A, Salvador J, Algaba F, Vicente J. Intravesical bacille Calmette–Guérin in the treatment of carcinoma in

situ or high-grade superficial bladder carcinoma after radiotherapy for bladder carcinoma. BJU Int 1999; 83: 429–31.

54. Quilty PM, Duncan W, Chisholm GD, et al. Results of surgery following radical radiotherapy for invasive bladder cancer. Br J Urol 1986; 58: 396–405.

55. Bloom HJ, Hendry WF, Wallace DM, Skeet RG. Treatment of T3 bladder cancer: controlled trial of pre-operative radiotherapy and radical cystectomy versus radical radiotherapy. Br J Urol 1982; 54: 136–51.

56. Shipley W, Kaufman D, Zehr E, et al. Selective bladder preservation by combined modality protocol treatment: long-term outcomes of 190 patients with invasive bladder cancer. Urology 2002; 60 :62–7.

57. Zietman A, Sacco D, Skowronski U, et al. Organ conservation in invasive bladder cancer by transurethral resection, chemotherapy and radiation: results of a urodynamic and quality of life study on long-term survivors. J Urol 2003; 170: 1772–6.

58. Coppin C, Gospodarowicz M, James K, et al. The NCI-Canada trial of concurrent cisplatin and radiotherapy for muscle invasive bladder cancer. J Clin Oncol 1996; 14: 2901–7.

59. Shearer RJ, Chilvers CED, Bloom HJG, et al. Adjuvant chemotherapy in T3 carcinoma of the bladder. A prospective trial: preliminary report. Br J Urol 1988; 62: 558–64.

60. Wallace DMA, Raghavan D, Kelly KA, et al. Neo-adjuvant (pre-emptive) cisplatin therapy in invasive transitional cell carcinoma of the bladder. Br J Urol 1991; 67: 608–15.

61. Shipley WU, Winter KA, Kaufman DS, et al. Phase III trial of neoadjuvant chemotherapy in patients with invasive bladder cancer treated with selective bladder preservation by combined radiation therapy and chemotherapy: initial results of Radiation Therapy Oncology Group 89-03. J Clin Oncol 1998; 16: 3576–83.

62. Sengelov L, von der Maase H, Lundbeck F, et al. Neoadjuvant chemotherapy with cisplatin and methotrexate in patients with muscle-invasive bladder tumours. Acta Oncol 2002; 41: 447–56.

63. Ghersi D, Stewart LA, Parmar KMB, et al. Neoadjuvant cisplatin, methotrexate, and vinblastine chemotherapy for muscle-invasive bladder cancer: a randomized controlled trial. Lancet 1999; 354: 533–40.

64. Farah R, Chodak GW, Vogelzang NJ, et al. Curative radiotherapy following chemotherapy for invasive bladder carcinoma (a preliminary report). Int J Radiat Oncol Biol Phys 1991; 20: 413–17.

65. Tester W, Caplan R, Heaney J, et al. Neoadjuvant combined modality program with selective organ preservation for invasive bladder cancer: results of Radiation Therapy Oncology Group phase II trial 8802. J Clin Oncol 1996; 14 : 119–26.

66. Wajsman Z, Marino R, Parsons J, Oblon D, McCarley D. Bladder-sparing approach in the treatment of invasive bladder cancer. Semin Urol 1990; 8(3): 210–15.

67. Advanced Bladder Cancer Meta-analysis Collaboration. Neoadjuvant chemotherapy in invasive bladder cancer: a systematic review and meta-analysis. Lancet 2003; 361: 1927–34.

68. Bristow RG, Hill RP. Molecular and cellular radiobiology. In Tannock IF, Hill RP, Harrington L, Bristow RG (eds): Basic Science of Oncology, 4th ed. New York: McGraw-Hill, 2005, Ch. 14.

69. Oxford G, Theodorescu D. The role of Ras superfamily proteins in bladder cancer progression. J Urol 2003; 170: 1987–93.

70. Raghavan D. Molecular targeting and pharmacogenomics in the management of advanced bladder cancer. Cancer 2003; 97: 2083–9.

71. Al-Sukhun S, Hussain M. Molecular biology of transitional cell carcinoma. Crit Rev Oncol Hematol 2003; 47: 181–93.

72. Faulhaber O, Bristow RG. Basis of cell kill following clinical radiotherapy. In Sluyser M (ed): Application of Apoptosis to Cancer Treatment. New York: Springer, 2005.

73. Wilson GD. Radiation and the cell cycle, revisited. Cancer Metastasis Rev 2004; 23: 209–25.

74. Cuddihy AR, Bristow RG. The p53 protein family and radiation sensitivity: Yes or no? Cancer Metastasis Rev 2004; 23: 237–57.

75. Doherty SC, McKeown SR, McKelvey-Martin V, et al. Cell cycle checkpoint function in bladder cancer. J Natl Cancer Inst 2003; 95: 1859–68.

76. Pollack A, Wu CS, Czerniak B, Zagars GK, Benedict WF, McDonnell TJ. Abnormal bcl-2 and pRb expression are independent correlates of

radiation response in muscle-invasive bladder cancer. Clin Cancer Res 1997; 3: 1823–9.

77. Bakkenist CJ, Kastan MB. Initiating cellular stress responses. Cell 2004; 118: 9–17.

78. Bristow RG, Hill RP. The scientific basis of clinical radiotherapy. In Tannock IF, Hill RP, Harrington L, Bristow RG (eds): Basic Science of Oncology, 4th ed. New York: McGraw-Hill, 2005, Ch. 15.

79. Mack PC, Gandara DR, Bowen C, et al. RB status as a determinant of response to UCN-01 in non-small cell lung carcinoma. Clin Cancer Res 1999; 5: 2596–604.

80. Chien M, Astumian M, Liebowitz D, Rinker-Schaeffer C, Stadler WM. In vitro evaluation of flavopiridol, a novel cell cycle inhibitor, in bladder cancer. Cancer Chemother Pharmacol 1999; 44: 81–7.

81. Bohm L, Roos WP, Serafin AM. Inhibition of DNA repair by pentoxifylline and related methylxanthine derivatives. Toxicology 2003; 193: 153–60.

82. Jones LA, Clegg S, Bush C, McMillan TJ, Peacock JH. Relationship between chromosome aberrations, micronuclei and cell kill in two human tumour cell lines of widely differing radiosensitivity. Int J Radiat Biol 1994; 66: 639–42.

83. Woudstra EC, Roesink JM, Rosemann M, et al. Chromatin structure and cellular radiosensitivity: a comparison of two human tumour cell lines. Int J Radiat Biol 1996; 70: 693–703.

84. Collis SJ, Sangar VK, Tighe A, et al. Development of a novel rapid assay to assess the fidelity of DNA double-strand-break repair in human tumour cells. Nucleic Acids Res 2002; 30: E1.

85. McKeown SR, Robson T, Price ME, Ho ET, Hirst DG, McKelvey-Martin VJ. Potential use of the alkaline comet assay as a predictor of bladder tumour response to radiation. Br J Cancer 2003; 89: 2264–70.

86. Moneef MA, Sherwood BT, Bowman KJ, et al. Measurements using the alkaline comet assay predict bladder cancer cell radiosensitivity. Br J Cancer 2003; 89: 2271–6.

87. Abraham RT. PI 3-kinase related kinases: 'big' players in stress-induced signaling pathways. DNA Repair 2004; 3: 883–7.

88. van Gent DC, Hoeijmakers JH, Kanaar R. Chromosomal stability and the DNA double-stranded break connection. Nat Rev Genet 2001; 2: 196–206.

89. Ortiz T, Lopez S, Burguillos MA, Edreira A, Pinero J. Radiosensitizer effect of wortmannin in radioresistant bladder tumoral cell lines. Int J Oncol 2004; 24: 169–75.

90. Siddik ZH. Cisplatin: mode of cytotoxic action and molecular basis of resistance. Oncogene 2003; 22: 7265–79.

91. Begg AC, Stewart FA, Dewit L, Bartelink H. Interactions between cisplatin and radiation in experimental rodent tumors and normal tissues. In Hill BT, Bellamy AS (eds): Antitumor Drug-Radiation Interactions. Boca Raton, FL: CRC Press, 2000, pp 153–70.

92. Wachters FM, van Putten JW, Maring JG, Zdzienicka MZ, Groen HJ, Kampinga HH. Selective targeting of homologous DNA recombination repair by gemcitabine. Int J Radiat Oncol Biol Phys 2003; 57: 553–62.

93. Pauwels B, Korst AE, Pattyn GG, et al. Cell cycle effect of gemcitabine and its role in the radiosensitizing mechanism in vitro. Int J Radiat Oncol Biol Phys 2003; 57: 1075–83.

94. Sangar VK, Cowan R, Margison GP, Hendry JH, Clarke NW. An evaluation of gemcitabine's differential radiosensitising effect in related bladder cancer cell lines. Br J Cancer 2004; 90: 542–8.

95. West CM. Invited review: intrinsic radiosensitivity as a predictor of patient response to radiotherapy. Br J Radiol 1995; 68: 827–37.

96. Moonen L, Ong F, Gallee M, et al. Apoptosis, proliferation and p53, cyclin D1, and retinoblastoma gene expression in relation to radiation response in transitional cell carcinoma of the bladder. Int J Radiat Oncol Biol Phys 2001; 49: 1305–10.

97. Wang S, El-Deiry WS. TRAIL and apoptosis induction by TNF-family death receptors. Oncogene 2003; 22: 8628–33.

98. Hussain SA, Ganesan R, Hiller L, et al. BCL2 expression predicts survival in patients receiving synchronous chemoradiotherapy in advanced transitional cell carcinoma of the bladder. Oncol Rep 2003; 10: 571–6.

99. Matsumoto H, Wada T, Fukunaga K, Yoshihiro S, Matsuyama H, Naito K. Bax to Bcl-2 ratio and Ki-67 index are useful predictors of neoadjuvant chemoradiation therapy in bladder cancer. Jpn J Clin Oncol 2004; 34: 124–30.

100. Ong F, Moonen LM, Gallee MP, et al. Prognostic factors in transitional cell cancer of the bladder: an emerging role for Bcl-2 and p53. Radiother Oncol 2001; 61: 169–75.

101. Qureshi KN, Griffiths TR, Robinson MC, et al. Combined p21WAF1/CIP1 and p53 overexpression predict improved survival in muscle-invasive bladder cancer treated by radical radiotherapy. Int J Radiat Oncol Biol Phys 2001; 51: 1234–40.

102. Rotterud R, Berner A, Holm R, Skovlund E, Fossa SD. p53, p21 and mdm2 expression vs the response to radiotherapy in transitional cell carcinoma of the bladder. BJU Int 2001; 88: 202–8.

103. Ribeiro JC, Barnetson AR, Fisher RJ, Mameghan H, Russell PJ. Relationship between radiation response and p53 status in human bladder cancer cells. Int J Radiat Biol 1997; 72: 11–20.

104. Rotterud R, Skomedal H, Berner A, Danielsen HE, Skovlund E, Fossa SD. TP53 and p21WAF1/CIP1 behave differently in euploid versus aneuploid bladder tumours treated with radiotherapy. Acta Oncol 2001; 40: 644–52.

105. Fechner G, Perabo FG, Schmidt DH, et al. Preclinical evaluation of a radiosensitizing effect of gemcitabine in p53 mutant and p53 wild type bladder cancer cells. Urology 2003; 61: 468–73.

106. Hinata N, Shirakawa T, Zhang Z, et al. Radiation induces p53-dependent cell apoptosis in bladder cancer cells with wild-type-p53 but not in p53-mutated bladder cancer cells. Urol Res 2003; 31: 387–96.

107. Pollack A, Czerniak B, Zagars GK, et al. Retinoblastoma protein expression and radiation response in muscle-invasive bladder cancer. Int J Radiat Oncol Biol Phys 1997; 39: 687–95.

108. Muro XGd, Condom E, Vigues F, et al. p53 and p21 Expression levels predict organ preservation and survival in invasive bladder carcinoma treated with a combined-modality approach. Cancer 2004; 100: 1859–67.

109. Wu CS, Pollack A, Czerniak B, et al. Prognostic value of p53 in muscle-invasive bladder cancer treated with preoperative radiotherapy. Urology 1996; 47: 305–10.

110. Rodel C, Grabenbauer GG, Rodel F, et al. Apoptosis, p53, bcl-2, and KI-67 in invasive bladder carcinoma: possible predictors for response to radiochemotherapy and successful bladder preservation. Int J Radiat Oncol Biol Phys 2000; 46: 1213–21.

111. Duggan BJ, Maxwell P, Kelly JD, et al. The effect of antisense Bcl-2 oligonucleotides on Bcl-2 protein expression and apoptosis in human bladder transitional cell carcinoma. J Urol 2001; 166: 1098–105.

112. Pagliaro LC, Keyhani A, Williams D, et al. Repeated intravesical instillations of an adenoviral vector in patients with locally advanced bladder cancer: a phase I study of p53 gene therapy. J Clin Oncol 2003; 21: 2247–53.

113. Slaton JW, Benedict WF, Dinney CP. P53 in bladder cancer: mechanism of action, prognostic value, and target for therapy. Urology 2001; 57: 852–9.

114. Bromfield GP, Meng A, Warde P, Bristow RG. Cell death in irradiated prostate epithelial cells: role of apoptotic and clonogenic cell kill. Prostate Cancer Prostatic Dis 2003; 6: 73–85.

115. Okada H, Mak TW. Pathways of apoptotic and non-apoptotic death in tumour cells. Nat Rev Cancer 2004; 4: 592–603.

116. Nakahata K, Miyakoda M, Suzuki K, Kodama S, Watanabe M. Heat shock induces centrosomal dysfunction, and causes non-apoptotic mitotic catastrophe in human tumour cells. Int J Hyperthermia 2002; 18: 332–43.

117. Altieri DC. Survivin, versatile modulation of cell division and apoptosis in cancer. Oncogene 2003; 22: 8581–9.

118. Schultz IJ, Kiemeney LA, Karthaus HF, et al. Survivin mRNA copy number in bladder washings predicts tumor recurrence in patients with superficial urothelial cell carcinomas. Clin Chem 2004; 50: 1425–8.

119. Swana HS, Grossman D, Anthony JN, Weiss RM, Altieri DC. Tumor content of the antiapoptosis molecule survivin and recurrence of bladder cancer. N Engl J Med 1999; 341: 452–3.

120. Ning S, Fuessel S, Kotzsch M, et al. siRNA-mediated down-regulation of survivin inhibits bladder cancer cell growth. Int J Oncol 2004; 25: 1065–71.

121. Fuessel S, Kueppers B, Ning S, et al. Systematic in vitro evaluation of survivin directed antisense oligodeoxynucleotides in bladder cancer cells. J Urol 2004; 171: 2471–6.

122. Glaser KB, Staver MJ, Waring JF, Stender J, Ulrich RG, Davidsen SK. Gene expression profiling of multiple histone deacetylase (HDAC) inhibitors: defining a common gene set produced by HDAC inhibition in T24 and MDA carcinoma cell lines. Mol Cancer Ther 2003; 2: 151–63.

123. Richon VM, Sandhoff TW, Rifkind RA, Marks PA. Histone deacetylase inhibitor selectively induces p21WAF1 expression and gene-associated histone acetylation. Proc Natl Acad Sci USA 2000; 97: 10014–19.

124. Duchesne GM, Hutchinson LK. Reversible changes in radiation response induced by all-trans retinoic acid. Int J Radiat Oncol Biol Phys 1995; 33: 875–80.

125. Milosevic M, Fyles A, Hedley D, Hill R. The human tumor microenvironment: invasive (needle) measurements of oxygen and interstitial fluid pressure. Semin Radiat Oncol 2004; 14: 249–58.

126. Brown JM, Wilson WR. Exploiting tumour hypoxia in cancer treatment. Nat Rev Cancer 2004; 4: 437–47.

127. Subarsky P, Hill RP. The hypoxic tumour microenvironment and metastatic progression. Clin Exp Metastasis 2003; 20: 237–50.

128. Hoskin P, Sibtain A, Daley F, Wilson G. GLUT1 and CAIX as intrinsic markers of hypoxia in bladder cancer: relationship with vascularity and proliferation as predictors of outcome of ARCON. Br J Cancer 2003; 89: 1290–7.

129. Fyles A, Milosevic M, Hedley D, et al. Tumor hypoxia has independent predictor impact only in patients with node-negative cervix cancer. J Clin Oncol 2002; 20: 680–7.

130. Brizel DM, Scully SP, Harrelson JM, et al. Tumor oxygenation predicts for likelihood of distant metastases in human soft tissue sarcoma. Cancer Res 1996; 56: 941–3.

131. Kaanders JH, Bussink J, van der Kogel AJ. ARCON: a novel biology-based approach in radiotherapy. Lancet Oncol 2002; 3: 728–37.

132. Chaudhary R, Bromley M, Clarke NW, et al. Prognostic relevance of micro-vessel density in cancer of the urinary bladder. Anticancer Res 1999; 19: 3479–84.

133. Sabichi AL, Lippman SM. COX-2 inhibitors and other nonsteroidal anti-inflammatory drugs in genitourinary cancer. Semin Oncol 2004; 31: 36–44.

134. Ma BB, Bristow RG, Kim J, Siu LL. Combined-modality treatment of solid tumors using radiotherapy and molecular targeted agents. J Clin Oncol 2003; 21: 2760–76.

135. Thames HD, Hendry JH. Fractionation in radiotherapy. London: Taylor and Francis, 1987, p 297.

136. Trott KR, Kummermehr J. What is known about tumour proliferation rates to choose between accelerated fractionation or hyperfractionation? Radiother Oncol 1985; 3: 1–9.

137. Hainau B, Dombernowsky P. Histology and cell proliferation in human bladder tumors. Cancer 1974; 33: 115–26.

138. Rew DA, Thomas DJ, Coptcoat M, Wilson GD. Measurement of in vivo urological tumour cell kinetics using multiplanar flow cytometry. Preliminary study. Br J Urol 1991; 68: 44–8.

139. Subarsky P, Hill R. The hypoxic tumour microenvironment and metastatic progression. Clin. Exp Metastasis 2003; 20: 237–50.

140. Majewski W, Maciejewski B, Majewski S, Suwinski R, Miszczyk L, Tarnawski R. Clinical radiobiology of stage T2–T3 bladder cancer. Int J Radiat Oncol Biol Phys 2004; 60: 60–70.

141. Cole DJ, Durrant KR, Roberts JT, Dawes PJ, Yosef H, Hopewell JW. A pilot study of accelerated fractionation in the radiotherapy of invasive carcinoma of the bladder. Br J Radiol 1992; 65: 792–8.

142. Pos F, Tienhoven Gv, Hulshof M, Koedooder K, Gonzalez DG. Concomitant boost radiotherapy for muscle invasive bladder cancer. Radiother Oncol 2003; 68: 75–80.

143. Yavuz A, Yavuz M, Ozgur G, et al. Accelerated superfractionated radiotherapy with concomitant boost for invasive bladder cancer. Int J Radiat Oncol Biol Phys 2003; 56: 734–45.

144. Zouhair A, Ozsahin M, Schneider D, et al. Invasive bladder carcinoma: a pilot study of conservative treatment with accelerated radiotherapy and concomitant cisplatin. Int J Cancer 2001; 96: 350–5.

145. Moonen L, van der Voet H, Horenblas S, Bartelink H. A feasibility study of accelerated fractionation in radiotherapy of carcinoma of the urinary bladder. Int J Radiat Oncol Biol Phys 1997; 37: 537–42.

146. Plataniotis G, Michalopoulos E, Kouvaris J, Vlahos L, Papavasiliou C. A feasibility study of partially accelerated radiotherapy for invasive bladder cancer. Radiother Oncol 1994; 33: 84–7.

147. Horwich A, Dearnaley D, Huddart R, et al. A trial of accelerated fractionation (AF) in T2/3 bladder cancer [abstract]. Eur J Cancer 1999; 35(Suppl 4): S342.

148. Naslund I, Nilsson B, Littbrand B. Hyperfractionated radiotherapy of bladder cancer. A ten-year follow-up of a randomized clinical trial. Acta Oncol 1994; 33: 397–402.

149. Goldobenko G, Matveev B, Shipilov V, Klimakov B, Tkachev S. Radiation treatment of bladder cancer using different fractionation regimens. Med Radiol (Mosk) 1991; 36: 14–16.

150. Stuschke M, Thames HD. Hyperfractionated radiotherapy of human tumors: overview of the randomized clinical trials. Int J Radiat Oncol Biol Phys 1997; 37: 259–67.

151. Dyrskjot L. Classification of bladder cancer by microarray expression profiling: towards a general clinical use of microarrays in cancer diagnostics. Expert Rev Mol Diagn 2003; 3: 635–47.

152. Ferguson RE, Selby PJ, Banks RE. Proteomic studies in urological malignancies. Contrib Nephrol 2004; 141: 257–79.

153. Sanchez-Carbayo M, Cordon-Cardo C. Applications of array technology: identification of molecular targets in bladder cancer. Br J Cancer 2003; 89: 2172–7.

154. Blankenberg FG. Recent advances in the imaging of programmed cell death. Curr Pharm Des 2004; 10: 1457–67.

155. Shah R, El-Deiry WS. p53-Dependent activation of a molecular beacon in tumor cells following exposure to doxorubicin chemotherapy. Cancer Biol Ther 2004; 3(9): 871–5.

156. Lewis JS, Welch MJ. PET imaging of hypoxia. Q J Nucl Med 2001; 45: 183–8.

19

Trimodality therapy in the management of muscle-invasive bladder cancer: a selective organ-preserving approach

John J Coen, Anthony L Zietman, Donald S Kaufman, Niall M Heney, Alex F Althausen, William U Shipley

Overview

Combined modality therapy with organ preservation has become standard therapy for a variety of solid tumors. Although radical cystectomy continues to be standard therapy for invasive bladder cancer, there is evidence to suggest that selective bladder preservation results in similar outcome with the opportunity to retain the native bladder. Older randomized trials have failed to demonstrate a survival advantage for immediate cystectomy as opposed to salvage cystectomy for recurrent disease in patients receiving radiation therapy. Selective bladder preservation using a trimodality approach, as commonly practiced in the US, affords an early cystectomy for patients who fail to respond to chemoradiation. Using this approach, a complete transurethral resection is performed. Following an induction course of concurrent chemotherapy and radiation, histologic response is evaluated by cystoscopy and rebiopsy. Clinical 'complete responders' (tumor site biopsy and urine cytology negative) continue with a consolidation course of chemotherapy and radiation, while others are encouraged to have an immediate cystectomy. Complete response rates of 65% to 80% can be achieved. Conserved bladders are closely followed by a urologist who will perform a prompt cystectomy if there is an invasive recurrence. Noninvasive recurrences can be managed by more conservative measures in a manner similar to a de novo tumor. Bladder conservation trials using this approach report 5-year survival rates of approximately 50%, with 80% of surviving patients retaining their bladder. Quality of life and urodynamic studies reveal good functional outcomes for patients with preserved bladders.

Introduction

The treatment options for muscle-invasive bladder cancer can be broadly divided into organ-sparing regimens and those that require immediate removal of the bladder. Radical cystectomy with surgical removal of the bladder, its adnexae, and the regional lymph nodes represents the most prevalent treatment offered in the US. Radiation therapy, the traditional bladder-sparing approach, has only been recommended for patients deemed 'unfit' for surgery secondary to advanced age, comorbidities or disease extent. Consequently, when comparisons of retrospective radiation and surgical series have been made, better outcomes for patients undergoing cystectomy are reported. This comparison is further confounded as an additional 15% of patients are excluded from cystectomy series secondary to intraoperative discovery of extravesical tumor extension, prompting abortion of the procedure. In contrast to historic series, modern bladder-sparing regimens do not consist of radiation monotherapy but are typified by a multimodality approach.

Nevertheless, radical cystectomy represents the standard against which bladder-conserving regimens must be measured. Pelvic recurrence rates between 5% and 30%, and overall 5-year survival between 45% and 60%, have been reported after cystectomy.[1-4] Following a radical cystectomy, a urinary diversion must be created which may be an incontinent or continent diversion. The ileal loop procedure allows urine to drain into an isolated segment of ileum which acts as a conduit to a stoma created at the skin surface. An appliance acts as an external reservoir to collect urine. Recent surgical advances offer the potential to make the loss of the native bladder more acceptable to the patient. For continent diversions, bowel segments are used to create internal reservoirs that are either intermittently catheterized by the patient through an abdominal wall stoma, or are anastomosed to the urethra (an orthotopic neobladder), allowing the patient to void more naturally. Although continent diversions are becoming more popular, they are still performed on less than half of patients undergoing radical cystectomy. They are also not without problems including enuresis, stenosis, mucosuria, alkalosis, and progressive renal impairment. Revision procedures may be required to resolve one or more of these problems. Despite the enthusiasm of the surgical community, the largest reported series looking at quality of life reported no increase in patient satisfaction with continent diversions as compared to an ileal conduit.[5] Although surgical advances are likely to continue, for the foreseeable future it is not expected that any internal reservoir will be created that functions as well as a preserved native bladder.

Multimodality organ-sparing treatment has become standard therapy for many solid malignancies, including those of the breast, anus, esophagus, and head and neck. Similar advances have been made in the treatment of muscle-invasive bladder cancer evolving into a trimodality approach involving cooperation between urologists, radiation oncologists, and medical oncologists. Modern bladder-sparing represents a selective bladder-preserving regimen where the primary goal is to cure the patient, using early cystectomy when necessary, with a secondary goal of conserving a well-functioning, tumor-free bladder in patients in whom avoidance of cystectomy does not compromise survival.

Evolution of the modern bladder-preserving approach

Randomized comparisons of external beam radiation with radical cystectomy

External beam radiation therapy represents the traditional alternative to radical cystectomy, with surgery reserved for salvage should there be any recurrence within the bladder. Urologists have feared that the delay of definitive surgery may compromise survival as the recurrent cancer has a second opportunity to metastasize.

By 1985, four randomized trials had been completed comparing external beam radiation with cystectomy reserved for salvage, with preoperative radiation plus immediate radical cystectomy[6-9] (Table 19.1) Miller et al reported the results of a randomized trial from the University of Texas M.D. Anderson Cancer Center for patients with clinical stage T3 tumors, demonstrating improved overall survival at 5 years for patients randomized to cystectomy as compared to radiation, 45% versus 22%.[6] This is the only trial that demonstrates a statistically significant benefit to early cystectomy; however; it included large T3 tumors unlikely to be adequately managed with radiation alone.

The Urologic Cooperative Group from the UK reported a larger randomized trial of 189 patients comparing radiation with cystectomy reserved for salvage with radiation plus immediate cystectomy.[7] The 5- and 10-year overall survival was 39% and 19% for patients randomized to immediate cystectomy, respectively. In patients randomized to radiation with salvage cystectomy, the 5- and 10-year overall survival was 28% and 15%, respectively. These differences were not statistically significant.

The Danish National Cancer Group also failed to demonstrate a significant overall survival difference at 5 years: 29% for cystectomy versus 23% for radiation and salvage cystectomy.[8] The local or pelvic failure was lower in patients randomized to immediate cystectomy as compared to radiation alone: 7% versus 35%, respectively. However, the incidence of metastatic disease was similar in both groups: 34% and 32% at 5 years, respectively.

The National Bladder Cancer Group performed a randomized trial of 72 patients.[9] There was no difference in the 5-year overall survival or distant metastasis rate in patients randomized to immediate cystectomy (27% and 38%, respectively) as compared to primary radiation and salvage cystectomy (40% and 31%, respectively).

These trials suggest that deferral of cystectomy until the time of local recurrence does not adversely influence overall survival or the incidence of metastatic disease after external beam radiation. Similarly, the Memorial Sloan-Kettering Cancer Center reported that deferring cystectomy in patients receiving neoadjuvant MVAC (methotrexate, vinblastine, doxorubicin [adriamycin], cisplatin) chemotherapy did not decrease overall survival at 5 years.[10] Thus, selective bladder preservation approaches with cystectomy offered for local tumor recurrence or persistence may be a safe alternative to radical cystectomy for invasive bladder cancer.

Monotherapy

Transurethral resection and chemotherapy provide a durable local control rate of less than 20% when used as monotherapy (Table 19.2). Although external beam radiation results in a higher local control rate, salvage cystectomy is still required for many of these patients. Compelled by the success of combined modality treatment as organ-preserving therapy in anal and breast cancer, efforts were made to establish a similar treatment approach in invasive bladder cancer. The complete response rate to transurethral resection followed by chemotherapy is nearly twice that achieved by chemotherapy alone, and is slightly greater than that achieved by radiation alone. Trimodality therapy achieves a complete response rate of more than 70%, far greater than that achieved with monotherapy (Table 19.3).

Table 19.1 Randomized trials of irradiation that did or did not defer radical cystectomy for salvage of recurrence

Treatment	No. pts	Clinical stage	5-year survival (%)	10-year survival (%)	Distant metastases (%)
M.D. Anderson Hospital[6]					
50 Gy + cystectomy	35	T3	46	–	–
60 Gy + salvage cystectomy	32	T3	22	–	–
UK Coop Group[7]					
40 Gy + radical cystectomy	98	T3	39	19	–
60 Gy + salvage cystectomy	91	T3	28	15	–
National Danish Trial[8]					
40 Gy + radical cystectomy	88	T3	29	–	34
60 Gy + salvage cystectomy	95	T3	23	–	32
National Bladder Cancer Group[9]					
40 Gy + radical cystectomy	37	T2–4a	27	–	38
S60 Gy + salvage cystectomy	35	T2–4a	40	–	31

Table 19.2 Success rates of bladder preservation with monotherapy

Treatment	No. of evaluated series	No. pts	% with bladder free of invasive recurrence
Transurethral resection alone*[35,36]	2	331	20‡
Radiation therapy alone†[37–41]	5	949	41
Chemotherapy alone†[42] (cisplatin + methotrexate)	1	27	19

*Used selectively as monotherapy, most patients at these centers had cystectomy.
†No transurethral resection of tumor.
‡Intravesical drug therapy often used for noninvasive recurrent tumors.

Table 19.3 Complete response rates after monotherapies and combined modality therapies

Treatment	No. of evaluated series	No. pts	Complete responses (%)
Radiation therapy alone[38,39,43,44]	4	721	45
Chemotherapy alone[45–50]	6	301	27
TURBT plus chemotherapy[51–55]	5	336	52
TURBT plus chemoradiotherapy[17,18,56,57]	4	218	71

TURBT, transurethral resection of bladder tumor.

Trimodality therapy

The combination of transurethral resection, chemotherapy, and radiation therapy may serve two purposes: 1) local control is enhanced as surgical debulking provides cytoreduction prior to radiation therapy; 2) concurrent chemotherapy with radiation-sensitizing agents such as cisplatin, 5-fluorouracil (5-FU) or taxol, increases cell death during radiation in a synergistic fashion. Thus, the probability of complete tumor eradication following radiation is maximized. Cytotoxic chemotherapy may also address micro-metastatic disease present at the time of local treatment.

The success of a bladder-preserving treatment approach rests on the ability to select patients for organ conservation based on the initial tumor response. This requires close cooperation with a urologist who is integral to the assessment of therapeutic response and who will perform a radical cystectomy if required. Commonly in the US, bladder conservation is reserved for patients found to have a complete clinical response mid-therapy[11,12] (Figure 19.1). Responders, who comprise more than two-thirds of patients, receive consolidation chemoradiation, and are followed indefinitely with regular cystoscopic examinations. Incomplete responders are encouraged to have an immediate cystectomy, thus averting further pelvic radiation which may complicate urinary diversion surgery. Prompt cystectomy is also recommended at the first sign of invasive recurrence for patients who have completed chemoradiation. Trimodality therapy with cystectomy when necessary results in overall survival rates comparable to radical cystectomy series when matched for age and clinical stage (49–63% at 5 years) (Table 19.4).

The potential success of trimodality therapy was exemplified in a study from the University of Paris. Transurethral resection of bladder tumor (TURBT) followed by concurrent cisplatin, 5-FU, and accelerated radiation was used initially as a precystectomy regimen. The first 18 patients demonstrated no residual tumor on cystoscopic examination and rebiopsy, but all underwent cystectomy as planned.[13] No patient had residual tumor identified in the

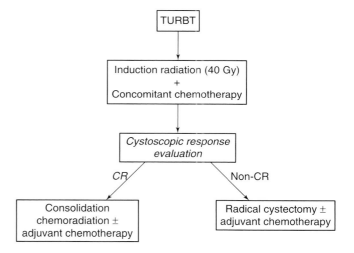

Figure 19.1
Selective bladder preservation treatment algorithm using trimodality therapy. (CR, complete response; TURBT, transurethral resection of bladder tumor.)

cystectomy specimen. Subsequently, patients with a clinical complete response were selected for bladder preservation.[13] Radical cystectomy was reserved for patients with a lesser response. In a series of 120 patients, they reported a complete response rate of 77% and a 5-year survival of 63%. A study of 93 patients treated with trimodality therapy at the University of Erlangen reported a clinical complete response rate of 85%. The 5-year overall survival was 61%, with 47% surviving with their native bladder.[14] An update of the Erlangen experience using combined modality treatment reported a clinical complete response rate of 72% in 415 treated patients (126 with radiation alone, 289 with chemoradiation).[15] The 10-year

Table 19.4 Recent results of TURBT and chemotherapy concurrent with radiation

Series (year)	Induction treatment	No. pts	5-year survival (%)	5-year survival with bladder preservation (%)
Dunst (1994)[57]	TURBT, cisplatin and XRT	79	52	41
RTOG (1993)[17]	Cisplatin and XRT	42	52	42
Shipley (2002)[11]	TURBT, MCV, cisplatin and XRT	190	54	46
RTOG (1998)[19]	TURBT, ± MCV, cisplatin and XRT	123	49	38
Paris (1997)[58]	TURBT, 5-fluorouracil, cisplatin and XRT	120	63	–

MCV, methotrexate, cisplatin, vinblastine; TURBT, transurethral resection of bladder tumor, XRT, external beam irradiation.

disease-specific survival was 42%, with 80% of survivors retaining their bladder. There was no decrement in survival for patients requiring a salvage cystectomy.

In the US, the Radiation Therapy Oncology Group (RTOG) has studied combined modality therapy in a multi-institutional setting, enrolling 415 patients on six prospective protocols over the last 15 years. Five of these protocols were phase I–II trials of concurrent chemoradiation, and one was a phase III trial that tested the efficacy of neoadjuvant chemotherapy with methotrexate, cisplatin, and vinblastine (MCV). These trials have shaped the manner in which combined modality therapy is administered in the US. Encouraged by the results reported by the National Bladder Cancer Group, the RTOG opened 85-12 which defined the RTOG paradigm for selective bladder preservation.[16] It evaluated trimodality therapy with cystectomy reserved for patients who failed to respond completely to 40 Gy with concurrent cisplatin.[17] Complete responders received consolidation therapy, with an additional 24 Gy delivered with concurrent cisplatin. The safety and efficacy of the regimen were demonstrated with a complete response rate of 66% and a 3-year survival rate of 64%. The subsequent protocol, RTOG 88-02, was a phase I–II trial which demonstrated that the addition of neoadjuvant MCV was well tolerated. It yielded a 75% response rate and a 62% 4-year survival rate in 91 entered patients.[18] This was followed by RTOG 89-03, a phase III trial to assess the efficacy of neoadjuvant MCV chemotherapy. It fell short of its accrual goals secondary to poor patient tolerance of the regimen. Toxicities consisted of severe leukopenia and sepsis. The 5-year overall survival rate in the 123 entered patients was 49% with no difference between treatment arms.[19] There was also no difference in the rate of distant metastasis or bladder preservation. Neoadjuvant chemotherapy was abandoned in future studies due to the toxicity and lack of therapeutic efficacy in this trial.

Beginning in 1995, the RTOG began a series of phase I–II protocols to evaluate accelerated radiation fractionation schemes in combination with concurrent outpatient chemotherapy. Protocol RTOG 95-06 evaluated the regimen piloted by the University of Paris using an outpatient regimen of 5-FU and cisplatin, concurrent with accelerated but hypofractionated radiation delivered over 17 days.[20] The eligibility criteria of this protocol were more stringent than prior RTOG studies. Patients with tumor-associated hydronephrosis were excluded because they were found to have lower complete response rates on previous trials. Among 34 evaluable patients, the complete response rate was 67% and overall survival was 83% at 3 years; however, there was a 21% rate of grade 3–4 hematologic toxicity. Subsequent trials included adjuvant chemotherapy after either selective bladder preservation or cystectomy. In RTOG 97-06, induction and consolidation chemoradiation included twice-daily radiation and outpatient cisplatin (30 mg/m^2)

given on the first three days of each week. Radiation doses of 1.8 Gy to the pelvis and 1.6 Gy to the tumor were given daily, with a 4–6 hour interval between treatments. After consolidation chemoradiation or cystectomy (depending on response), each patient received three cycles of MCV chemotherapy. Only 11% of patients experienced grade 3–4 toxicity during induction and consolidation chemoradiation.[21] The complete response rate was 71%. Only 40% of patients received a full three cycles of adjuvant MCV, and 35% of patients developed grade 3 toxicity. The development of metastasis may have been decreased by this regimen. The 2-year incidence of metastasis was 18%, which compares favorably to the arm of RTOG 89-03 that did not receive adjuvant chemotherapy. In the subgroup that did not have tumor-associated hydronephrosis, the 2-year incidence of distant metastasis was 31%. RTOG 99-06 included two innovative changes:

- the inclusion of an adjuvant chemotherapy regimen of cisplatin and gemcitabine. In the metastatic setting, this regimen has demonstrated efficacy with lesser toxicity than MVAC.[22–24]
- the inclusion of paclitaxel as a radiation-sensitizing agent during the induction and consolidation schedules.[25,26]

The trial has been closed, but the outcomes have not yet been reported.

In addition to the efforts made refining the combined modality regimen, the RTOG, through the Genitourinary Translational Research Group, has also made efforts to better delineate the molecular biology of bladder cancer and its response to therapy. They have assessed the significance of overexpression of p53, p21, pRb, p16, Erb1 (EGFR), and Erb2 (Her2) as measured by immunohistochemical staining in 73 patients treated on protocols RTOG 88-02, 89-03, 95-06, and 97-06.[27] Multivariate analysis revealed that p53, p21, pRb, and p16 fail to predict complete response rate, overall survival or disease-specific survival. Overexpression of Her2 was associated with a reduced complete response rate (50% versus 81%, $p = 0.026$). EGFR positivity was associated with improved disease-specific survival. These preliminary data will need to be confirmed in larger data sets and evaluated on prospective trials. Delineation of the role of individual markers in the biology of bladder cancer and its response to therapy may lead to the rational development of targeted therapies.

The RTOG has refined the selective bladder-preserving approach as it is currently practiced in the US. These trials will continue to optimize radiation and chemotherapy schedules to maximize response to therapy and make bladder preservation more likely. The study of adjuvant chemotherapy regimens may also increase the survival rate of all patients with invasive bladder cancer regardless of local therapy.

Urologic concerns about bladder-sparing approach

Despite the success of selective bladder preservation reported in retrospective series and phase II trials, its acceptance in the urologic community has been limited. Urologists have several concerns regarding leaving the diseased bladder in situ.

Does an incomplete turbt preclude bladder preservation?

While it is evident that a complete TURBT improves the complete response rate after chemoradiation, inability to perform a complete TURBT is not a contraindication to selective bladder preservation. The Erlangen experience revealed that completeness of TURBT and early tumor stage were the most important factors predicting complete response and overall survival.[15] They reported complete response rates of 90%, 77%, and 54% for visibly and microscopically complete (R0), visibly but not microscopically complete (R1), and visibly incomplete (R2) responses, respectively. The 10-year overall survival rates were 76%, 52%, and 34%, respectively. Although this series demonstrated TURBT extent as independent from tumor stage as a prognostic indicator for survival, it included superficial tumors whose clinical stage is more reliable and which are more apt to have R0 resections. Less complete TURBT may still serve as a marker for more advanced disease in the muscle-invasive tumors. It cannot be concluded that patients with incomplete TURBT gain a survival benefit from immediate cystectomy. In the Massachusetts General Hospital (MGH) experience, which included only muscle-invasive disease, there is no significant disease-specific survival detriment in patients with less than a visibly complete TURBT.[28] At 5 years, the rates were 69% and 58% for visibly complete and less than complete resections, respectively (log-rank, p=0.24). Furthermore, there was no demonstrated survival detriment for salvage as compared to immediate cystectomy in the series as a whole or in patients with lesser resections. However, the crude rate of cystectomy by last follow-up was higher for less than complete resections as compared to visibly complete resections, 50% versus 29%, respectively. For muscle-invasive bladder cancer, visibly complete TURBT increases the likelihood of bladder preservation, but inability to obtain a complete resection does not preclude selective bladder preservation. At MGH, the complete response rate for patients with less than a complete resection was 63%, and 74% of responders maintained their native bladder at 5 years.

Is Cystectomy frequently required for superficial relapse?

Bladder cancer is often associated with a field change which leaves the conservatively treated patient at risk for a superficial relapse. A risk of 9% to 28% at 5 years has been reported. Zietman et al reported a 26% (32 recurrences in 121 patients) rate of superficial recurrence among complete responders to trimodality therapy.[29] Of the 32 recurrences, 27 patients were managed with transurethral resection and intravesical therapy and tolerated it well. Cystectomy was ultimately required in 31% (10 of 32 cases), for additional superficial recurrence in seven patients and invasive recurrence in three. There was no survival decrement associated with superficial relapse. With routine urologic surveillance, superficial recurrences can be detected promptly, and salvage cystectomy averted in the majority of cases.

Is Bladder function poor after trimodality therapy?

Many urologists believe that an irradiated bladder is functionally worthless as it is prone to bleeding and contracture. Recent reports contradict this assumption for patients receiving modern radiation therapy. In the Erlangen experience, only three cystectomies were required for bladder contracture in 186 preserved bladders for an incidence of 2%.[15] In that series, 3% of patients had a reduced bladder capacity and 10% reported mild urinary symptoms including frequency, urgency, and dysuria. In the MGH experience, none of the 190 patients treated on selective bladder preservation protocols has required a cystectomy because of bladder morbidity.[11] A British quality of life analysis of 72 patients treated to 60 Gy in 30 fractions reported no difference in urinary and rectal function as compared to an age- and sex-matched control group.[30] More recently, Zietman et al reported the results of an urodynamic and quality of life study performed on 49 patients with preserved bladders several years after treatment at MGH.[31] Urodynamic studies demonstrated that 77% (24/31) of patients had normal bladder function by sex and age. Bladder outlet obstruction was demonstrated in 33% of men, and 30% of the studied women had involuntary detrusor contractions. Bladder symptoms were uncommon with the exception of urinary control. Overall, 19% of patients reported control problems, with 11% wearing pads. All pad wearers were women. Only 6% of patients reported moderate or higher urinary distress, and 14% reported distress over bowel urgency. Sexual function was maintained in the majority of the men studied, with 54% reporting satisfactory erections. Comparative quality of life studies from Denmark and Italy suggest an advantage to bladder preservation using chemoradiation over cystectomy with regards to urinary and sexual function.[32,33] Trimodality therapy, as practiced today, results in a well-functioning bladder and maintenance of sexual function in the majority of patients.

Is Uncontrolled pelvic disease common after trimodality therapy?

Local control rates of 40% achieved in radiation monotherapy series are inferior to those obtained with radical cystectomy. The poor results do not apply to patients treated with trimodality therapy if a prompt cystectomy is performed in less than complete responders. Invasive relapse rates of 9% to 17% have been reported after trimodality therapy. At MGH, 66 of 190 patients treated on selective bladder preservation protocols (35%) required a cystectomy: 41 for a less than complete response and 25 for recurrent tumors.[11] In this series, the rate of pelvic recurrence was 8.4%. A rate of 12% was reported by the RTOG for 123 patients treated on multi-institutional selective bladder preservation protocols. These rates compare favorably to the 9% pelvic recurrence rate reported for patients

Table 19.5 Survival in contemporary cystectomy and selective bladder preservation series

Series (year)	Stages	No. pts	5-year survival (%)	10-year survival (%)
Cystectomy				
USC (2001)[59]	P2–4A	633	48	32
MSKCC (2001)[60]	P2–4A	181	36	27
Selective bladder preservation				
Erlangen (2002)[15]	cT2–4	326	45	29
MGH (2002)[11]	cT2–4a	190	54	36
RTOG (1998)[19]	cT2–4a	123	49	–

receiving a contemporary radical cystectomy for bladder cancer at the University of Southern California.[34] Chemoradiation does not result in a high rate of pelvic recurrence; however, close urologic surveillance should be pursued in order to detect invasive recurrences while they are still confined to the bladder.

Does delaying cystectomy decrease survival?

Multiple randomized trials demonstrate that delayed cystectomy does not result in inferior survival after radiation as compared to immediate surgery. Comparison of modern cystectomy and modern trimodality series demonstrate that, when matched for tumor stage, selective preservation results in comparable survival rates while preserving the bladder in the majority of patients. For T2–4a bladder cancer, 5-year overall survival rates of 45% to 50% have been reported after selective bladder preservation as compared to 36% to 58% after contemporary radical cystectomy (Table 19.5).

Care must be taken when comparing surgical series to bladder preservation series as several biases exist. Cystectomy series do not report by 'intention to treat', and exclude patients where the procedure is abandoned secondary to intraoperative findings such as node positivity or unresectable disease. Conversely, trimodality series include patients that fail to respond to chemoradiation and require cystectomy. Also, many surgical series do not have preoperative proof of muscle-invasive disease. Cystectomy series commonly include less than P2 stage tumors in 25% to 40% of patients.

Conclusion

Bladder preserving treatment for invasive bladder cancer in patients selected on the basis of their response to transurethral resection, concurrent chemotherapy, and radiation results in overall survival and freedom from disease comparable to radical cystectomy. This approach results in 5-year survival of approximately 50%, with 80% of these patients retaining their native bladder. Despite these results, the acceptance of this approach in the urologic community has been limited due to the following concerns addressed in this chapter:

1. The inability to obtain a visibly complete transurethral resection, which does result in a higher cystectomy rate, has a 63% complete response rate, and does not preclude selective bladder preservation.

2. Superficial relapse, which may occur in 26% of patients after bladder preservation, is adequately managed by transurethral resection and intravesical therapy in the majority of patients.
3. Quality of life and urodynamic studies demonstrate that preserved bladders function well.
4. Pelvic recurrence rates after selective bladder preservation are comparable to rates seen after cystectomy.
5. Several randomized trials demonstrate no survival detriment to delayed cystectomy for patients receiving radiation therapy.

Selective bladder preservation using trimodality therapy represents a cooperative effort between the treating urologist, radiation oncologist, and medical oncologist. Bladder conservation trials have demonstrated results comparable to radical cystectomy with a high rate of bladder preservation.

References

1. McDougal WS. Continent urinary diversion. In Osterling JE, Richie JP (eds): Urologic Oncology. Philadelphia: WB Saunders, 1997, pp 336–40.
2. Greven KM, Spera JA, Solin LJ, Morgan T, Hanks GE. Local recurrence after cystectomy alone for bladder carcinoma. Cancer 1992; 69: 2767–70.
3. Martinez-Pineiro JA, Gonzalez Martin M, Arocena F, et al. Neoadjuvant cisplatin chemotherapy before radical cystectomy in invasive transitional cell carcinoma of the bladder: a prospective randomized phase III study. J Urol 1995; 153: 964–73.
4. Pressler LB, Petrylak DP, Olsson CA. Invasive transitional cell carcinoma of the bladder: prognosis and management. In Osterling JE, Richie JP (eds): Urologic Oncology. Philadelphia: WB Saunders, 1997, pp 275–91.
5. Hart S, Skinner EC, Meyerowitz BE, Boyd S, Lieskovsky G, Skinner DG. Quality of life after radical cystectomy for bladder cancer in patients with an ileal conduit, cutaneous or urethral Kock pouch [comment]. J Urol 1999; 162: 77–81.
6. Miller LS. Bladder cancer: superiority of preoperative irradiation and cystectomy in clinical stages B2 and C. Cancer 1977; 39: 973–80.
7. Bloom HJ, Hendry WF, Wallace DM, Skeet RG. Treatment of T3 bladder cancer: controlled trial of pre-operative radiotherapy and radical cystectomy versus radical radiotherapy. Br J Urol 1982; 54: 136–51.
8. Sell A, Jakobsen A, Nerstrom B, Sorensen BL, Steven K, Barlebo H. Treatment of advanced bladder cancer category T2, T3 and T4a. A randomized multicenter study of preoperative irradiation and cystectomy versus radical irradiation and early salvage cystectomy for residual tumor. DAVECA protocol 8201. Danish Vesical Cancer Group. Scand J Urol Nephrol 1991; 138(Suppl): 193–201.
9. Cutler SD. National Cancer Institute, unpublished observations, 1983.
10. Schultz PK, Herr HW, Zhang ZF, et al. Neoadjuvant chemotherapy for invasive bladder cancer: prognostic factors for survival of patients

treated with M-VAC with 5-year follow-up [comment]. J Clin Oncol 1994;12:1394–1401.

11. Shipley WU, Kaufman DS, Zehr E, et al. Selective bladder preservation by combined modality protocol treatment: long-term outcomes of 190 patients with invasive bladder cancer. Urology 2002; 60: 62–67; discussion 67–68.

12. Shipley WU, Kaufman DS, Tester WJ, et al. Overview of bladder cancer trials in the Radiation Therapy Oncology Group. Cancer 2003; 97: 2115–19.

13. Housset M, Maulard C, Chretien Y, et al. Combined radiation and chemotherapy for invasive transitional-cell carcinoma of the bladder: a prospective study. J Clin Oncol 1993; 11: 2150–7.

14. Sauer R, Birkenhake S, Kuhn R, Wittekind C, Schrott KM, Martus P. Efficacy of radiochemotherapy with platin derivatives compared to radiotherapy alone in organ-sparing treatment of bladder cancer. Int J Radiat Oncol Biol Phys 1998; 40: 121–7.

15. Rodel C, Grabenbauer GG, Kuhn R, et al. Combined-modality treatment and selective organ preservation in invasive bladder cancer: long-term results [comment]. J Clin Oncol 2002; 20: 3061–71.

16. Shipley WU, Prout GR Jr, Einstein AB, et al. Treatment of invasive bladder cancer by cisplatin and radiation in patients unsuited for surgery. JAMA 1987;258(7):931–935.

17. Tester W, Porter A, Asbell S, et al. Combined modality program with possible organ preservation for invasive bladder carcinoma: results of RTOG protocol 85-12. Int J Radiat Oncol Biol Phys 1993; 25: 783–90.

18. Tester W, Caplan R, Heaney J, et al. Neoadjuvant combined modality program with selective organ preservation for invasive bladder cancer: results of Radiation Therapy Oncology Group phase II trial 8802. J Clin Oncol 1996; 14: 119–26.

19. Shipley WU, Winter KA, Kaufman DS, et al. Phase III trial of neoadjuvant chemotherapy in patients with invasive bladder cancer treated with selective bladder preservation by combined radiation therapy and chemotherapy: initial results of Radiation Therapy Oncology Group 89-03 [comment]. J Clin Oncol 1998; 16: 3576–83.

20. Kaufman DS, Winter KA, Shipley WU, et al. The initial results in muscle-invading bladder cancer of RTOG 95-06: phase I/II trial of transurethral surgery plus radiation therapy with concurrent cisplatin and 5-fluorouracil followed by selective bladder preservation or cystectomy depending on the initial response. Oncologist 2000; 5: 471–6.

21. Hagan MP, Winter KA, Kaufman DS, et al. RTOG 9706: initial report of a phase I/II trial of bladder-conservation employing TURB, twice daily accelerated irradiation sensitized with cisplatin followed by adjuvant MCV combination chemotherapy. Int J Radiat Oncol Biol Phys 2003; 57: 665–72.

22. Moore MJ, Winquist EW, Murray N, et al. Gemcitabine plus cisplatin, an active regimen in advanced urothelial cancer: a phase II trial of the National Cancer Institute of Canada Clinical Trials Group. J Clin Oncol 1999; 17: 2876–81.

23. Kaufman D, Raghavan D, Carducci M, et al. Phase II trial of gemcitabine plus cisplatin in patients with metastatic urothelial cancer. J Clin Oncol 2000; 18: 1921–7.

24. von der Maase H, Hansen SW, Roberts JT, et al. Gemcitabine and cisplatin versus methotrexate, vinblastine, doxorubicin, and cisplatin in advanced or metastatic bladder cancer: results of a large, randomized, multinational, multicenter, phase III study [comment]. J Clin Oncol 2000; 18: 3068–77.

25. Roth BJ. The role of paclitaxel in the therapy of bladder cancer. Semin Oncol 1995; 22: 33–40.

26. Dreicer R, Manola J, Roth BJ, Cohen MB, Hatfield AK, Wilding G. Phase II study of cisplatin and paclitaxel in advanced carcinoma of the urothelium: an Eastern Cooperative Oncology Group Study. J Clin Oncol 2000; 18 :1058–61.

27. Chakravarti A, Winter K, Wu CL. Expression of EGFR is associated with improved outcome in muscle invading bladder cancer: An RTOG study. Proceedings of the American Society of Clinical Oncology (ASCO) Meeting, Orlando, FL. J Clin Oncol 2002; 179a: Abstract 713.

28. Coen JJ, Heney NM, Althausen AF, Zietman AL, Kaufman DS, Shipley WU. An update of selective bladder preservation using combined modality treatment in invasive bladder cancer: long term outcome

29. Zietman AL, Grocela J, Zehr E, et al. Selective bladder conservation using transurethral resection, chemotherapy, and radiation: management and consequences of Ta, T1, and Tis recurrence within the retained bladder. Urology 2001; 58: 380–5.

30. Lynch WJ, Jenkins BJ, Fowler CG, Hope-Stone HF, Blandy JP. The quality of life after radical radiotherapy for bladder cancer. Br J Urol 1992; 70: 519–21.

31. Zietman AL, Sacco D, Skowronski U, et al. Organ-conservation in invasive bladder cancer by transurethral resection, chemotherapy, and radiation: results of a urodynamic and quality of life study on long-term survivors. J Urol 2003; 170(5): 1772–6.

32. Caffo O, Fellin G, Graffer U, Luciani L. Assessment of quality of life after cystectomy or conservative therapy for patients with infiltrating bladder carcinoma. A survey by a self-administered questionnaire [erratum appears in Cancer 1996;78(5):2037]. Cancer 1996; 76(9): 1089–97.

33. Henningsohn L, Steven K, Kallestrup EB, Steineck G. Distressful symptoms and well-being after radical cystectomy and orthotopic bladder substitution compared with a matched control population. J Urol 2002; 168: 168–74; discussion 174–175.

34. Stein JP, Lieskovsky G, Cote R, et al. Radical cystectomy in the treatment of invasive bladder cancer: long-term results in 1,054 patients. J Clin Oncol 2001; 19: 666–75.

35. Henry K, Miller J, Mori M, Loening S, Fallon B. Comparison of transurethral resection to radical therapies for stage B bladder tumors. J Urol 1988; 140: 964–7.

36. Herr HW. Conservative management of muscle-infiltrating bladder cancer: prospective experience. J Urol 1987; 138: 1162–3.

37. De Neve W, Lybeert ML, Goor C, Crommelin MA, Ribot JG. Radiotherapy for T2 and T3 carcinoma of the bladder: the influence of overall treatment time. Radiother Oncol 1995; 36: 183–8.

38. Gospodarowicz MK, Hawkins NV, Rawlings GA, et al. Radical radiotherapy for muscle invasive transitional cell carcinoma of the bladder: failure analysis. J Urol 1989; 142: 1448–53; discussion 1453–1454.

39. Jenkins BJ, Caulfield MJ, Fowler CG, et al. Reappraisal of the role of radical radiotherapy and salvage cystectomy in the treatment of invasive (T2/T3) bladder cancer. Br J Urol 1988; 62: 343–6.

40. Mameghan H, Fisher R, Mameghan J, Brook S. Analysis of failure following definitive radiotherapy for invasive transitional cell carcinoma of the bladder. Int J Radiat Oncol Biol Phys 1995; 31: 247–54.

41. Shearer RJ, Chilvers CF, Bloom HJ, Bliss JM, Horwich A, Babiker A. Adjuvant chemotherapy in T3 carcinoma of the bladder. A prospective trial: preliminary report. Br J Urol 1988; 62: 558–64.

42. Hall RR. Transurethral resection for transitional cell carcinoma. Prob Urol 1992; 6: 460–70.

43. Quilty PM, Duncan W. Primary radical radiotherapy for T3 transitional cell cancer of the bladder: an analysis of survival and control. Int J Radiat Oncol Biol Phys 1986; 12: 853–60.

44. Smaaland R, Akslen LA, Tonder B, Mehus A, Lote K, Albrektsen G. Radical radiation treatment of invasive and locally advanced bladder carcinoma in elderly patients. Br J Urol 1991; 67: 61–9.

45. Farah R, Chodak GW, Vogelzang NJ, et al. Curative radiotherapy following chemotherapy for invasive bladder carcinoma (a preliminary report). Int J Radiat Oncol Biol Phys 1991; 20: 413–17.

46. Hall RR, Roberts JT. Neoadjuvant chemotherapy, a method to conserve the bladder? Proceedings of the 6th European Cancer Conference on Oncology and Cancer Nursing, Florence, Italy, 1991. Eur J Cancer 1991; 27(Suppl 2):Abstract 144.

47. Keating JP, Zincke H, Hahn RG, Morgan WR. Extended experience of neo-adjuvant M-VAC chemotherapy for T1–4 N0 M0 transitional cell carcinoma of the urinary bladder. Progr Clin Biol Res 1990; 353: 119–27.

48. Kurth KH, Splinter TA, Jacqmin D. Transitional cell carcinoma of the bladder: a phase II study of chemotherapy in T3–4 N0 M0 of the EORTC GU group. In Alderson AR, Oliver RT, Hanham IW, Bloom HJ (eds): Urologic Oncology Dilemmas and Developments. New York: Wiley-Liss, 1991, pp 115–128.

49. Maffezzini M, Torelli T, Villa E, et al. Systemic preoperative chemotherapy with cisplatin, methotrexate and vinblastine for locally advanced bladder cancer: local tumor response and early followup results. J Urol 1991; 145: 741–3.

50. Roberts JT, Fossa SD, Richards B, et al. Results of Medical Research Council phase II study of low dose cisplatin and methotrexate in the primary treatment of locally advanced (T3 and T4) transitional cell carcinoma of the bladder. Br J Urol 1991; 68: 162–8.

51. Hall RR, Newling DW, Ramsden PD, Richards B, Robinson MR, Smith PH. Treatment of invasive bladder cancer by local resection and high dose methotrexate. Br J Urol 1984; 56: 668–72.

52. Parsons JT, Million RR. Bladder cancer. In: Perez CA, Brady IW (eds): Principles and Practice of Radiation Oncology. Philadelphia: Lippincott, 1991, pp 1036–1058.

53. Prout GR Jr, Shipley WU, Kaufman DS, et al. Preliminary results in invasive bladder cancer with transurethral resection, neoadjuvant chemotherapy and combined pelvic irradiation plus cisplatin chemotherapy. J Urol 1990; 144: 1128–34; discussion 1134–6.

54. Scher HI, Herr HW, Sternberg C, Fair W, Bosl G, Sogani P. Neoadjuvant chemotherapy for invasive bladder cancer: experience with the MVAC regimen. Br J Urol 1989; 64: 250–6.

55. Herr HW, Bajorin DF, Scher HI. Neoadjuvant chemotherapy and bladder-sparing surgery for invasive bladder cancer: ten-year outcome. J Clin Oncol 1998; 16(4): 1298–301.

56. Cervak J, Cufer T, Marolt F. Combined chemotherapy and radiotherapy in muscle-invasive bladder carcinoma. Complete remission results. Proceedings of the 6th European Conference on Oncology and Cancer Nursing, Florence, Italy, 1991. Eur J Cancer 1991; 27(Suppl 2): Abstract 561.

57. Dunst J, Sauer R, Schrott KM, Kuhn R, Wittekind C, Altendorf-Hofmann A. Organ-sparing treatment of advanced bladder cancer: a 10-year experience. Int J Radiat Oncol Biol Phys 1994; 30: 261–6.

58. Housset M, Dufour B, Maulard C. Concomitant 5-fluorouracil–cisplatin and bifractionated split course radiation therapy for invasive bladder cancer. Proc Am Soc Clin Oncol 1997; 16: 319a.

59. Stein JP, Lieskovsky G, Cote R, et al. Radical cystectomy in the treatment of invasive bladder cancer: long-term results in 1,054 patients. J Clin Oncol 2001; 19: 666–75.

60. Dalbagni G, Genega E, Hashibe M, et al. Cystectomy for bladder cancer: a contemporary series. J Urol 2001; 165: 1111–6.

Section 4

Urinary tract reconstruction

20

Orthotopic neobladder

Richard E Hautmann

Introduction

Urinary diversion has reached a new level. The ultimate goal of urinary reconstruction has become not only to create a means to divert urine and protect the upper urinary tract, but also to provide patients with a continent means to store urine and allow for volitional voiding through the native urethra. These advances in urinary diversion have been made in an effort to give patients a normal lifestyle with a positive self-image following removal of the bladder. We and others have been dedicated to the continued improvement of lower urinary tract reconstruction, and believe that the neobladder represents the most ideal form of urinary diversion.[1–4] Orthotopic reconstruction was proposed by Tizzoni and Foggi in 1888.[5] They replaced the bladder in one female dog by an isoperistaltic ileal segment. In 1951 Couvelaire reactivated this idea.[6]

During the past 15 years orthotopic reconstruction has evolved from 'experimental surgery' to 'standard of care at larger medical centers' and to the 'preferred method of urinary diversion' in both sexes. The ileal conduit was described 1950 by Bricker and has remained the standard urinary diversion against which others have to be judged.[7] During the last decade, use of the time-honored conduit has given way to the increasingly frequent use of orthotopic reconstruction.

Indication: substantial change in paradigm for urinary diversion

The goal of patient counseling about urinary diversion should be to find the method that would be the safest for cancer control, has the fewest complications in both the short and long term, and provides the easiest adjustment for the patient's lifestyle, i.e. supporting the best quality of life. The paradigm for choosing a urinary diversion has changed substantially. Today, all cystectomy patients are candidates for a neobladder, and we should identify patients in whom orthotopic reconstruction may be less than ideal. The proportion of cystectomy patients receiving a neobladder has increased at medical centers from 50% to 90%.[8–11]

Patient selection criteria

Absolute and relative contraindications

Absolute contraindications to continent diversion of any type are compromised renal function as a result of long-standing obstruction or chronic renal failure, with serum creatinine >150–200 μmol/l. Severe hepatic dysfunction is also a contraindication to continent diversion. Patients with compromised intestinal function, particularly inflammatory bowel disease, may be better served by a bowel conduit. Orthotopic reconstruction is absolutely contraindicated in all patients that are candidates for simultaneous urethrectomy because of their primary tumor.[12,13]

The role of relative contraindications and comorbidity is steadily decreasing. However, mental impairment, external sphincter dysfunction, or recurrent urethral strictures deserve serious consideration.

Patient factors: pros

The primary patient factor is the 'patient's desire for a neobladder'. The patient needs a certain motivation to tolerate the initial and sometimes lasting inconveniences of nocturnal incontinence associated with a neobladder. Most patients readily accept some degree of nocturnal incontinence for the benefit of avoiding an external stoma and pouch. However, not all patients do, and realistic expectations of the functional outcome are essential for both the surgeon and the patient. The psychological damaging stigma to the patient who enters surgery expecting a neobladder, but awakens with a stoma, plays an increasing role. It should always be remembered that in many parts of the world a bag may be either socially unacceptable or economically unrealistic as a long-term solution. These pressures may drive the urologist toward some form of continent urinary diversion, and although rectal pouches have been utilized widely as an alternative to conduits, continent catheterizable reservoirs, and orthotopic bladder substitutes in particular, represent attractive alternative options.

Patient factors: cons

There are still patients that are better served with a conduit. Patient factors arguing against a neobladder include the following:

- If the patient's main motivation is to 'get out of the hospital as soon as possible' and resume normal, rather sedentary activities. Many frail patients undergoing cystectomy will have less disruption of normal activities with a well-functioning conduit than with an orthotopic reservoir associated with less than ideal continence.
- If the patient is an elderly person.
- If the patient is not concerned about body image. Most older patients do not have the same 'body image' concerns that a younger patient might have, and their main goal is returning to their previous lifestyle, which is often quite sedentary.[14]

Oncologic factors

Following cystectomy the rhabdosphincter must remain intact. Nevertheless, the cancer operation must not be compromised. This concern applies to urethral tumor recurrence in men and the use of orthotopic replacement in women. One of the initial deterrents to orthotopic diversion is the risk for urethral recurrence of cancer. Historically this risk following cystectomy was 10%.[15] The best predictor of the risk for urethral disease is the presence and extent of carcinoma in situ (CIS) in the prostatic urethra, ducts, or stroma. If there is diffuse CIS in the ducts and invasion of the stroma, the risk for urethral disease historically has been 25% to 35%,[16] a risk that discouraged use of the urethra. Lesser amounts of CIS confer a lesser degree of risk. Our aggressive approach to neobladder diversion relies only on a frozen section of the urethral margin at the time of surgery. A conservative approach would disqualify a patient with any prostatic involvement. In our view, neither multifocal bladder tumors nor CIS of the bladder are indications for urethrectomy. The frequency of urethral recurrence after orthotopic diversions is much less than anticipated. Freeman et al[15] and others[8,9] provide data on a 2% to 4% frequency of urethral recurrence after orthotopic diversion.

Orthotopic bladder substitution for women with invasive bladder cancer has recently become popular.[17–19] Analysis of pathologic specimens has supported its use in women who have no evidence of tumor at the bladder neck.[20,21] Indeed, the majority of the invasive cancers are located in the area of the trigone, making a wide excision—together with the anterosuperior part of the vagina and the dorsomedial bladder pedicle in the paravaginal region—necessary.

Increasing experience with orthotopic reconstruction has fostered less restrictiveness for patient selection based on tumor stage. Should extensive pelvic disease, a palpable mass, or positive but resectable lymph nodes preclude a neobladder because of the high propensity for a pelvic recurrence or distant relapse?

We have studied local recurrence and diversion-related complications in a series of 435 patients. The local recurrence rate was the expected 10%. Interference of a local recurrence with the neobladder occurred in 11 patients only: infiltration of the neobladder occurred in 6 patients and obstruction was the problem in the remaining 5. There is no convincing evidence that a patient with an orthotopic diversion tolerates adjuvant chemotherapy less well or that a pelvic recurrence is any more difficult to manage with a neobladder than after an ileal conduit.

Patients can anticipate normal neobladder function until the time of death.[22]

Adjuvant chemotherapy may substantially weaken the patient and prolong the time for neobladder maturation. Nevertheless, our philosophy respects the patient's desire for a neobladder if the patient is strongly motivated. Even though the patient has a poor prognosis and relapse is likely to occur, we still try to construct the diversion they want. Previous radiation therapy, especially with an advanced cancer, usually mitigates against an orthotopic diversion but does not absolutely preclude it. However, all patients should be informed that diversion to the skin, either by a continent reservoir or an ileal conduit, may be necessary because of unexpected tumor extent, and there should be an appropriate stoma site marked on the abdominal wall beforehand.

Current practice

Despite the fact that orthotopic bladder replacement provides the ideal method of urinary diversion after cystectomy, many patients treated outside of centers that are dedicated to neobladder reconstruction receive an ileal conduit. In addition, patients selected for a conduit are frequently older patients with more comorbidity, and more previous cancer therapy, including patients with previously deemed unresectable cancers undergoing desperation cystectomy or after failed previously combined radiation therapy and chemotherapy regimens.[14]

Thus, despite our strong desire to offer orthotopic diversion whenever possible, some patients do not qualify on the basis of current clinical judgment. An ileal conduit remains an expedient, safe, and appropriate method of diversion in these patients. Many factors go into the decision to perform a urinary diversion and must be kept paramount in discussing the pros and cons of each method with the patient and the family.

Comparison of ileal, ileocolic, right colic and sigmoid reservoirs

There are clear differences between ileum and colon in regard to metabolic consequences (see section 'Gut mucosa as a substitute for urothelium'). But this is only one consideration when planning orthotopic reconstruction. Because of the reduced absorption of electrolytes in ileal urinary reservoirs, ileum seems to be preferable to large bowel for storing urine, at least in patients with decreased kidney function and increased risk for metabolic disorders.[23,24]

An obvious advantage of the sigmoid reservoir is its ease of accessibility. However, there is the substantial disadvantage of high reservoir pressures as compared to cecum or ileum that is confirmed by most urodynamic studies.[25–27] We, like others, use a sigmoid reservoir only in cases in which ileum or right colon is not available.[11] An advantage of the ileocolonic reservoir is its initial volume. However, it requires mobilization of the entire right colon and is potentially the most tedious procedure to perform.[28] The greatest disadvantage of the procedure is the loss of the ileocecal valve. There is also a greater risk of vitamin B_{12} deficiency secondary to resection of terminal ileum and the ileocecal valve. Most investigators have reported on one single type of diversion. Santucci et al performed six different continent urinary reservoir operations and revealed remarkably different continence rates and urodynamic data.

Their experience suggests that neobladders composed of stomach or sigmoid should be used only under unusual circumstances because of the high rates of incontinence.[27]

Ileal reservoirs are the most common form of neobladders used worldwide. There are three major categories:

- The Hemi Kock was originally developed by Kock and popularized by Skinner and associates.[29,30] The most recent modification (T pouch) is technically complex, unnecessarily time consuming, and has yet to be widely adopted.[10]
- The ileal reservoir initially described by Studer et al has the advantage of an afferent limb that facilitates placement of the ileoureterostomies but without any valve formation.[3]
- The ileal neobladder is a W-shaped reservoir described by Hautmann and coworkers.[1,2,31] Its obvious advantage is the high continence rates as a consequence of having the greatest volume of all reservoirs. Both the incorporation of an afferent or efferent limb for ureteral anastomosis, and orthotopic anastomosis of the ureters directly into the reservoir, with or without antireflux technique, is feasible.[11,31–33] In our experience, difficulty reaching the urethral remnant occurs less often with this type of reservoir.

Of course, other patient and surgeon issues might supersede these guidelines. Surgeon's preference, length of surgery, ease of construction, potential need for revision, differences in body image, and other patient characteristics are among the many factors that must be considered when choosing which type of orthotopic reconstruction to provide for each individual patient.

Reflux prevention in neobladders

Controversy exists about the importance of an antireflux mechanism,[7,10,13,34] and the benefits are not easy to define. It is clear that the need for reflux prevention is not the same as in ureterosigmoidostomy conduit or continent diversion. Many reports have revealed a high incidence (13–41%) of renal deterioration associated with a refluxing ileal conduit, as evaluated using serum creatinine and urography.[35,36] After long-term follow-up (mean 13 years) in patients with colonic conduits, significantly more renal units not showing reflux on the loopogram remained normal on urography than did units with reflux.[37]

Conduits are not low-pressure systems[38] because of distal obstruction at the level of the fascia immediately superficial to the external oblique muscle. This, coupled with the very frequent presence of infected urine, means that high-pressure reflux may occur. This reflux, or alternatively, ureteroileal obstruction, may contribute to the gradual deterioration in renal function in these patients that has become apparent over the past two decades.

The rationale for implanting the ureters in an antireflux fashion into orthotopic bladder substitutes or continent reservoirs is to prevent the upper urinary tract from retrograde hydrodynamically transmitted pressure peaks and from ascending bacteriuria. However, the routine of antireflux ureter implantation into intestinal urinary reservoirs was born in the era before creation of designated low-pressure reservoirs.

Glomerular filtration pressure is calculated to 25–30 cm of water, and the amplitude of the peristaltic waves in the ureters is normally less than 10 cm. In view of these figures, long-lasting periods with pressure exceeding about 25 cm of water in the urinary receptacle, in the long run, will probably impair renal function by impeding the urine flow. Patients with a continent ileal reservoir for urinary diversion utilize approximately 60% of the maximal volume capacity during the daytime, i.e. about 300–500 ml. At this reservoir volume, the pressure exceeds zero by more than 25 cm water only during about 2 min/hour.[39]

Reflux prevention in neobladders is even less important than in a normal bladder: 1) there are no coordinated contractions during micturition; 2) a simultaneous pressure increase in neobladder, abdomen, and kidney pelvis during the Valsalva maneuver; and 3) the ileourethrostomy provides a true leak point. When nonrefluxing techniques are used, the risk of obstruction is at least twice that of a direct anastomosis, irrespective of the type of bowel segment used. Half of these strictures require secondary procedures.[9]

In a recent study, the reported obstruction rate following direct anastomoses was 1.7%, and was significantly lower than the 13% rate for nonrefluxing techniques.[40] Of the latter techniques, the LeDuc is associated with the highest postoperative stricture rate. Studer et al reported a 3% obstruction rate using ureteral direct anastomoses as opposed to 13% postoperative strictures in patients in whom Coffey flap valves were used.[40]

Roth et al reported 3.6% and 20.4% obstruction rates respectively when ureteral direct anastomoses to an afferent loop were compared with the LeDuc antireflux anastomoses.[41] Moreover, the reported obstruction rate was 3.8% for the nipple valve of the Kock pouch,[42] but 9.3% for the LeDuc antireflux anastomoses of the Hautmann neobladder.[9] For the latter antireflux technique, an obstruction rate of up to 29% has been reported.[43]

We conclude that obstruction from anastomotic strictures is a greater potential source of short- and long-term morbidity than reflux. Direct techniques are easier to use and preserve renal function equally as well as nonrefluxing methods. We see no justification for any antireflux mechanism in neobladders.

Since 1996 we have been using a freely refluxing open end-to-side ureteroileal anastomosis which is the simplest small bowel surgery (Figure 20.1).[31] Our 9.5% stenosis rate associated with LeDuc (first 363 patients) went down to 1.0% (patient numbers 364–558).

Further advantages of this chimney modification are:[7]

- extra length to reach the ureteral stump
- ease of surgery far outside the pelvic cavity
- a tension-free anastomosis
- no risk of ureteral angulation with neobladder filling
- a simplified flank access for revisional surgery.[31–33]

Intestinal tissues as a substitute for the bladder

It would be ideal if, over time, the transposed gut segment lost its own organization and intrinsic control, and the smooth muscle changed properties to become more like normal detrusor, being reinnervated through the sacral parasympathetic micturition pathway so that it could contribute to bladder emptying.

Potentially the greatest difference between conduit and neobladder is that the conduit functions as a somewhat longer ureter, whereas a neobladder is a substitute for the detrusor. Understanding orthotopic bladder replacement in full means understanding the phenomenon of maturation, i.e. unlike a conduit, the motor and pharmacologic responses of a neobladder change dramatically towards that of the original bladder. Maturation of a neobladder takes anywhere from a few weeks to over several months up to 8 years.[7] Approximately 4–6 weeks after surgery conduit patients are usually into a well-established routine.

Gut as a substitute for the detrusor

Structural changes
Interstitial cells of Cajal (ICC), so named for their identification with the interstitial cells observed by Cajal in the mammalian small intestine,[44] possess a morphology and location specific for each of

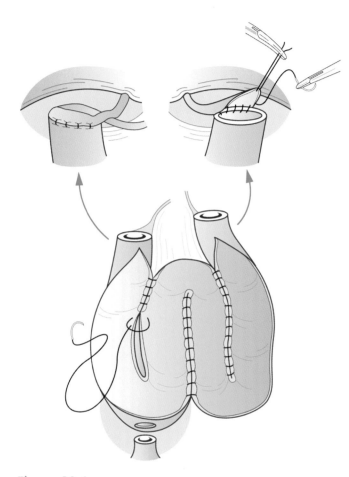

Figure 20.1
Refluxing ileoureteral anastomosis using chimneys of a 3–5 cm afferent limb on each side.

the specialized regions of the gastrointestinal tract.[45,46] ICC are considered of primary importance for gastrointestinal motility, and are accepted as the intestinal pacemaker cells. In the small intestines of humans, ICC are located at two different muscle coat areas.[47] One population (the ICC-MP) is located between the longitudinal and circular muscle layers and has a relationship to the myenteric plexus (MP). The presence of this cell type has been correlated with slow-wave activity, and found to be of fundamental importance for the occurrence of normal peristalsis.[48] The second ICC population (the ICC-DMP) is specific for the small intestine. It is located between the innermost inner circular muscle layer (ICL) and outermost subdivisions of the circular muscle layer, in association with the deep muscular plexus (DMP), and its role might be related to motility that is specific to this gut area.

Faussone-Pellegrini and coworkers[49] have studied motor patterns, intraluminal pressures, volume capacity, and histoanatomic characteristics in full-thickness specimens from orthotopic ileal bladders removed during corrective surgery. The ICC-MP were scarce in the detubularized segments 1–6 years after reconstruction, and intact ICC-DMP cells and DMP nerve fibers were not seen. Furthermore, the innermost circular muscular layer could not be identified. This loss of structural organization was associated with a better functional outcome. In contrast, the tubular segments (the ICC-MP, ICC-DMP, and circular muscle layer) retained normal features for up to 3 years. After this, ICC-DMP was lost, DMP nerve fibers were scant, the circular muscle layer appeared to degenerate but the ICC-MP remained intact. It was apparent that those reservoirs maintaining a normal ICC-MP population developed pressure waves and those segments with intact ICC-DMP had a contractile response to distension. Whether these physiologic changes are a result of the ileal segment chronically functioning as a reservoir, or are the product of the surgical interruption of myoneural networks and the ICC syncytium, is unclear (Table 20.1).[49]

Pharmacologic changes
In experimental animals, it has been possible to follow the changes in function of implanted segments after their incorporation into the bladder, to see if they do indeed become more like detrusor in their function. Batra et al[50] have looked in detail at the changes in the pharmacologic properties of muscle strips taken from the ileal segment of augmentation cystoplasty in rabbit models. The contractile response of the ileal segment changed from the response typical of normal ileum to a phasic response more characteristic of detrusor.

Table 20.1 Distribution of ICC in ileal reservoirs (humans) and motor response characteristics

	Tubular Early (<3 years)	Late (3–8 years)	Detubularized Early + late
ICC-MP	Retained	Retained	Scarce
ICC-DMP	Retained	Lost	Lost
DMP nerve fibers	Retained	Scant	Disappeared
Inner circular muscle layer	Retained	Scant	Disappeared
Pressure	High	High	Low
Peristaltic activity	Normal	Normal	Absent
Contractile activity			
Low filling	Present		
Increased filling		Present	
Capacity	Low	Increased	High

Based on data from Faussone-Pellegrini et al.[49]
DMP, deep muscular plexus; ICC, interstitial cells of Cabal; MP, myenteric plexus.

Furthermore, the normal ileal relaxation reverses to a contractile response similar to that seen in the detrusor, after incorporation into the cystoplasty. The number of muscarinic receptors in the ileal segment decreased after incorporation. Further experiments comparing strip responses from tubular and detubularized segments showed that these changes were more profound in detubularized cystoplasties. This observation was compatible with the concept that the surgical interruption of myoneural networks is the primary signal for the transformation from ileal-type to detrusor-type responses, as opposed to exposure to urine or chronic functioning as a reservoir.

Detubularization

Although it would be ideal if the bowel segment could contribute to voluntary voiding, in reality this does not seem to happen, and a highly compliant neobladder is the desired outcome.[51] Detubularized bowel segments provide greater capacity at lower pressure and require a shorter length of intestine than do intact segments. Four factors account for their superiority:

- their configuration takes advantage of the geometric fact that volume increases by the square of the radius so that a pouch has a larger diameter than a tube
- they accommodate to filling more readily because, as Laplace's law states, the container with the greater radius—and, thus, the lower mural tension—will hold larger volumes at lower pressure
- compliance is superior to that of the tubular bowel
- contractile ability is blunted by the failure of contractions to encompass the entire circumference.[52]

These theoretical considerations are consistent with clinical observations showing that detubularization substantially increases reservoir capacity and delays the onset and reduces the amplitude of the pressure rise produced by contractions. These findings account for the markedly improved initial nocturnal incontinence (80% versus 17% at 2 years), the longer voiding intervals (2.5 hours initial versus 4 hours at 1 year), and the predisposition to urinary retention (0% initial versus 25% at 1 year) with detubularized bladder substitution. Altering the shape of a reservoir from spherical to ellipsoid is calculated to have only a slight effect on its mechanical characteristics. Consequently, the essence of detubularization is to create a reservoir with high capacity, while shape is of secondary importance.[53]

Capacity and pressure characteristics of reservoirs (Table 20.2)[39,53–55]

Berglund et al have studied the volume capacity and the pressure characteristics of three types of intestinal reservoir—the continent ileostomy, the continent ileal urostomy, and the continent cecostomy—in patients at intervals after surgical construction of the reservoirs. The volume increases of the ileostomy and the urostomy reservoirs were almost identical but were significantly greater than those of the cecal reservoir. The basal pressure was low in all types of reservoir, although somewhat higher in the cecal reservoir at greater filling volumes. In the ileal reservoirs, motor activity appeared at a filling volume of about 40% of the maximal capacity, whereas in the cecal reservoir motor activity was recorded at all filling levels. The motor activity increased with greater volumes. The amplitude of the highest pressure wave in the cecal reservoir was twice as high as that of the ileal reservoirs. The motor activity of the cecal reservoir, calculated in two different ways, was 10–20 times greater than in the ileal reservoirs.[39]

An interesting comparison of the properties of different gut smooth muscles was made by Hohenfellner et al who examined the ileal and cecal segments incorporated into a canine model of the Mainz bladder substitution. Sonomicrometry transducers were implanted in the circular and longitudinal muscular layers to allow measurements of their properties. It was found that the circular ileal layer was most distensible, followed by the colonic circular and longitudinal ileal layers. The longitudinal layer of the colonic segment was relatively indistensible.[54]

Clinically significant cystoplasty contractions are arbitrarily defined as those 40 cmH$_2$O in amplitude or higher that begin to occur at low volumes (<200 ml). The incidence of such contractions was 70% for tubular ileocystoplasties, 36% for tubular right colon, 10% for detubularized colon, and none in patients with detubularized ileocystoplasties.[55]

Table 20.2 Capacity and pressure characteristics of reservoirs

	Ileum	Colon
Volume increase		
Initially		Advantage
Late	Advantage	
Capacity		
First contraction	Advantage	
Maximum contraction	Advantage	
Involuntary contractions: maximum amplitude	Advantage	
Motor activity (calculated)		10–20× higher
Distensibility: ileum (ICL) >colon (CCL) >ileum (ILL) >colon (CLL)	Advantage	
Compliance	Advantage	

Based on data from Berglund et al,[39] Colding-Jørgensen et al,[53] Hohenfellner et al,[54] Goldwasser et al.[55]
CCL, colonic circular layer; CLL, colonic longitudinal layer; ICL, ileal circular layer; ILL, ileal longitudinal layer.

The detubularized ileal reservoir for either continent stomal diversion or bladder replacement would seem to constitute the ideal low-pressure reservoir.

Gut mucosa as a substitute for urothelium

Most research on transposed gut segments has focused on the potential for malignancy arising in the reconstructed bladder substitute, a contingency that will not be discussed here.

Structural/ultrastructural changes in neobladder mucosa

Systematic follow-up of the effects of the ileal mucosa in patients with continent reservoirs results in constant and homogeneous changes. They seem to be directly related to the time from surgery and can be subdivided into early and late. From these observations and those published previously, it seems evident that when the ileum is removed from its absorptive function and must respond to a chronic irritative stimulus, the result is biphasic; the first inflammatory phase is followed by a second regressive phase in which the epithelium tends to assume a morphology similar to that of the urothelium, better adapted for coating and protective functions than for absorption. Therefore, it is not surprising that it should be the structures responsible for absorption (brush border and villi) that suffer the most damage. Considering that in a normal ileum the villi increase the absorptive surface eightfold in comparison to a flat surface, their atrophy greatly reduces the area of absorption and, consequently, the risk of metabolic alterations. Paneth's cells (which produce digestive enzymes) and goblet cells seem more tolerant of the prolonged contact with urine, and the regressive phenomena appear significantly later. Because the villi and crypta are markedly shorter, the ileal mucosa tends to become linear (Box 20.1).[56] This also explains the alternation of areas in which cells with few microvilli (corresponding to the primitive surface epithelium) are predominant, with others in which goblet cells (corresponding to the primitive glandular epithelium) are predominant.

After 4 years of follow-up, the areas of villous atrophy predominate; Paneth's and goblet cells are scanty, and only few residual glands are visible. The resulting epithelium has lost its absorptive and secretive functions to acquire the function of a urinary reservoir. Electron microscopy and enzyme histochemistry in the epithelial cells also showed that there was a reduction in the number of cell organelles and also a decreased metabolic activity.[57]

Progressive mucosal atrophy has been observed in continent colonic reservoirs. They show similar, although much less severe, changes of the microvilli.[56,58] Follow-up studies in patients with ileal conduit also showed atrophic changes with reduction of the villous height, although there are wide variations between different authors and individual patients.[59]

Biologic consequences of exposing gut mucosa to urine

Intestinal segments vary in handling of solutes. Length of bowel segment, surface area, duration of urinary exposure, solute concentration, pH, renal function, and urine osmolality all play a role. The reservoir surface is exceedingly difficult to estimate. There is no difference between ileal and colonic mucosa in regard to sodium-absorbing capacity. However, in the colon, chloride absorption and bicarbonate excretion are more pronounced, and there is increasing evidence to suggest that inherent chloride absorption is maintained when in contact with urine.[23,57] Therefore, it may be preferable to use ileum rather than colon for bladder reconstruction to reduce the risk of hyperchloremic acidosis, particularly in the presence of renal impairment.

The final result of the process of maturation can be summarized as follows:

- Structure and pharmacologic response of the implanted ileum (not colon) change to detrusor-like responses.
- Structural and ultrastructural changes in ileal (not colonic) mucosa lead to a primitive surface and glandular epithelium similar to urothelium.
- The transformation of the ileal mucosa minimizes the risk of metabolic complications.

Consequently, Mother Nature has engineered a new bladder almost as good as the one given initially.

Box 20.1 Structural and ultrastructural changes in ileal neobladder mucosa

1. Early (<1 year): inflammatory
   - Infiltration of lamina propria
   - Rarefaction of terminal web
   - Goblet cell hyperplasia
   - Reduction of microvilli:
     a. Toxic effect of urine
     b. Low pH
     c. Ischemia
     d. Lack of contact with intestinal content
2. Late (1–4 years): regressive
   - Villous atrophy
   - Shortening of crypts
   - Goblet cells decreased (>4 years)
   - Flat mucosa
   - Stratified epithelium

Based on data from Aragona et al.[56]

Upper urinary tract preservation

In a prospective, randomized study of patients undergoing conduit or continent reservoir diversion, renal function was evaluated after a mean follow-up of 10 years.[60] Patients scheduled for conduit diversion were randomized as to the type of intestinal segment and technique for ureterointestinal anastomosis. There was a moderate decrease in the preoperative total glomerular filtration rate (GFR) in the ileal and colonic conduit groups (17 and 19 ml/min, respectively).

Part of the change in GFR is probably a normal age-related decrease, which has been estimated to be about 1 ml/min/year at ages >50 and 0.5 ml/min/year in younger people.[61] If ≥25% fall in GFR is defined as renal deterioration, then this occurred in 34% of patients after a conduit diversion (40% colonic, 28% ileal) and in 28% of those with a continent cecal reservoir. Similar results were reported in patients with a Kock pouch observed for 5–11 years and in patients with an ileal bladder substitute.[8,62]

In a recent report on upper tract preservation, Jonsson et al describe 25 years of follow-up on kidney function in 126 patients with a Kock reservoir.[63] They reach two significant conclusions: kidney function is not impaired by the diversion per se, provided stenosis is recognized and managed; the patient's health status is influenced more by the underlying disease than by the diversion.

Voiding dysfunction

When voiding dysfunction occurs after orthotopic bladder substitution, quality of life is no better than after failure of alternative forms of diversion. Functional results should be reported in accordance with the International Continence Society standards established for intestinal urinary reservoirs.[64]

A comparison of the severity and prevalence of voiding dysfunction in many surgical series is confounded by variability in endpoints, definitions, length of follow-up, patient age and sex, and surgical technique. Moreover, lower urinary tract symptoms, incontinence, or retention rarely have been assessed with validated outcome instruments and/or voiding diaries. Despite these obvious limitations, some general observations can be made and are reviewed in this report.

Failure to store

Daytime incontinence

In a review of 2238 patients, with a follow-up of 26 ± 18 months, daytime incontinence occurs in 13.3 ± 13.6% of patients.[65] Functional urethral length does not correlate with daytime urinary incontinence. Rather, there is a trend for a lower maximal urethral closure pressure in patients that complain of stress urinary incontinence. More importantly, a suboptimal neobladder capacity is found in many patients with incontinence. Because the neobladder enlarges over time, these patients may become continent 6 months to a year after surgery. Evaluation should be postponed until after this period.

Risk factors for the development of daytime urinary incontinence include advanced patient age, the use of colonic segments, and, in some series, a lack of nerve-sparing techniques.[66,67]

Daytime continence rates decreased gradually 4–5 years after bladder substitution.[68] One factor is a declining external urethral sphincter function with age.[68] The importance of age is underlined by the fact that, at 5 and 10 years after surgery, the mean age of the patients was 68 years and 73 years, respectively. It is noteworthy that in this age group 10% to 15% of healthy men already report urinary incontinence.[69] Urethral sensitivity, which generally decreases after radical cystectomy, might be an additional factor. Hugonnet et al demonstrated that the sensory threshold in the membranous urethra was lower in incontinent patients.[70] It was suggested that the conscious or unconscious sensation of urine leakage in the membranous urethra, which normally produces either a reflex or voluntary contraction or increased tonus of the external urethral sphincter, is impaired.

Nocturnal leakage

Some degree of nocturnal leakage is a constant finding in most reports, even despite a technically sound operation. Nocturnal incontinence following replacement cystoplasty, which is more common and lasts longer than daytime incontinence, is a feature shared by all forms of neobladders. Nocturnal enuresis plagues nearly 28% (range 0–67%) of patients.[65] Similar to daytime incontinence, night-time incontinence resolves as the functional capacity increases over time. Unlike patients after radical prostatectomy, those with an orthotopic bladder substitute have no detrusor–sphincteric reflex that increases urethral closure pressure as bladder pressure increases. Also, unlike a normal bladder, there are no sensory vesical fibers allowing feedback to the brain to alert the patient when the reservoir is full, particularly at night (overflow incontinence). As long as the functional capacity is lower than the (increased) nocturnal urinary output, the use of an alarm clock at night is recommended until the patient has learned to be awaked by the new sensation of bladder fullness. Apart from the same mechanisms responsible for the gradual decline in daytime continence with age, increased night-time diuresis and shift of free water into the concentrated urine are additional factors.[54,71] Nocturnal incontinence may be related to the physiologic circadian rhythm of arginine vasopressin (AVP) secretion and an interdependence among urine osmolality, distensibility, and peristaltic contractions of the intestinal segments of a pouch, and the generation of pressure waves. Nocturnal antidiuresis with subsequently increased urine osmolality may reduce compliance and increase pressure waves, a phenomenon that may be reversed by the topical application of oxybutynin.[54]

Sensory innervation of the urethra from the intrapelvic branches of the pudendal nerve or branches of the pelvic plexus may also have a role in preventing urinary leakage. Division of these nerves may result in loss of the afferent innervation of the external sphincter guarding reflex stimulated by urinary leakage into the proximal urethra.[72]

Failure to empty

From 4% to 25% of male patients must perform intermittent self-catheterization for incomplete emptying of the neobladder.[65] The reported functional outcome in female patients differs among series, particularly in regard to voiding ability. Some reported a 53%[19] and 41%[73] rate of intermittent catheterization, whereas others noted a much lower rate of 0%[74] and 3%.[75] The precise pathogenesis of urinary retention, or elevated residual urine requiring intermittent self-catheterization, remains uncertain. Angulation of the urethra is the most common basis for obstruction.[76,77] An attempt to preserve continence by lengthening the bladder neck anastomosed to the urethra can cause obstruction.[78] The angle of the reservoir with the urethra and the supporting system is highly important for emptying of the neobladder. Comparing good voiders with poor voiders, Mikuma et al found no differences of intrareservoir pressure. Instead, they demonstrated two findings in poor voiders: 1) the neobladder outlet was not located at the bottom of the pouch; and 2) funneling of the bladder outlet was not seen even on abdominal straining.[79] A preserved but dysfunctional bladder neck may result in obstructed voiding; a denervated floppy proximal urethra may lead to ineffective active relaxation, or simply kinking, during voiding, and, thus, incomplete emptying.[80,81]

In the postoperative period, voiding re-education is of paramount importance. Patients must clearly understand the principle that lowering outlet resistance is the key to success.

Increasing intra-abdominal pressure alone does not allow voiding. Instruction on pelvic floor relaxation, regular voiding to prevent overdistension, and regular follow-up are essential.[82] In some patients, incomplete voiding is associated with an inability to sustain abdominal straining.

Complications

The complications of both continent catheterizable reservoirs and orthotopic bladder substitutes in the hands of the most experienced surgeons have been considered in detail.[83] Reoperation for early complications overall occurred in 3% of continent catheterizable reservoirs and 7% of orthotopic bladder substitutions. Reoperation for late complications overall occurred in about 30% of continent catheterizable reservoirs and 13% of orthotopic bladder substitutions. We believe that the morbidity of orthotopic bladder substitutes is actually similar to, or lower than, the true rates of morbidity after conduit formation, contrary to the popular view that conduits are simple and safe.[84–87]

There are several new complications unknown during the conduit era: incisional hernias as a consequence of the Valsalva maneuver, neobladder–intestinal and neobladder–cutaneous fistulas, mucus formation, and neobladder rupture. The secretion of mucus can be dramatically increased.[88] The constant exposure of the neobladder to urine is a chronic irritation and leads to morphologic changes in the reservoir mucosa (see section 'Intestinal tissues as a substitute for the bladder. Gut mucosa as a substitute for urothelium'). A relative increase in goblet cell number was evident after 6 months, continued in the following 8 years, and stopped thereafter. This confirms the clinical observation that, on long-term follow-up, mucus secretion tends to be constant. The increase of goblet cells results in a shift in the secretive pattern towards sialomucins.[89] Probably this shift makes the mucus less viscous and therefore N-acetyl-L-cystein is not necessary for most of the patients after 6–18 months.

Spontaneous late rupture of neobladders is a rare, but potentially life-threatening, complication. In the majority of cases it is secondary to acute or chronic overdistension and bacterial infection. Other factors are minor blunt abdominal trauma or urethral occlusion. Chronic ischemic changes of the neobladder wall, possibly facilitated by detubularization and the variability of the mesenteric circulation, are additional factors that lead to perforation. The rupture site is typically the upper part of the right side of the reservoir. This is the most mobile part of the reservoir, and it undergoes the most marked distension during overfilling, which may constitute an additional factor for perforation in this location.[7]

There is no reliable procedure to establish the diagnosis. Cystography is misleading in three out of four patients with neobladder rupture. A high index of suspicion and early aggressive operative treatment in patients suspected of having a neobladder rupture are instrumental in providing a successful outcome. (*Editor's note*: We have managed three patients with neobladder rupture, and no evidence of an acute abdomen, conservatively with Foley catheter drainage without surgical intervention.) Prevention of neobladder rupture requires careful monitoring of neobladder emptying.[90] Physicians must be aware of the risk of rupture. Patients must be encouraged to void regularly, especially at bedtime, and to perform clean intermittent self-catheterization to avoid chronic reservoir overdistension. In the event that an anesthetic is required, proper bladder drainage should be performed.

Medical advantages of neobladder urinary diversion versus conduit diversion

Orthotopic bladder replacement stimulates earlier cystectomy at a time when the potential for cure is highest. When orthotopic reconstruction was considered experimental surgery, we offered cystectomy patients the choice of a neobladder versus a conduit. We evaluated the intervals from the primary diagnosis of bladder cancer, the diagnosis of invasive cancer, and the recommendation of cystectomy to cystectomy, as well as the number of previous transurethral resections of bladder tumor. Our data clearly suggest that the option of the neobladder may decrease physician and patient reluctance early in the disease process, thus increasing the survival rate significantly.[91]

The overall incidence and impact of ureterointestinal leakage remains rather constant, regardless of the form of urinary diversion used. However, if a bag leaks, it does so to a substantial degree that cannot be easily disguised. This contrasts with leakage of orthotopic bladder substitutes, which tend to be a little more than a few drops or milliliters, and thus can be controlled with a pad.

Upper tract safety

See section 'Reflux prevention in neobladders'.

Metabolic safety

Metabolic and nutritional complications of urinary diversions through bowel segments are common but, fortunately, not often severe. When metabolic abnormalities are problematic, deterioration or baseline insufficiency in renal function is the most likely cause. Deterioration is most commonly associated with obstruction or infection.[24,92–94] The urologist should be acutely aware of the potential for metabolic derangements when the prediversion creatinine is greater than 2.0 mg/dl. The more ileum used for reservoir construction, the higher the incidence of postoperative metabolic acidosis. This leads to the greatest advantage a conduit has over a neobladder.

Quality of life

Some quality of life studies suggest that patients tolerate the orthotopic bladder better than an ileal conduit.[95] However, other outcome studies have pointed out that the orthotopic neobladder fails to provide increased quality of life compared to an ileal conduit when patients experience voiding dysfunction. The patient satisfaction rate is high with either type of diversion, thus requiring the surgeon to provide a full and informed consent regarding all of the diversion options.[96–98]

In fact, ileal conduit patients may find life with an ileal conduit better than anticipated in terms of satisfaction, whereas continent diversion patients, if they anticipated their internal reservoir to work as well as their original bladder, may be dissatisfied. Patient satisfaction depends on the anticipated results—this is largely a function of informed consent and a realistic preparation by the clinician and enterostomal therapist in explaining, before surgery, the physical and lifestyle changes required postoperatively.

The effects on sexual function of radical cystectomy and the accompanying urinary diversion may be difficult to separate. The presence of an external appliance may impose additional barriers to sexual function for both men and women and their partners.

Other advantages of a neobladder are superior cosmetic appearance, and the potential for normal voiding function and continence. There is no need for an abdominal stoma, and therefore no need for a stomal appliance.

Conclusion

The disadvantages of conduits stimulated the development of orthotopic bladder substitutes. The early and late complication rates of orthotopic bladder substitutes are actually similar to, or lower than, the true rates of morbidity after conduit formation, contrary to the popular view that conduits are simple and safe. The experience with orthotopic bladder substitution has shown that patients who are well motivated and carefully selected can obtain outstanding outcomes.[7,9,10,11,89,99] For these patients, life is similar to that with a native lower urinary tract. Enthusiasm for the use of orthotopic reconstruction, however, should be tempered by an understanding of its indications and how not to contravene them.

References

1. Hautmann RE, Egghart G, Frohneberg D, et al. The ileal neobladder. J Urol 1988; 139: 39–42.
2. Hautmann RE. The ileal neobladder to the female urethra. Urol Clin North Am 1997; 24: 827–35.
3. Studer UE, Danuser H, Merz VW, et al. Experience in 100 patients with an ileal low pressure bladder substitute combined with an afferent tubular isoperistaltic segment. J Urol 1995; 154: 49–56.
4. Stein JP, Grossfeld GD, Freeman JA, et al. Orthotopic lower urinary tract reconstruction in women using the Kock ileal neobladder: updated experience in 34 patients. J Urol 1997; 158: 400–5.
5. Tizzoni G, Foggi A. Die Wiederherstellung der Harnblase. Zentralbl Chir 1888; 15: 921–4.
6. Couvelaire R. Le réservoir iléale de substitution après la cystectomie totale chez l'homme. J Urol (Paris) 1951; 57: 408–17.
7. Hautmann RE. Review article: Urinary diversion: ileal conduit to neobladder. J Urol 2003; 169: 834–42.
8. Studer UE, Zingg EJ. Ileal orthotopic bladder substitutes. What we have learned from 12 years' experience with 200 patients. Urol Clin North Am 1997; 24: 781–93.
9. Hautmann RE, Petriconi de R, Gottfried HW, et al. The ileal neobladder: complications and functional results in 363 patients after 11 years of followup. J Urol 1999; 161: 422–8.
10. Stein JP, Skinner DG. Application of the T-mechanism to an orthotopic (T-pouch) neobladder: a new era of urinary diversion. World J Urol 2000; 18: 315–23.
11. Montie JE, Wei JT. Formation of an orthotopic neobladder following radical cystectomy: historical perspective, patient selection and contemporary outcomes. J Pelvic Surg 2002; 8: 141–7.
12. Skinner DG, Studer UE, Okada K, et al. Which are suitable for continent diversion or bladder substitution following cystectomy or other definitive local treatment? Int J Urol 1995; 2(Suppl 2): 105–12.
13. Studer UE, Hautmann RE, Hohenfellner M, et al. Indications for continent diversion after cystectomy and factors affecting long-term results. Urol Oncol 1998; 4: 172–82.
14. Montie JE. Ileal conduit diversion after radical cystectomy. Pro Urology 1997; 49: 659–62.
15. Freeman JA, Tarter TA, Esrig D, et al. Urethral recurrence in patients with orthotopic ileal neobladders. J Urol 1996; 156: 1615–19.
16. Hardeman SW, Soloway MS. Urethral recurrence following radical cystectomy. J Urol 1990; 144: 666–9.
17. Stein JP, Stenzl A, Esrig D, et al. Lower urinary tract reconstruction following cystectomy in women using the Kock ileal reservoir with bilateral ureteroileal urethrostomy: initial clinical experience. J Urol 1994; 152: 1404–8.
18. Stenzl A, Draxl H, Posch K, et al. The risk of urethral tumors in female bladder cancer: can the urethra be used for orthotopic reconstruction of the lower urinary tract? J Urol 1995; 153: 950–5.
19. Hautmann RE, Paiss T, Petriconi de R. The ileal neobladder in women: 9 years of experience with 18 patients. J Urol 1996; 155: 76–81.
20. Groshen S, Skinner EC, Boyd SD, et al. Indications for lower urinary tract reconstruction in women after cystectomy for bladder cancer: a pathological review of female cystectomy specimens. J Urol 1995; 54: 1329–33.
21. Coloby PJ, Kakizoe T, Tobisu K, et al. Urethral involvement in female bladder cancer patients: mapping of 47 consecutive cystourethrectomy specimens. J Urol 1994; 152: 1438–42.
22. Hautmann RE, Simon J. Ileal neobladder and local recurrence of bladder cancer: patterns of failure and impact on function in men. J Urol 1999; 162: 1963–6.
23. Åkerlund S, Forssell-Aronsson E, Jonsson O, et al. Decreased absorption of 22Na and 36Cl in ileal reservoirs after exposure to urine. An experimental study in patients with continent ileal reservoirs for urinary or fecal diversion. Urol Res 1991; 19: 249–52.
24. Mills RD, Studer UE. Metabolic consequences of continent urinary diversion. J Urol 1999; 161: 1057–66.
25. Lytton B, Green DF. Urodynamic studies in patients undergoing bladder replacement surgery. J Urol 1989; 141: 1394–7.
26. Koraitim MM, Atta MA, Foda MK. Early and late cystometry of detubularized and nondetubularized intestinal neobladders: new observations and physiological correlates. J Urol 1995; 154: 1700–2; discussion 1702–3.
27. Santucci RA, Park CH, Mayo ME, et al. Continence and urodynamic parameters of continent urinary reservoirs: comparison of gastric, ileal, ileocolic, right colon, and sigmoid segments. Urology 1999; 54: 252–2.
28. Kolettis PN, Klein EA, Novick AC, et al. The Le Bag orthotopic urinary diversion. J Urol 1996; 156: 926–30.
29. Skinner DG, Boyd SD, Lieskovsky G, et al. Lower urinary tract reconstruction following cystectomy: experience and results in 126 patients using the Kock ileal reservoir with bilateral ureteroileal urethrostomy. J Urol 1991; 146: 756–60.
30. Stein JP, Lieskovsky G, Ginsberg DA, et al. The T pouch: an orthotopic ileal neobladder incorporating a serosal lined ileal antireflux technique. J Urol 1998; 159: 1836–42.
31. Hautmann RE. The ileal neobladder. Atlas Urol Clin North Am 2001; 9: 85.
32. Hollowell CMP, Christiano AP, Steinberg GD. Technique of Hautmann ileal neobladder with chimney modification: interim results in 50 patients. J Urol 2000; 163: 47–51.
33. Lippert MC, Theodorescu D. The Hautmann neobladder with a chimney: a versatile modification. J Urol 1997; 158: 1510–12.
34. Studer UE, Spiegel T, Casanova GA, et al. Ileal bladder substitute: antireflux nipple or afferent tubular segment? Eur Urol 1991; 20: 315–26.
35. Pernet FP, Jonas U. Ileal conduit urinary diversion: early and late results of 132 cases in a 25-year period. World J Urol 1985; 3: 140–4.
36. Orr JD, Shand JE, Watters DA, Kirkland IS. Ileal conduit urinary diversion in children. An assessment of long-term results. Br J Urol 1981; 53: 424–7.
37. Elder DD, Moisey CU, Rees RW. A long-term follow-up of the colonic conduit operation in children. Br J Urol 1979; 51: 462–5.
38. Dybner R, Jeter K, Lattimer JK. Comparison of intraluminal pressures in ileal and colonic conduits in children. J Urol 1972; 108: 477–9.
39. Berglund B, Kock NG. Volume capacity and pressure characteristics of various types of intestinal reservoirs. World J Surg 1987; 11: 798–803.

40. Pantuck AJ, Han KR, Perrotti M. Ureteroenteric anastomosis in continent urinary diversion: long-term results and complications of direct versus nonrefluxing techniques. J Urol 2000; 163: 450–5.

41. Roth S, Ahlen van H, Semjonow A, et al. Does the success of ureterointestinal implantation in orthotopic bladder substitution depend more on surgeon level of experience or choice of technique? J Urol 1997; 157: 56–60.

42. Elmajian DA, Stein JP, Esrig D, et al. The Kock ileal neobladder: updated experience in 295 male patients. J Urol 1996; 156: 920–5.

43. Shaaban AA, Gaballah MA, el-Diasty TA, Ghoneim MA. Urethral controlled bladder substitution: a comparison between the intussuscepted nipple valve and the technique of Le Duc as antireflux procedures. J Urol 1992; 148: 1156–61.

44. Cajal SR. Los Gangliosy Plexos Nerviosos del intestino de las Mammiferos. Madrid Moya 1893; 1.

45. Faussone-Pellegrini MS. Histogenesis, structure and relationship of interstitial cells of Cajal (ICC): from morphology to functional interpretation. Eur J Morphol 1992; 30: 137–48.

46. Thuneberg L. Interstitial cells of Cajal. In Handbook of Physiology. The Gastrointestinal System. Motility and Circulation. Bethesda: American Physiological Society, 1989, Sect. 5, 1: 349.

47. Rumessen JJ, Mikkelsen HB, Thuneberg L. Ultrastructure of interstitial cells of Cajal associated with deep muscular plexus of human small intestine. Gastroenterology 1992; 102: 56–68.

48. Huizinga JD, Thuneberg L, Kluppel M, et al. Gene acquired for interstitial cells of Cajal and for intestinal pacemaker activity. Nature 1995; 373: 347–9.

49. Faussone-Pellegrini MS, Serni S, Carini M. Distribution of ICC and motor response characteristics in urinary bladders reconstructed from human ileum. Am J Physiol 1997; 273: G147–157.

50. Batra AK, Hanno PM, Ruggieri MR. Detubularization-induced contractile response change of the ileum following ileocystoplasty. J Urol 1992; 148: 195–9.

51. Moore JA, Brading AF. Gastrointestinal tissue as a substitute for the detrusor. World J Urol 2000; 18: 305–14.

52. Hinman F Jr. Selection of intestinal segments for bladder substitution: physical and physiological characteristics. J Urol 1988; 139: 519–23.

53. Colding-Jørgensen M, Poulsen AL, Steven K. Mechanical characteristics of tubular and detubularised bowel for bladder substitution: theory, urodynamics and clinical results. Br J Urol 1993; 72: 586–93.

54. Hohenfellner M, Burger R, Schad H. Reservoir characteristics of Mainz pouch studied in animal model. Osmolality of filling solution: an effect of oxybutinin. Urology 1993; 42: 741–6.

55. Goldwasser B, Madgar I, Hanani Y. Urodynamic aspects of continent urinary diversion, Review Scand J Urol Nephrol 1987; 21: 245–53.

56. Aragona F, De Caro R, Parenti A. Structural and ultrastructural changes in ileal neobladder mucosa: a 7-year follow up. Br J Urol 1998; 81: 55–61.

57. Philipson B, Hockenstrom T, Akerlund S. Biological consequences of exposing ileal mucosa to urine. World J Surg 1987; 11: 790–7.

58. Carlén B, Willen R, Mansson W. Mucosal ultrastructure of continent cecal reservoir for urine and its ileal nipple valve 2–9 years after construction. J Urol 1990; 143: 372–6.

59. Deane AM, Woodhouse CR, Parkinson MC. Histological changes in ileal conduits. J Urol 1984; 132: 1108–11.

60. Kristiánsson A, Wallin L, Mánsson W. Renal function up to 16 years after conduit (refluxing or anti-reflux anastomosis) or continent urinary diversion. 1. Glomerular filtration rate and patency of ureterointestinal anastomosis. Br J Urol 1995; 76: 539–45.

61. Granerus G, Aurell M. Reference values for 51Cr-EDTA clearance as a measure of glomerular filtration rate. Scand J Clin Lab Invest 1981; 41: 611–16.

62. Studer UE, Danuser H, Möhrle K, et al. Results in the upper urinary tract in 220 patients with an ileal low pressure bladder substitute combined with an afferent tubular segment. J Urol 1999; 161: 91.

63. Jonsson O, Olofsson G, Lindholm E, et al. Long-time experience with the Kock ileal reservoir for continent urinary diversion. Eur Urol 2001; 40: 632–40.

64. Thüroff JW, Mattiasson A, Andersen JT, et al. The standardization of terminology and assessment of functional characteristics of intestinal urinary reservoirs. Br J Urol 1996; 78: 516–23.

65. Steers WD. Voiding dysfunction in the orthotopic neobladder. World J Urol 2000; 18: 330–7.

66. Park JM, Montie JE. Mechanisms of incontinence and retention after orthotopic neobladder diversion. Urology 1998; 51(4): 601–9.

67. Porru D, Madeddu G, Campus G. et al. Urodynamic analysis of voiding dysfunction in orthotopic ileal neobladder. World J Urol 1999; 17(5): 285–9.

68. Hammerer P, Michl U, Meyer-Moldenhauer WH, et al. Urethral closure pressure changes with age in men. J Urol 1996; 156: 1741–3.

69. Temml C, Haidinger G, Schmidbauer J, et al. Urinary incontinence in both sexes: prevalence rates and impact on quality of life and sexual life. Neurourol Urodyn 2000; 19: 259–71.

70. Hugonnet, CL, Danuser H, Springer JP, et al. Decreased sensitivity in the membranous urethra after orthotopic ileal bladder substitute. J Urol 1999; 161: 418–21.

71. Jagenburg R, Kock NG, Norlen L, et al. Clinical significance of changes in composition of urine during collection and storage in continent ileum reservoir urinary diversion. Scand J Urol Nephrol 1978; 49: 43–8.

72. Garry RC, Roberts TD, Todd JK. Reflexes involving the external urethral sphincter in the cat. J Physiol 1953; 149: 653.

73. Linn JF, Hohenfellner M, Roth S, et al. Treatment of interstitial cystitis: comparison of subtrigonal and supratrigonal cystectomy combined with orthotopic bladder substitution. J Urol 1998; 159: 774–8.

74. Ghoneim MA. Orthotopic bladder substitution in women following cystectomy for bladder cancer. Urol Clin North Am 1997; 24: 225–39.

75. Stenzl A, Colleselli K, Bartsch G. Update for urethra-sparing approaches in cystectomy in women. World J Urol 1997; 15: 134–8.

76. Ali-El-Dein B, El-Sobky E, Hohenfellner M, et al. Orthotopic bladder substitution in women: functional evaluation. J Urol 1999; 161: 1875–80.

77. Fujisawa M, Isotani S, Gotoh A, et al. Voiding dysfunction of sigmoid neobladder in women: a comparative study with men. Eur Urol 2001; 40: 191–5.

78. Smith E, Yoon J, Theodorescu D. Evaluation of urinary continence and voiding function: early results in men with neo-urethral modification of the Hautmann orthotopic neobladder. J Urol 2001; 166: 1346–9.

79. Mikuma M, Hirose T, Yokoo A, et al. Voiding dysfunction in ileal neobladder. J Urol 1997; 158: 1365–8.

80. Aboseif SR, Borirakchanyavat S, Lue TF, et al. Continence mechanism of the ileal neobladder in women: a urodynamic study. World J Urol 1998; 16: 400–4.

81. Arai Y, Okubo K, Konami T, et al. Voiding function of orthotopic ileal neobladder in women. Urology 1999; 54: 44–49.

82. Mills RD, Studer UE, Female orthotopic bladder substitution: a good operation in the right circumstances. J Urol 2000; 163: 1501–4.

83. Rowland RG. Complications of continent cutaneous reservoirs and neobladders—series using contemporary technique. AUA Update Ser 1995; 14(Lesson 25): 201.

84. Turner WH, Bitton A, Studer UE. Reconstruction of the urinary tract after radical cystectomy: the case for continent urinary diversion [editorial]. Urology 1997; 49: 663–7.

85. Benson MC, Slawin KM, Wechsler MH, Olsson CA. Analysis of continent versus standard urinary diversion. Br J Urol 1992; 69: 156–62.

86. Gburek BM, Lieber MM, Blute ML. Comparison of Studer ileal conduit diversion with respect to perioperative outcome and late complications. J Urol 1998; 160: 721–3.

87. Jahnson S, Pedersen J. Cystectomy and urinary diversion during twenty years—complications and metabolic implications. Eur Urol 1993; 24: 343–9.

88. Leibovitch IJ, Ramon J, Chaim JB, et al. Increased urinary mucus production: a sequela of cystography following enterocystoplasty. J Urol 1991; 145: 736–7.

89. Gatti R, Ferretti S, Bucci G, et al. Histological adaptation of orthotopic ileal neobladder mucosa: 4-year follow-up of 30 patients. Eur Urol 1999; 36: 588–94.

90. Nippgen JBW, Hakenberg OW, Manseck A, et al. Spontaneous late rupture of orthotopic detubularized ileal neobladders: report of five cases. Urology 2001; 58: 43–6.

91. Hautmann RE, Paiss T. Does the option of the ileal neobladder stimulate patient and physician decision towards earlier cystectomy? [abstract]. J Urol 1996; 155(Suppl): 437A.

92. Stampfer DS, McDougal WS, McGovern FJ. Metabolic and nutritional complications. Urol Clin North Am 1997; 24: 715–22.

93. Kristjánsson A, Davidsson T, Månsson W. Metabolic alterations at different levels of renal function following continent urinary diversion through colonic segments. J Urol 1997; 157: 2099–103.

94. Chang SS, Koch MO. Metabolic complications of urinary diversion. Urol Oncol 2000; 5: 60–70.

95. Hobisch A, Tosun K, Kinzl J, et al. Quality of life after cystectomy and orthotopic neobladder versus ileal conduit urinary diversion. World J Urol 2000; 18: 338–44.

96. Hart S, Skinner EC, Meyerowitz BE, et al. Quality of life after radical cystectomy for bladder cancer in patients with an ileal conduit, or cutaneous or urethral Kock pouch. J Urol 1999; 162: 77–81.

97. Månsson Å, Johnson G, Månsson W. Quality of life after cystectomy. Comparison between patients with conduit and those with continent caecal reservoir urinary diversion. Br J Urol 1988; 62: 240–5.

98. Henningsohn L, Wijkström H, Dickman PW, et al. Distressful symptoms after radical cystectomy with urinary diversion for urinary bladder cancer: a Swedish population-based study. Eur Urol 2001; 40: 151–62.

99. Abol-Enein H, Ghoneim MA. Functional results of orthotopic ileal neobladder with serous-lined extramural ureteral reimplantation: experience with 450 patients. J Urol 2001; 165: 1427–32.

21

Continent cutaneous diversion

Christoph Wiesner, Randall G Rowland, Joachim W Thüroff

Introduction

Kock devised the first continent ileostomy reservoir for proctocolectomized patients in 1969. It was used first in 1975 for continent cutaneous urinary diversion.[1] Since that time, several surgical procedures for continent cutaneous diversion have been developed using different bowel segments for reservoir construction. Numerous modifications of reservoir construction have been established as well as surgical techniques for ureteral implantation and for construction of a continence mechanism.

In bladder cancer patients, in whom orthotopic diversion is not feasible, continent cutaneous diversion provides a catheterizable low-pressure reservoir, which contributes to an increased quality of life and body image.

Indications and patient selection

Indications for continent cutaneous diversion are cystourethrectomy for bladder cancer, when preservation of the sphincter and urethra are not possible due, for example, to positive urethral biopsies or positive intraoperative surgical margins. In addition, orthotopic bladder substitution should not be recommended for patients with incontinence due to urethral sphincter incompetence.

Careful patient selection for motivation, compliance and manual dexterity to perform self-catheterization is necessary to ensure success of the continent diversion in the long term. Patients with previous irradiation encompassing bowel segments required to construct the reservoir, bowel resection, and chronic inflammatory bowel disease (Crohn's disease, ulcerative colitis) should be excluded.

Contraindications for continent cutaneous diversion are inadequate manual dexterity to perform self-catheterization and reduced intellectual capacity of understanding the reservoir and its function. Furthermore, renal function must be adequate to compensate for reabsorption of acids and liquids from the intestinal reservoir (clearance >50% of age-specific norm, serum creatinine <2.0 mg/dl).

Preoperative preparation

Preoperative radiographic imaging includes intravenous pyelography (IVP) for exclusion of upper tract urothelial cancer. If upper tract dilation is present, a radioisotope study should be performed to ensure adequate renal function. If large bowel is used for reservoir construction, a colonic contrast study or colonoscopy to check for bowel polyps and diverticulosis is recommended.

For bowel preparation a liquid diet is given the day before surgery. For bowel cleansing, 3–4 liters of hyperosmotic solution are administered. Subcutaneous prophylaxis for deep vein thrombosis is started the evening before surgery and antithrombotic stockings are used perioperatively. Patients are shaved just before surgery. Patient positioning for surgery is supine with some hyperextension.

Postoperative care

Full parenteral nutrition is administered until regular bowel movements are encountered. Antibiotic therapy includes metronidazole for 5 days and amoxicillin until removal of the ureteral stents. The reservoir is irrigated twice a day with saline to avoid mucus formation and catheter blockage. The ureteral stents are usually removed between days 8 and 10 after surgery. After removal of the ureteral stents, drainage of the upper urinary tract is studied by ultrasound or IVP. Before removal of the indwelling catheter, 3 weeks postoperatively, a pouchogram is performed to check for extravasation and ureteral reflux. Patients are then instructed to perform intermittent self-catheterization. The interval between catheterization should not exceed 2 hours initially, and is to be stepwise increased until the pouch capacity reaches 500–600 ml.

Follow-up

When the indwelling pouch catheter is removed about 3 weeks postoperatively, and urine storage is initiated in an intestinal urinary reservoir, patients are at risk of developing metabolic acidosis. Close follow-up of the acid–base balance from capillary blood gas analysis is required. Acid–base balance may vary between −2.5 and +2.5 mmol/l; acid–base balance below −2.5 mmol/l should be corrected by alkali substitution.

Serum creatinine and electrolytes should be obtained every 3 months in the first postoperative year.

Renal ultrasound is essential to check for postoperative hydronephrosis and should be obtained every 3 months within the first year after surgery. The interval can be prolonged to every 6 months in the second year and to once a year after 3 years. If hydronephrosis is diagnosed, diuretic radioisotope studies (e.g. MAG-III clearance) are recommended for differentiation between dilation and obstruction.

Patients with continent urinary diversion are at theoretical risk of developing cancer at the site of the ureteral implantation.

Hence pouchoscopy starting 5 years postoperatively is recommended once a year.

Surgery

The basic principles of continent cutaneous diversion focus on creation of a high-capacity and low-pressure reservoir, which can easily be emptied by intermittent self-catheterization, preserves the upper urinary tract, and provides continence by its specific outlet. A variety of surgical techniques using different bowel segments have been established. Numerous variants of pouch formation, ureteral implantation, and outlet construction have been introduced and combined in modifications of original techniques to reduce the risk of complications and to optimize clinical outcome.

Kock pouch

Kock was the first to present a continent ileal reservoir for urinary diversion using 60–70 cm of ileum for pouch formation and construction of two valves (Figure 21.1). At the proximal and distal ends of the ileum, which has been excluded from the fecal stream for pouch formation, 10–12 cm of bowel each are left intact for creation of the afferent and efferent valves. The remaining 40 cm of ileum is incised antimesenterically, sutured side-to-side in a U-shape, folded over, and closed to a spherical pouch (Figures 21.2, 21.3). For the final position, the reservoir is rotated in such a manner that the posterior aspect is brought anteriorly (Figure 21.4). Strips of fascia from the anterior rectus sheath or of Marlex mesh are used around the base of the intussusception to secure the afferent antirefluxing valve and the efferent continence valve. The ureters are implanted end-to-side into the afferent ileum. The nipple valves are intussuscepted over a length of 5 cm and fixed by four rows of staples (Figure 21.5). The technique was later modified with a longer ileal intussusception by placing three staple rows at the 6, 10 and 2 o'clock positions and fixation of the nipple by inserting fibrin glue and several sutures at the intussusception.[2]

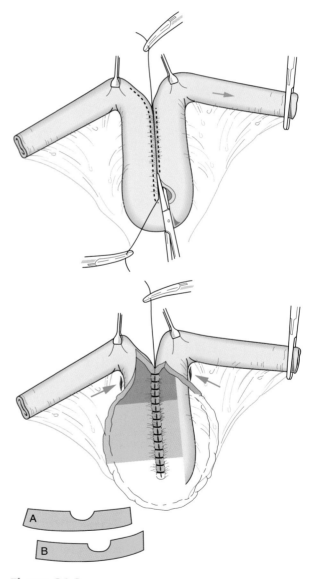

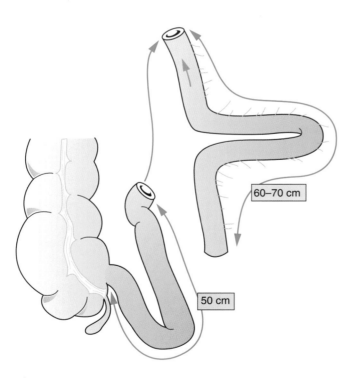

Figure 21.1
Kock pouch cutaneous diversion. 60–70 cm of ileum are isolated approximately 50 cm above the ileocecal valve. The bowel is positioned in a U-shape. Adapted from Kock NG, Nilson LD, Nilson LJ, Philipson BM. Urinary diversion via a continent ileal reservoir: Clinical results in 12 patients. J. Urol 1982;128:469–475.

Figure 21.2
Kock pouch cutaneous diversion. The ileum is incised along its antimesenteric border and sutured side-to-side in a U-shape. Adapted from Kock NG, Nilson LD, Nilson LJ, Philipson BM. Urinary diversion via a continent ileal reservoir: Clinical results in 12 patients. J. Urol 1982;128:469–475.

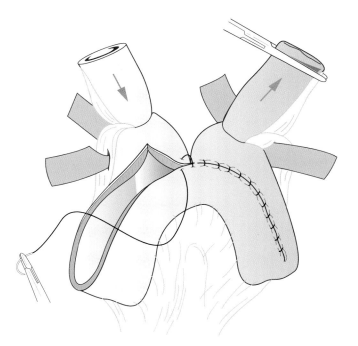

Figure 21.3
Kock pouch cutaneous diversion. Closure of the reservoir is performed by two inverting running sutures. Adapted from Kock NG, Nilson LD, Nilson LJ, Philipson BM. Urinary diversion via a continent ileal reservoir: Clinical results in 12 patients. J. Urol 1982;128:469–475.

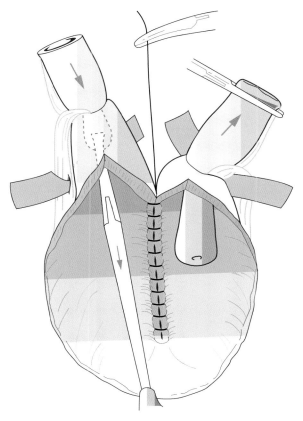

Figure 21.5
Kock pouch cutaneous diversion. The nipple valves are fixed by ileal intussusception with three rows of staples. The afferent valve serves as antireflux mechanism to ureteral implantation, the efferent valve as the continent outlet. The valves are secured by strips of fascia or Marlex mesh, which are positioned around the base of each valve. Adapted from Kock NG, Nilson LD, Nilson LJ, Philipson BM. Urinary diversion via a continent ileal reservoir: Clinical results in 12 patients. J. Urol 1982;128:469–475.

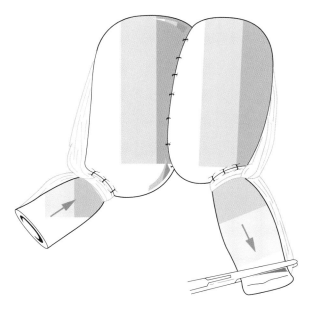

Figure 21.4
Kock pouch cutaneous diversion. For the final positioning, the reservoir is rotated in such a manner that the posterior aspect is brought anteriorly. Adapted from Kock NG, Nilson LD, Nilson LJ, Philipson BM. Urinary diversion via a continent ileal reservoir: Clinical results in 12 patients. J. Urol 1982;128:469–475.

Complication rates

Complications with the need for surgical reintervention range between 32% and 53%.[2–8] In a series of 40 patients with Kock pouch diversion, early pouch-related complications were encountered in 25%, including two patients with reoperation for pouch rupture and pinhole fistula at the efferent segment.[2] Eight patients were re-hospitalized, seven because of pouch sepsis, which was associated with transient acidosis, and one with a pelvic abscess.

Late complications were most frequently associated with dysfunction of the efferent segment including stomal incontinence (17–23%), nipple prolapse/nipple gliding (7–10%), stomal stenosis (0–10%), or calculus formation (8–15%). Complications of the afferent segment are rare and comprise mostly strictures of the ureteroileal anastomosis (2–5%), ureteral reflux (2–13%), afferent nipple stones (5.2%), or afferent limb stenosis in 4.3%.[8] Continence rates vary between 78% and 94%.

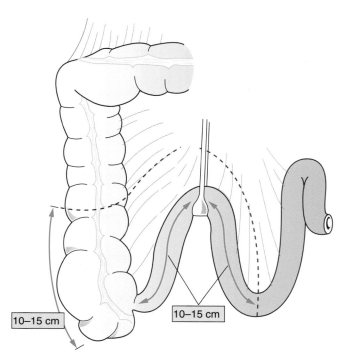

Figure 21.6
Mainz pouch diversion. 10–15 cm of cecum and ascending colon and two ileal segments of the same length are used for reservoir construction.

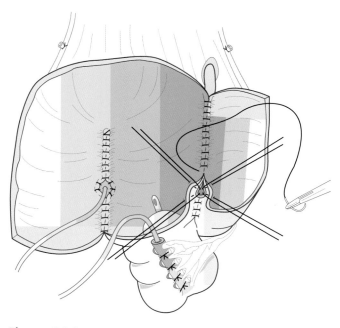

Figure 21.8
Extramural serosa lined tunnel. After the ureters have been positioned into the serosa bed, the tunnel is closed by closing the bowel margins over it using a running absorbable suture.

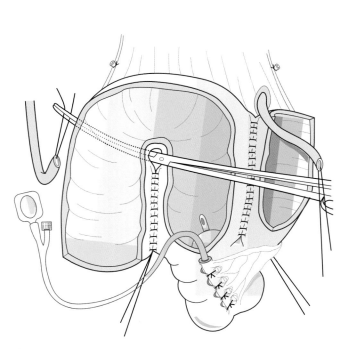

Figure 21.7
Implantation of the ureters by extramural serosa lined tunnel technique. The serosa of the adjacent bowel segments is sutured approximately 2 cm from the margins by a nonabsorbable running suture for construction of the bed of the tunnel.

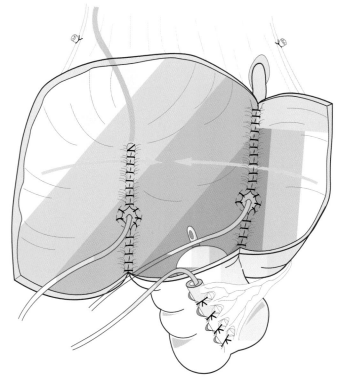

Figure 21.9
Extramural serosa lined tunnel. The neo-orifices are created by 6-0 sutures of the ureter with the intestinal mucosa.

Mainz pouch and alternative/modified procedures

The Mainz pouch I procedure was established in 1983 using 10–15 cm of cecum and ascending colon and two terminal ileal segments of equal length for reservoir construction (Figure 21.6).[9] The surgical procedure comprises antimesenteric incision of ileum, cecum, and ascending colon, and side-to-side anastomosis of the ascending colon with the terminal ileal loop, and of the latter with the proximal ileal loop. The anterior wall of the pouch is closed by a single row of running sutures.

A

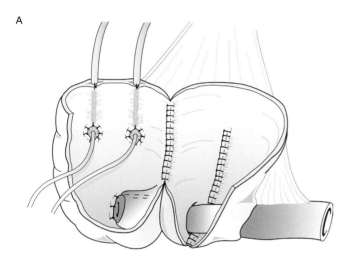

B

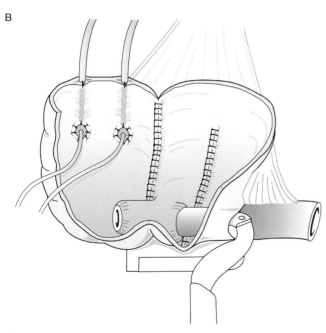

Figure 21.10
Intussuscepted ileal nipple. (A) 12–15 cm of terminal ileum are used for construction of the intussuscepted ileal nipple valve. The ileum is left tubularized and intussuscepted isoperistaltically through the ileocecal valve and secured by three rows of metal staples. (B) One row of staples fixes the nipple to the reservoir wall.

Both ureters are implanted in an antirefluxing manner into the large bowel using the submucosal tunnel technique described by Goodwin et al.[10] Alternatively, the Aboul-Enein technique is performed for preoperatively dilated ureters in order to avoid postoperative obstruction (Figures 21.7–21.9).[11] The technique entails fashioning of two serosa lined extramural tunnels, and was first applied to the W-shaped ileal neobladder. The 'buttonhole' technique implies direct refluxing ureteral implantation.[12]

Originally, the continent outlet was created using 12–15 cm of terminal ileum, which was left intact and was intussuscepted isoperistaltically over a length of about 5 cm through the ileocecal valve. Fixation of the segment was performed by three rows of metal staples, one of which fixed the nipple to the reservoir wall (Figure 21.10). Since 1990, the submucosally embedded in-situ appendix is increasingly used for construction of the continent outlet.[13] The submucosal tunnel is created by seromuscular incision of the tenia libra (Figure 21.11). The appendix is flipped over into the submucosal bed and the seromuscularis layer is closed over it (Figure 21.12).

The seromuscular and full-thickness bowel flap tubes were presented in 1995 as an alternative procedure for patients in whom the appendix was not available.[14] For the seromuscularis bowel flap tube, a 3 × 5 cm pedicled flap is created by an inverted U-shaped incision along the tenia libra and then tubularized. The bowel flap tube is embedded submucosally by closing the lateral margins of the seromuscular incisions over it. In the full-thickness bowel flap tube technique, the pedicled bowel flap is excised from the anterior tenia

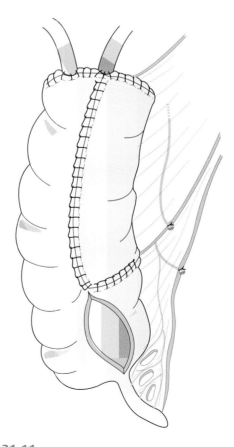

Figure 21.11
Appendiceal stoma. The seromuscularis is incised along the tenia libra.

A

B

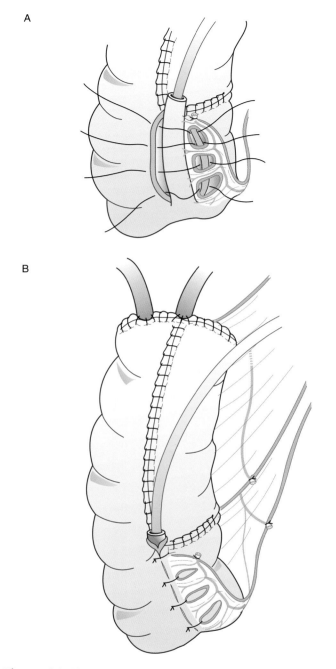

Figure 21.12
Appendiceal stoma. (A) The appendix is flipped over into the submucosal bed. (B) The tunnel is finished by closure of the seromuscularis over the appendix.

A

B

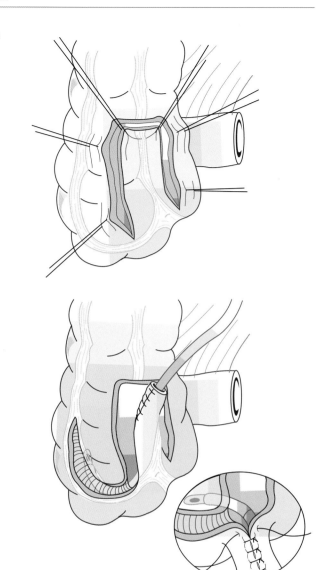

Figure 21.13
Full-thickness bowel flap tube. (A) A flap is created by an inverted U-shaped incision along the tenia libra of the cecum and tubularized (B).

and embedded into a submucosal tunnel at the tenia omentalis (Figures 21.13 and 21.14).

The transverse colonic pouch (Mainz pouch III, transverse ascending or transverse descending pouch) was created for continent urinary diversion in patients with previous pelvic irradiation.[15] A total of 15–17 cm of transverse colon and either ascending or descending colon are used (Figure 21.15). The outlet is created by tapering a 5–7 cm tubular colonic segment into a tube, which is embedded into a serosal or submucosal tunnel (Figure 21.16). The

ureteral implantation follows the Goodwin technique or the serosal extramural tunnel technique (Figure 21.17).

Complication rates

Since the creation of the Mainz pouch, several techniques for outlet construction and ureteral implantation have been developed. The initial complication rates for sutured and stapled ileoileal intussusception nipples of 45% decreased to 10% for nipples with additional fixation to the ileocecal valve.[16,17] Minor complications of the intussuscepted ileal nipple are calculus formation (3–5.5%) and stoma stenosis (1.9–11.7%)[18,19]; major complications were nipple necrosis (3.8%) and nipple prolapse/nipple gliding (6.6%).[18]

Stoma stenosis is the most frequent complication of the appendix outlet, ranging from 14.6% to 21%.[17–20] Development of calculi is

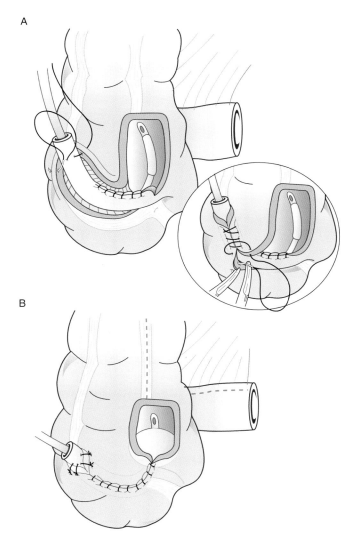

A

B

Figure 21.14
Full-thickness bowel flap tube. (A) The tube is embedded into a submucosal tunnel at the tenia omentalis. (B) The tunnel is finished by closing the lateral margins of the seromuscularis.

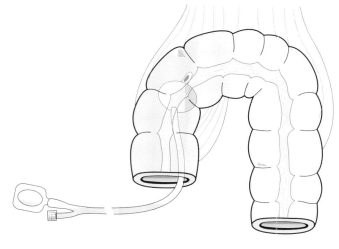

Figure 21.15
Transverse colon pouch diversion (Mainz III). The colonic pouch (Mainz III) is constructed by a 15–17 cm segment of transverse colon and either ascending or descending colon. Adapted from Leissner J, Black P, Fisch M, Hockel M, Hohenfellner R. Colon pouch (Mainz pouch III) for continent urinary diversion after pelvic irradiation. Urology 2000;56:798–802.

incontinence required surgical revision by creating a new outlet. Patients with stoma stenosis were treated by endoscopic scar incision (67%) or by open surgical YV-plasty (33%).

rare. Major complications were appendiceal necrosis (2.1–2.5%) with the consequence of surgical revision and replacement by an ileal nipple.[18,20] Continence rates of the appendix outlet range between 98% and 100%.[18–20]

Stoma stenoses were seen in 11% of patients with a full-thickness bowel flap tube.[21] Antirefluxing ureteral implantation with a submucosal tunnel was associated with a 5.7% ureteral obstruction rate for preoperatively nondilated ureters, and a 16% obstruction rate for preoperatively dilated systems at long-term follow-up.[22] Direct ureterointestinal implantation was performed in 30 patients with Mainz pouch diversion.[12] The technique was used for primary anastomosis in 20 patients, and for reimplantation in cases of stenosis of the ureterointestinal anastomosis in another 10 patients. At follow-up there was no deterioration of kidney function and no evidence of obstruction; reflux occurred in one renal unit only without necessity for intervention.

Complication rates (18%) of the transverse colonic pouch (Mainz III) were related to the tapered colonic efferent segment with stoma incontinence in 5% and stoma stenosis in 14%.[15] Stoma

Indiana pouch

The Indiana pouch was developed in 1984 as a modification of the Gilchrist procedure.[23] Up to 8–10 cm of terminal ileum and 25–30 cm of cecum and ascending colon are isolated and opened along the antimesenteric border (Figure 21.18A). The distal end of the opened colon is folded down to the apex of the incision. The reservoir is closed with a single layer of sutures (Figure 21.18B,C). If the reservoir was to be constructed by mechanical stapling, a 2–3 cm incision at the antimesenteric border of the cecum opposite to the ileocecal valve is performed. The distal end of the colonic segment is folded down to the cecal incision, fixed by holding sutures, cut open and stapled between the holding sutures using the GIA stapler with absorbable staples until complete detubularization of the colonic segment is achieved. The edges of the opposing colonic segments are finally closed by absorbable Ta 55 staples. Originally, ureteral implantation was performed through a T-shaped incision of the colonic tenia, leaving the mucosa intact (Figure 21.19A). The ureteral neo-orifice was established after mucosal incision (Figure 21.19B), and the submucosal tunnel was closed by a running suture of the incised seromuscularis (Figure 21.19C, D). Currently a refluxing end-to-side direct anastomosis is used. The efferent segment is constructed by tapered ileum. The antimesenteric portion of the terminal ileum is tapered using metal GIA staples, leaving a residual caliber of ileum that allows easy passage of an 18 Fr. catheter. The outlet is imbricated and secured by sutures at the junction of ileum and cecum to create a functional continence mechanism (Figure 21.20).

A

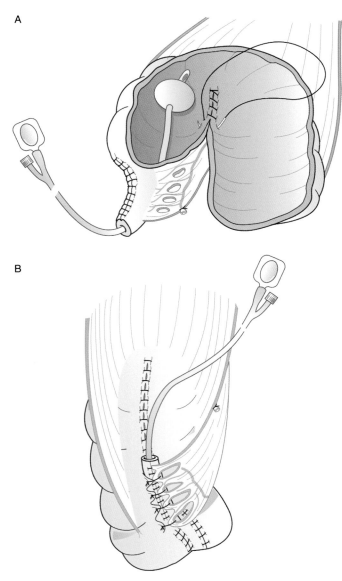

B

Figure 21.16
Transverse colon pouch diversion (Mainz III). (A) The outlet is created by tapering a 5–7 cm tubular colonic segment into a tube, which is embedded into a serosal tunnel (B). Adapted from Leissner J, Black P, Fisch M, Hockel M, Hohenfellner R. Colon pouch (Mainz pouch III) for continent urinary diversion after pelvic irradiation. Urology 2000;56:798–802.

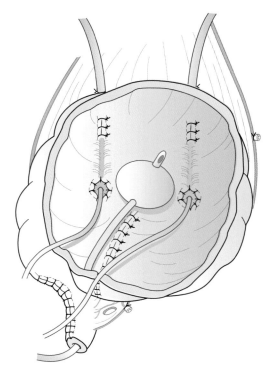

Figure 21.17
Transverse colon pouch diversion (Mainz III). The ureters are implanted by the Goodwin technique, or by an extramural serosal tunnel. Adapted from Leissner J, Black P, Fisch M, Hockel M, Hohenfellner R. Colon pouch (Mainz pouch III) for continent urinary diversion after pelvic irradiation. Urology 2000;56:798–802.

rate of surgical reinterventions ranging between 10.8% and 52.0%.[25–27] Pouch-related complications were pouch rupture (2.5–3.2%) and calculus formation (3.7–10.5%). Complications of the efferent segment were stoma stenosis (3.7–15.2%) and stoma incontinence (1.2–28.2%). Obstruction of the ureteral anastomosis was recognized in 0% to 7.2%. Preoperative radiotherapy did influence postoperative outcome negatively.

Complication rates of 130 patients, including 34 (26%) patients with preoperative pelvic irradiation, were reported, in whom the Indiana pouch was performed for urinary diversion.[28] The overall complication rate was 12%; ureteral obstruction was seen in 15% of the patients with preoperative irradiation and in 4% without preoperative irradiation. Stoma incontinence developed in 4% of the patients, all of whom had undergone preoperative radiotherapy.

The procedure was modified by Managadze, who embedded the tapered ileum segment into a submucosal tunnel by incision of the seromuscularis between the tenia libra and the tenia mesocolica of the cecum.[24]

Complication rates

Complication rates of urinary diversion using the Indiana pouch procedure were investigated in several studies and revealed a total

Florida pouch

In 1987 Lockhart described an alternative colonic reservoir (Florida pouch) that included cecum, ascending colon, one-third of the right transverse colon, and 10–12 cm of the terminal ileum for the outlet.[29] The colon is U-folded, fully detubularized, and closed by a locked running suture. Ureteral implantation was originally performed using the Le Duc antirefluxing ureteroileal implantation by ureteral fixation in a mucosal sulcus,[30] or by the Goodwin technique (described above).[10] It was later modified into a direct anastomosis

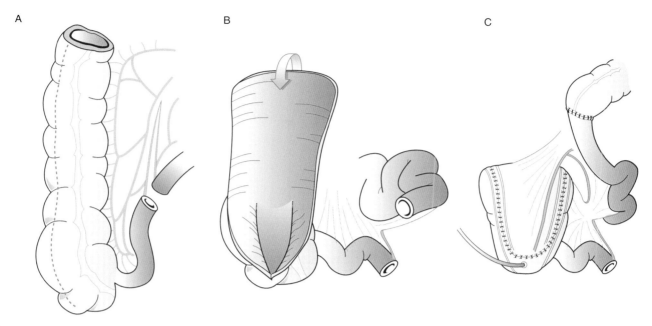

Figure 21.18
Indiana pouch diversion. (A) 8–10 cm of terminal ileum and 25–30 cm of cecum and ascending colon are used for construction of the Indiana pouch and opened along the antimesenteric border. (B) The distal end of the opened colon is folded down to the apex of the incision, and closed with a single layer of sutures (C). Adapted from Rowland RG. Present experience with the Indiana Pouch. World J Urol 1986;14:92–98.

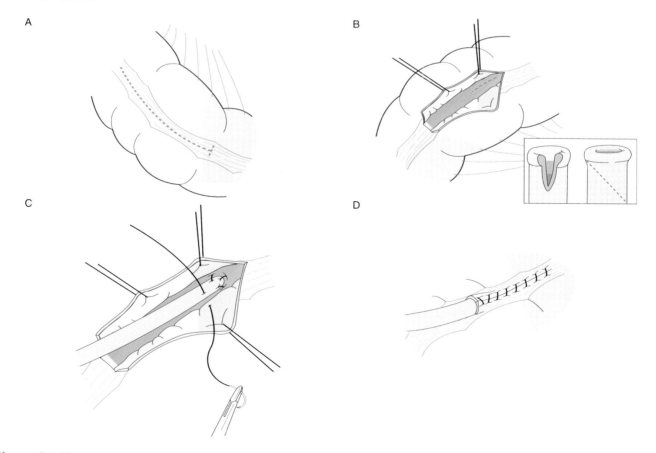

Figure 21.19
Indiana pouch diversion. (A) Ureteral implantation is performed through a T-shaped incision of the colonic tenia leaving the mucosa intact. (B) The ureteral orifice is established after mucosal incision. (C) The spatulated ureter is anastomosed to the bowel mucosa by single sutures and D the seromuscularis is closed over it. As an alternative, a direct end-to-side anastomosis can be performed. Adapted from Rowland RG. Present experience with the Indiana Pouch. World J Urol 1986;14:92–98.

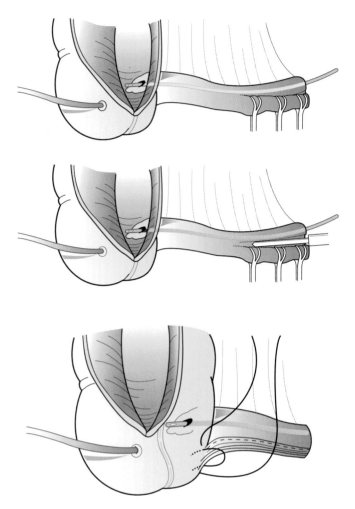

Figure 21.20
Indiana pouch diversion. The efferent segment is established by tapering the terminal ileum using metal GIA staples leaving a caliber of ileum for passage of 18 Fr. catheter. The outlet is imbricated by sutures at the junction of the ileum and cecum to create the continence mechanism. Adapted from Rowland RG. Present experience with the Indiana Pouch. World J Urol 1986;14:92–98.

of the ureters to the colon, avoiding an antirefluxing implantation.[31] The ureteral adventitia is fixed to the seromuscularis of the bowel with four quadrant sutures, and the spatulated ureter is sutured to the bowel mucosa. The terminal ileum is used as the efferent segment. The ileum is left attached to the reservoir and plicated with two parallel rows of sutures, placed longitudinally into the ileum and ileocecal valve.

Complication rates

Complication rates of ureter implantation were evaluated concerning the ureteral implantation technique (tunneled by Le Duc/Goodwin or nontunneled end-to-side anastomosis).[31,32] Ureteral obstruction was noted in 13.3% with tunneled implantation, and in 4.9% with end-to-side implantation of the ureters; however, the rate of refluxing units was higher in the latter group (7.0%

versus 3.3%). Complications of the efferent segment were stoma incontinence in 3.0% to 6.7%, and stoma stenosis in 4.0% to 10.0%.[17,30] Pouch stones were seen in 3.0% to 5.4%.[6,33]

Conclusion

Continent cutaneous diversion with a catheterizable abdominal wall stoma is a reproducible and safe alternative for patients in whom orthotopic urinary diversion is not feasible. To ensure success of continent cutaneous diversion, careful patient selection is required prior to surgery.

Several techniques using only small bowel, small and large bowel segments, or large bowel only have been developed for creation of a high-capacity and low-pressure reservoir, which contribute to an increased quality of life and body image of the patients. Numerous surgical techniques and modifications referring to reservoir construction, ureteral implantation, and creation of the outlet have been established in the past. Variations of procedures and growing experience with bowel reservoirs have led to a reduction of their specific complication rates in the long run. Most of the complications are related to the reservoir outlet and can be treated by minor surgical interventions. Postoperatively, a close follow-up including acid–base balance, serum creatinine, serum electrolytes, and ultrasound of the upper urinary tract are essential. Pouchoscopy, starting 5 years postoperatively, is recommended once a year to check for tumor development.

References

1. Kock NG, Nilson AR, Norlen L, Sundin T, Trasti H. Urinary diversion via a continent ileum reservoir: clinical experience. Scand J Urol Nephrol Suppl 1978; 49: 23.
2. Soulie M, Seguin P, Martel P, Vazzoler N, Mouly P, Plante P. A modified intussuscepted nipple in the Kock pouch urinary diversion: assessment of perioperative complications and functional results. Br J Urol 2002; 90: 397–402.
3. Jonsson O, Olofsson G, Lindholm E, Törnquist H. Long time experience with Kock ileal reservoir for continent urinary diversion. Eur Urol 2001; 40: 632–40.
4. Skinner DG, Lieskovski G, Boyd S. Continent urinary diversion. J Urol 1989; 141: 1323–7.
5. Okada Y, Shichiri Y, Terai A, et al. Management of late complications of continent urinary diversion using the Kock pouch and the Indiana pouch procedures. Int J Urol 1996; 3: 334–9.
6. Carr LK, Webster GD. Kock versus right colon continent urinary diversion: comparison of outcome and reoperation rate. Urology 1996; 48: 711–14.
7. Bander NH. Initial results with slightly modified Kock pouch. Urology 1991; 37: 100–5.
8. Stein JP, Freeman JA, Esrig D, et al. Complications of the afferent antireflux valve mechanism in the Kock ileal reservoir. J Urol 1996; 155: 1579–84.
9. Thüroff JW, Alken P, Riedmiller H, Engelmann U, Jacobi GH, Hohenfellner R. The Mainz pouch (mixed augmentation ileum and cecum) for bladder augmentation and continent diversion. J Urol 1986; 136: 17–26.
10. Goodwin WE, Winter CC, Turner RD. Replacement of ureter by small intestine: clinical application and results of the 'ileal ureter'. J Urol 1959; 81: 406–18.
11. Aboul-Enein H, Ghoneim MA. A novel uretero-ileal re-implantation technique: the serous lined extramural tunnel. A preliminary report. J Urol 1994; 151: 1193–8.

12. Hohenfellner R, Black P, Leissner J, Allhoff EP. Refluxing ureteroin-testinal anastomosis for continent cutaneous urinary diversion. J Urol 2002; 168: 1013–17.

13. Riedmiller H, Bürger R, Müller S, Thüroff JW, Hohenfellner R. Continent appendix stoma: a modification of the Mainz pouch technique. J Urol 1990; 143: 1115–16.

14. Lampel A, Hohenfellner M, Schultz-Lampel D, Thüroff JW. In situ tunneled bowel flap tubes: 2 new techniques of a continent outlet for Mainz pouch cutaneous diversion. J Urol 1995; 153: 308–15.

15. Leissner J, Black P, Fisch M, Höckel M, Hohenfellner R. Colon pouch (Mainz pouch III) for continent urinary diversion after pelvic irradiation. Urology 2000; 56: 798–802.

16. Thüroff JW, Alken P, Riedmiller H, Jacobi GH, Hohenfellner R. 100 cases of Mainz pouch: continuing experience and evolution. J Urol 1988; 140: 283–8.

17. Lampel A, Fisch M, Stein R, Schultz-Lampel D, Hohenfellner M, Thüroff JW. Continent diversion with the Mainz pouch. World J Urol 1996; 14: 85–91.

18. Gerharz EW, Köhl U, Weingärtner K, Melekos MD, Bonfig R, Riedmiller H. Complications related to different continence mechanisms in ileocecal reservoir. J Urol 1997; 158: 1709–13.

19. Fichtner J, Fisch M, Hohenfellner R. Appendiceal continence mechanisms in continent urinary diversion. World J Urol 1996; 14: 105–7.

20. Gerharz EW, Köhl UN, Melekos MD, Bonfig R, Weingärtner K, Riedmiller H. Ten years' experience with the submucosally embedded in situ appendix in continent urinary diversion. Eur Urol 2001; 40: 625–31.

21. Roth S, Weining C, Hertle L. Continent cutaneous urinary diversion using the full thickened bowel flap tube as continence mechanism: a simplified tunnel technique. J Urol 1996; 156: 1922–5.

22. Stein R, Pfitzenmaier J, Behringer M, Hohenfellner R, Thüroff JW. The long-term results (5–16 years) of Mainz pouch I technique at a single institution. J Urol 2001; 165(Suppl): 88.

23. Rowland RG, Mitchell ME, Bihrle R, Kahnoski RJ, Piser JE. Indiana continent urinary reservoir. J Urol 1987; 137: 1136–9.

24. Chanturaia Z, Pertia A, Managadze G, Khvadagiani G, Chigogidze L, Managadze L. Right colonic reservoir with submucosally embedded tapered ileum—'Tiflis pouch'. Urol Int 1997; 59: 113–18.

25. Rowland RG. Present experiences with the Indiana pouch. World J Urol 1996;14:92–98.

26. Holmes DG, Trasher JB, Park GY, Kueker DC, Weigel JW. Long term complications related to the modified Indiana pouch. Urology 2002; 60: 603–6.

27. Aria Y, Kawakita M, Terachi T, et al. Long-term followup of the Kock and Indiana pouch procedures. J Urol 1993; 150: 51–5.

28. Wilson TG, Moreno JG, Weinberg A, Ahlering TE. Late complications of the modified Indiana pouch. J Urol 1994; 151: 331–4.

29. Lockhart JL. Remodeled right colon: an alternative urinary reservoir. J Urol 1987;138:730–34.

30. Le Duc A, Camey M, Teillac P, An original antireflux ureteroileal implantation technique: long term follow-up. J Urol 1987; 137: 1156–8.

31. Helal M, Pow-Sang J, Sanford E, Figueroa E, Lockhart J. Direct (non tunneled) ureterocolonic reimplantation in association with continent reservoirs. J Urol 1993; 150: 835–7.

32. Lockhart JL, Pow-Sang JM, Persky L, Kahn P, Helal M, Sanford E. A continent colonic urinary reservoir: the Florida pouch. J Urol 1990; 144: 864–7.

33. Webster C, Bukkapatnam R, Seigne JD, et al. Continent colonic urinary reservoir (Florida pouch): long term surgical complications (greater than 11 years). J Urol 2003;169:174–6.

22

Noncontinent urinary diversion

Wiking Månsson, Fredrik Liedberg, Roland Dahlem, Margit Fisch

Introduction

Noncontinent urinary diversion remains the most commonly used method for reconstructing the lower urinary tract in conjunction with radical cystectomy. Thus, in 2002 in Sweden, 64% of all patients undergoing cystectomy within 3 months of diagnosis received a noncontinent form of reconstruction, while 13% got a continent cutaneous diversion and 21% an orthotopic bladder substitute. Data were missing for 3%.[1] This is not surprising considering the high age of the patients at cystectomy. It is our impression that older patients are, in general, little interested in continent reconstruction, although there are exceptions. Most of them want a simple system with low risk of early and late complications and a short hospital stay. We believe that 80 years of age is an arbitrary upper limit for recommending continent reconstruction. In fact, many patients above the age of 70 settle for an ileal conduit at the final counseling after having been informed about pros and cons, read some literature and, if possible, having met patients with different types of reconstruction. In addition, when a malignant disease is present, there seem to be no major differences in the quality of life when comparing patients with incontinent diversion and those with continent diversion.[2]

Other facts that contribute to a high incidence of noncontinent diversion are that a substantial number of patients turn out to have very advanced disease at laparotomy, and that a considerable number of cystectomies are performed outside major centers. Improvements in the quality of the appliances and the development of enterostomal therapy into a specific field of its own have been important for the acceptance of noncontinent diversion. Marking the site of the stoma and managing stomal complications are today carried out in close cooperation between the urologist and the stoma therapist.

Patient preparation

Together with the stoma therapist, the urologist should mark the site of the stoma prior to surgery. It should be placed in an area free of scars and skin folds, and most often it will be slightly below a line between the umbilicus and the anterior superior iliac spine. The adhesive portion of the appliance is usually a quadrant with the side 7–8 cm, which will influence position with regard to the umbilicus and the iliac spine. The patient should wear the appliance for a day or two preoperatively.

When a colonic conduit is planned, imaging with water-soluble contrast media should be performed in order to exclude polyps and diverticula. Bowel preparation is important in order to reduce infectious complications and for ease of working with the bowel intraoperatively. There are many suggestions as to how to prepare the bowel. Most common seems to be intake of polyethylene glycol or phospho-soda preparations. Alternatively, the intestine can be irrigated with 8–10 liters of Ringer's lactate solution via a gastric tube. Intraoperatively, broad-spectrum antibiotics such as cefoxitin or tetracycline together with metronidazole are usually given.

Surgical techniques

Cutaneous ureterostomy

This method of diversion is infrequently used today, and there are few reports in the literature during the past 10 years. The main indication has been palliation in advanced stages of bladder cancer. However, the current method of diversion of urine is usually through percutaneous nephrostomy tube. Cutaneous ureterostomy is associated with less risk of early complications than conduit diversion. Thus, Martinez-Pineiro et al[3] reported an incidence of 7% of such complications after cystectomy, whereas it was three times higher if a conduit was created. Stomal stenosis is a frequent problem, especially in nondilated ureters. However, high patency rates have been reported following primary plasty of the ureterocutaneous junction.[4,5] In addition, new materials allow for leaving indwelling single J-shaped stents in cases of ureterocutaneous obstruction for long periods of time with little tendency for infection and encrustation.

In certain cases cutaneous ureterostomy can be combined with a transureteroureterostomy with acceptable results. However, there is a risk with this procedure of urine pendulating from one ureter to the other—the 'yo-yo phenomenon'—due to disrupted ureteric peristalsis. In order to diminish this risk, the recipient ureter should be mobilized only to the level where the anastomosis will be performed.[6] The end of the nondilated donor ureter is cut obliquely and sutured without tension end-to-side to the recipient ureter, which is usually dilated.

Conduit diversion

Conduits can be constructed from stomach, jejunum, ileum, and colon, and there are specific indications for each conduit.

A   B

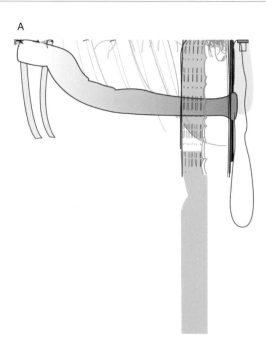

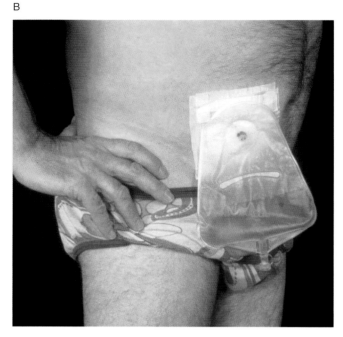

Figure 22.1
(A) Ileal conduit. (B) Patient with ileal conduit diversion.

Ileal conduit

This is the most common form of urinary diversion in conjunction with radical cystectomy. A 15–20 cm long distal ileal segment is isolated and the ureters implanted in the proximal end, most usually with a refluxing technique (Figure 22.1). There are many techniques described, the 'classical' ones being a Nesbit-like technique as used in Bricker's original publication[7] and the Wallace technique[8] (Figure 22.2). In Lund, the standard method is the open technique described by Sundin and Pettersson[9] (Figure 22.3). The stoma is usually below and to the right of the umbilicus.

Although originally described in the early 1930s, the ileal conduit did not attain clinical popularity until 20 years later, after the publications by Eugene Bricker.[7,10,11] It quickly replaced ureterosigmoidostomy as the preferred method for urinary diversion with a lower incidence of metabolic disturbances, the most common being hyperchloremic acidosis. The technique has a low degree of complexity and a vast experience of ileal conduit has been gained. However, few publications have appeared during the last decade, when instead the focus has been on continent reconstruction.

Is radical cystectomy associated with fewer complications when combined with an ileal conduit than in conjunction with continent reconstruction? Some studies have failed to find such differences when stratifying, according to the comorbidity index.[12–15] The authors are skeptical as to whether these findings have general applicability within this field: the more complicated the surgery, the higher the likelihood of complications, early as well as late. This should also be part of the preoperative information provided to the patient.

Jejunal conduit

The jejunal conduit received a bad reputation because of several reports in the 1970s on 'the jejunal conduit syndrome', characterized by hypochloremia, hyponatremia, and hyperkalemia and by acidosis, caused by the inherent absorptive characteristics of the jejunum. The clinical signs are dehydration and lethargy; treatment is by intravenous sodium chloride, which often has to be followed by oral salt supplementation for some period of time.[16,17] However, a recent report expressed satisfaction with this type of diversion and found a low incidence of electrolyte problems.[18] The authors stressed that a short conduit should be used. A possible indication is when the distal ileum cannot be used, as in radiation enteritis.

Gastric conduit

The gastric conduit can be used in exceptional cases. The good blood supply, relatively poorly absorbing mucosa, and acidification of urine have been considered advantageous.[19] In Lund, we have experience with four patients, three of whom had severely reduced renal function and required diversion. The conduit was created from the gastric antrum using the GIA instrument and we have seen no early or late complications. However, ulcer formation with perforation and subsequent death has been described.[20]

Colonic conduit diversion

In 1952, Übelhör described the use of a colonic segment for conduit urinary diversion.[21] Later reports by Mogg in 1967[22] and Morales and Golimbu in 1975[23] confirmed the usefulness of a sigmoid conduit. Today the sigmoid conduit is used mainly for intermediate diversion in children.[24,25] The transverse colonic conduit described by Hohenfellner and Wulff in 1970[26] has been increasingly used in patients with bladder cancer or gynecologic malignancies in whom radiotherapy has been given.[27,28] With its cranial position in the abdominal cavity, the transverse colon is outside the irradiation field

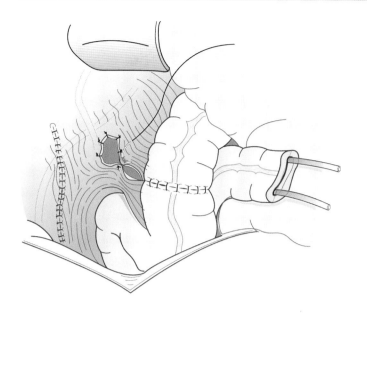

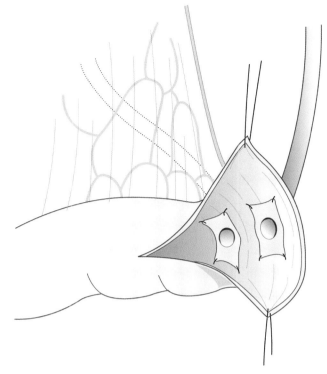

Figure 22.3
Ureteric implantation according to Sundin and Pettersson.[9]

A

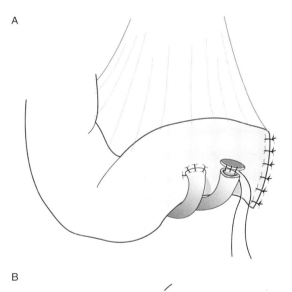

B

Figure 22.2
(A) Nesbit type of ureteric implantation as used by Bricker.
(B) Ureteric implantation, 'head-to-tail', according to Wallace.[8]

used for pelvic malignancies, and the long mesentery enables individual adaptation.

Both the sigmoid and the transverse colon offer the possibility of antirefluxing ureteral implantation, and these segments are less prone to stomal stenosis than the ileum. A direct anastomosis of the conduit to the renal pelvis represents an option in patients with total damage to the ureters by irradiation or retroperitoneal fibrosis, and in patients with recurrent superficial urothelial tumor in a single kidney.[29]

Sigmoid conduit

A 12–15 cm segment is isolated, respecting the blood supply. Bowel continuity is established using one-layer seromuscular single sutures. The ureters can be implanted directly (Nesbit technique) or via a submucous tunnel using an open end-to-side or 'buttonhole' technique. The conduit is usually placed lateral to the remaining sigmoid colon, probably with less risk of postoperative intra-abdominal complications (Figure 22.4).

Transverse conduit

A more extensive bowel mobilization including the hepatic and splenic colon flexure is required for this type of diversion. The

Figure 22.4
Sigmoid conduit.

omentum should be dissected off the transverse colon. Subsequently, the desired segment is isolated. Ureteral implantation is identical to the techniques used for a sigmoid conduit (Figure 22.5). For the direct anastomosis of the renal pelvis to the ureters, the latter are divided at the ureteropelvic junction and the renal pelvis is spatulated longitudinally. The right renal pelvis is anastomosed end-to-end to the aboral end of the conduit, whereas an end-to-side technique is used for the left renal pelvis.

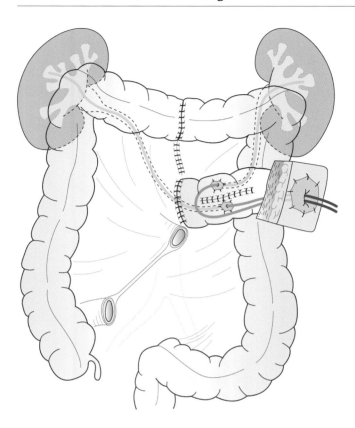

Figure 22.5
Transverse colonic conduit.

Complications

Long-term follow-up complications of ileal conduit diversion are frequent, the most common being stomal/peristomal problems, parastomal hernia, conduit stenosis, and upper tract deterioration. The incidence of these correlates with length of follow-up.[30]

Stomal and peristomal complications

These include erythematous/erosive, pseudoverrucous skin lesions, fungal infections, and stenosis, and retraction of the stoma. The skin lesions are often a consequence of inappropriate construction of the stoma, such as a flush stoma (Figure 22.6). Other causative factors may be allergic reaction to, or poor fit of, appliances and alkaline urine. These complications jeopardize adherence of the plate of the appliance to the skin and thus entail risk of urine leakage. It should be remembered that the stoma is the only part of the diversion that the patient can see and actively take care of. A spout at least 2 cm in length should be fashioned, which will decrease the risk of parastomal complications. The spout should protrude into the appliance bag. The appliance will fit much better and there will be less risk of urine leakage. Studies show that stomal and peristomal problems are common, being reported in up to 30%.[30,31] Such complications may secondarily affect the patient's lifestyle and also cause emotional and psychosocial problems, aspects of urinary diversion that have increasingly attracted interest. The quality of life issue is covered in Chapter 60.

Parastomal hernia

This occurs in 5% to 15% of patients.[30,32] Parastomal hernias are rather large, and although the majority of patients are asymptomatic, some need surgery (Figure 22.7). There is a high recurrence rate requiring reoperation if the repair is done in situ without relocating the stoma.[32] For first-time parastomal hernia repairs, stoma relocation is probably superior to fascial repair.[33] We have seen infections with erosions and fistulas using synthetic mesh, which usually is employed in recurrent hernia repair. Newer techniques with the incision placed lateral and far away from the stoma, with closure of the fascial defect and using mesh material as an onlay, have been reported to give good results.[34,35]

Conduit stenosis

Conduit stenosis seems to be unique to ileal conduits. This condition has never been described in colonic conduits. The whole, or part, of the conduit is transformed into a thick-walled tube without peristaltic activity (Figure 22.8). The pathogenesis of this disorder, which usually manifests late after diversion, is obscure. Chronic inflammation and/or vascular insufficiency have been suggested. The clinical picture is colicky flank pain and/or fever and is produced by upper urinary tract obstruction. Treatment is by removal of the conduit or partial resection, with or without ureteric reimplantation.[36]

Upper urinary tract deterioration

Numerous retrospective studies during the 1970s and 1980s revealed a high incidence (13–41%) of renal deterioration associated with a refluxing ileal conduit.[37–40] These figures are not substantially different from recent long-term follow-up reports,[30,32,41] although some study in patients with jejunal conduit gives more favorable results.[18] The generally dismal results provided the background for the recommendation of nonrefluxing ureterointestinal anastomosis and a more favorable result was reported in nonrefluxing ileal conduit diversion.[42] It is, however, difficult to evaluate these different studies in relation to each other as they are all retrospective with differences regarding age, follow-up, underlying conditions, and pre- and postoperative techniques and routines.

Another problem relates to the methods of measuring renal function after urinary diversion. Most reports have relied upon serum creatinine and intravenous urography (IVP); however, both are imprecise for this purpose. In a prospective randomized study evaluating type of conduit (ileal versus colonic) and method of ureteric implantation (refluxing versus antirefluxing), total and separate glomerular filtration rate (GFR) was assessed using ^{51}Cr-EDTA[43] and renal scarring was assessed using renal scintigraphy.[44] No statistically significant differences were found with regard to symptomatic urinary tract infection, number of ureterointestinal anastomotic strictures, and incidence of GFR deterioration. With a mean follow-up of 10 years, mean GFR fell from 88 to 71 ml/min in ileal conduit patients and from 88 to 65 ml/min in colonic conduit patients. Corresponding figures for patients with continent diversion were 100 and 85 ml/min, respectively.

Scarring was more common in refluxing units than in antirefluxing units, supporting the role of reflux from the conduit in which pressure may be intermittently high.[45]

A

B

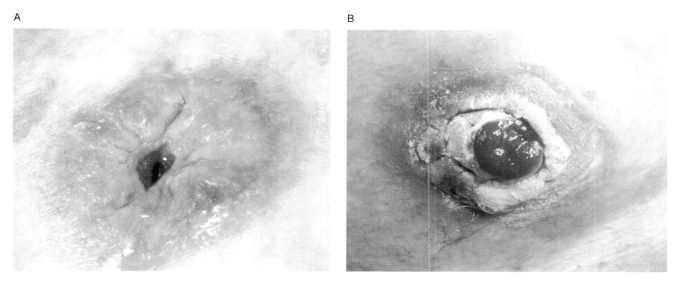

Figure 22.6
(A) Parastomal pseudoverrucous skin lesion. (B) Parastomal Candida infection.

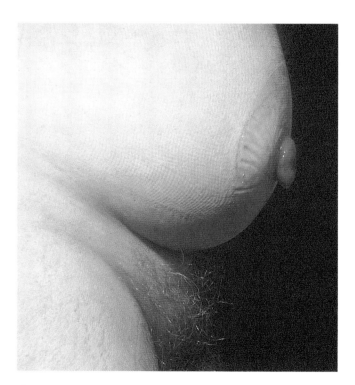

Figure 22.7
Parastomal hernia.

Follow-up of patients with conduit diversion

Due to the increasing incidence of complications seen with longer follow-up, it is essential that patients with urinary diversion are subjected to indefinite follow-up. This should include regular visits to the stomal therapist. In our opinion, follow-up should include periodic upper tract imaging studies. There are reasons to question the

A

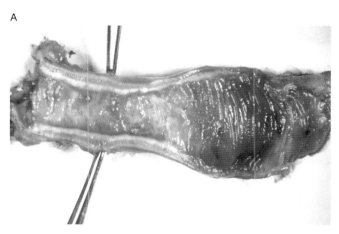

B

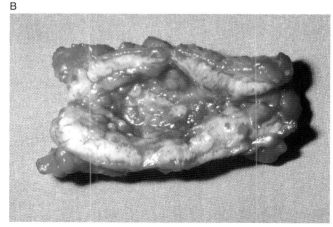

Figure 22.8
(A) Stenosis of proximal part of ileal conduit. (B) Extensive ileal conduit stenosis.

recommendations in the European Association of Urology guidelines,[46] in which follow-up is by ultrasonography and plain film. Ultrasonography can never be a substitute for IVP as obstruction can be present without gross dilation and vice versa. In addition, ultrasonography is user-dependent. In most cases serum creatinine can be used for following the patient's renal function. As tubular damage precedes glomerular damage from postrenal causes, estimation of α_1-microglobulin in urine can be a suitable marker for tubular dysfunction.[47] If in doubt about true renal function, there is no substitute for estimation of GFR. Electrolytes should be assessed, particularly when renal function is affected.

Conclusion

Even though several forms of continent urinary tract reconstruction are available today, urinary diversion via a conduit has a firm place in clinical urology. The low rate of surgical complexity, probably accompanied by less risk of complications compared to continent reconstruction, makes this type of diversion the most suitable for the majority of elderly patients undergoing radical cystectomy. Good quality appliances and access to a stoma therapist contribute to high patient acceptance.

References

1. National Bladder Cancer Registry in National Health Care Quality Registries in Sweden 2002, Information Dept. The Federation of Swedish County Councils, Stockholm, 2004, p 25.
2. Gerharz EW, Månsson Å, Hunt S, Månsson W. Is there any evidence that patients with continent reconstruction after radical cystectomy have better quality of life than conduit patients? In: Dawson C, Muir G (eds): The Evidence for Urology. London: TFM Publishing, 2005.
3. Martinez-Pineiro L, Julve E, Garcia Cardoso JV, Madrid J, de la Pena J, Martinez-Pineiro JA. Review of complications of urinary diversions performed during a 6-year period in the era of orthotopic neobladders. Arch Esp Urol 1997; 50: 433–45.
4. Yoshimura K, Maekawa S, Ichioka K, Terada N, Matsuta Y, Okubo K, Arai Y. Tubeless cutaneous ureterostomy: the Toyoda method revisited. J Urol 2001; 165: 785–88.
5. Kearney GP, Docimo SG, Doyle CJ, Mahoney EM. Cutaneous ureterostomy in adults. Urology 1992; 40: 1–6.
6. Lindstedt E, Månsson W. Transureteroureterostomy with cutaneous ureterostomy for permanent urinary diversion. Scand J Urol Nephrol 1983; 17: 205–7.
7. Bricker EM. Bladder substitution after pelvic evisceration. Surg Clin North Am 1950; 30: 1511–21.
8. Wallace DM. Uretero-ileostomy. Br J Urol 1970; 42: 529–34.
9. Sundin T, Pettersson S. Open technique for ureteric implantation in ileal conduits. Urol Int 1974; 29: 369–74.
10. Eiseman B, Bricker EM. Electrolyte absorption following bilateral ureteroenterostomy into an isolated intestinal segment. Ann Surg 1952; 136: 761–69.
11. Bricker EM, Butcher H, McAfee CA. Late results of bladder substitution with isolated ileal segments. Surg Gynec Obstet 1954; 99: 469–82.
12. Gburek BM, Lieber MM, Blute ML. Comparison of Studer ileal neobladder and ileal conduit urinary diversion with respect to perioperative outcome and late complications. J Urol 1998; 160: 721–3.
13. Parekh DJ, Gilbert WB, Koch MO, Smith JA Jr. Continent urinary reconstruction versus ileal conduit: a contemporary single-institution comparison of perioperative morbidity and mortality. Urology 2000; 55: 852–5.
14. Malavaud B, Vaessen C, Mouzin M, Rischmann P, Sarramon JP, Schulman C. Complications of radical cystectomy. Impact of the American Society of Anesthesiologists score. Eur Urol 2001; 39: 79–84.
15. Chang SS, Cookson MS, Baumgartner RG, Wells N, Smith JA. Analysis of early complications after radical cystectomy: results of a collaborative care pathway. J Urol 2002; 167: 2012–16.
16. Golimbu M, Morales P. Electrolyte disturbances in jejunal urinary diversion. Urology 1973; 1: 432–38.
17. Månsson W, Lindstedt E. Electrolyte disturbances after jejunal conduit urinary diversion. Scand J Urol Nephrol 1978; 12: 17–21.
18. Fontaine E, Barthelemy Y, Houlgatte A, Chartier E, Beurton D. Twenty-year experience with jejunal conduits. Urology 1997; 50: 207–13.
19. Leong CH. Use of stomach for bladder replacement and urinary diversion. Ann R Coll Surg Engl 1978; 60: 283–89.
20. Tainio H, Kylmala T, Tammela TL. Ulcer perforation in gastric urinary conduit: never use a gastric segment in the urinary tract if there are other options available. Urol Int 2000; 64: 101–102.
21. Übelhör R. Die Darmblase. Langenbecks Arch Klein Chir 1952; 271: 202–05.
22. Mogg RA. Urinary diversion using the colonic conduit. Br J Urol 1967; 39: 687–92.
23. Morales P, Golimbu M. Colonic urinary diversion: 10 years of experience. J Urol 1975; 113: 302–7.
24. Skinner DG, Gottesmann JE, Ritchie JP. The isolated sigmoid segment: its value in temporary urinary diversion and reconstruction. J Urol 1975; 113: 614–8.
25. Hendren WH. Exstrophy of the bladder—an alternative method of management. J Urol 1975; 115: 195–202.
26. Hohenfellner R, Wulff HD. Zur Harnableitung mittels ausgeschalteter Dickdarmsegmente. Akt Urol 1970; 1: 18–27.
27. Alken P, Jacobi GH, Thüroff J, Walz P, Hohenfellner R. Transversumconduit, Bericht über das 7. Klinische Wochenende der Urologischen Universitätskliniken Mainz, Bern, Berlin-Charlottenburg 1984, pp 157–71.
28. Altwein JE, Hohenfellner R. Use of the colon as a conduit for urinary diversion. Surg Gynecol Obstet 1975; 140: 33–38.
29. Lindell O, Lethonen T. Rezidivierende urotheliale Tumoren in Einzelnieren mit Anschluss eines Kolonsegments an das Nierenbecken. Akt Urol 1988; 19: 130–3.
30. Madersbacher S, Schmidt J, Eberele JM, Thoeny HC, Burkhard F, Hochreiter W, Studer UE. Long-term outcome of ileal conduit diversion. J Urol 2003; 169: 985–90.
31. Nordström GM, Borglund E, Nyman CR. Local status of the urinary stoma—the relation to peristomal skin complications. Scand J Urol Nephrol 1990; 24: 117–22.
32. Singh G, Wilkinson JM, Thomas DG. Supravesical diversion for incontinence: a long-term follow-up. BJU Int 1997; 79: 348–53.
33. Rubin MS, Schoetz DJ Jr, Matthews JB. Parastomal hernia. Is stoma relocation superior to fascial repair? Arch Surg 1994; 129: 413–18.
34. Amin SN, Armitage NC, Abercrombie JF, Scholefield JH. Lateral repair of parastomal hernia. Ann R Coll Surg Engl 2001; 83: 206–9.
35. Franks ME, Hrebinko RL Jr. Technique of parastomal hernia repair using synthetic mesh. Urology 2001; 57: 551–3.
36. Magnusson B, Carlen B, Bak-Jensen E, Willen R, Mansson W. Ileal conduit stenosis—an enigma. Scand J Urol Nephrol 1996; 30: 193–7.
37. Schmidt JD, Hawtrey CE, Flocks RH, Culp DA. Complications, results and problems of ileal conduit diversion. J Urol 1973; 109: 210–16.
38. Pitts WR, Muecke A. A 20-year experience with ileal conduits: the fate of the kidneys. J Urol 1979; 122: 154–7.
39. Philip NH, Williams JL, Byers CE. Ileal conduit urinary diversion: long-term follow-up in adults. Br J Urol 1980; 52: 515–19.
40. Pernet FP, Jonas U. Ileal conduit urinary diversion: early and late results in 132 cases in a 25-year period. World J Urol 1985; 3: 140–44.
41. Iborra I, Casanova JL, Solsona E, Ricos JV, Monros J, Rubio J, Dumont R. Tolerance of external urinary diversion (Bricker) followed for more than 10 years. Eur Urol 2001; 39(Suppl 5): 146.
42. Starr A, Rose DH, Cooper JF. Antireflux ureteroileal anastomoses in humans. J Urol 1975; 113: 170–4.

43. Kristjánsson A, Wallin L, Mansson W. Renal function up to 16 years after conduit (refluxing or anti-reflux anastomosis) or continent urinary diversion 1. Glomerular filtration rate and patency of ureterointestinal anastomosis. Br J Urol 1995; 76: 539–45.

44. Kristjánsson A, Bajc M, Wallin L, Willner J, Mansson W. Renal function up to 16 years after conduit (refluxing or anti-reflux anastomosis) or continent urinary diversion. Renal scarring and location of bacteriuria. Br J Urol 1995; 76: 546–50.

45. Neal DE. Urodynamic investigation of the ileal conduit: upper tract dilatation and the effects of revision of the conduit. J Urol 1989; 142: 97–100.

46. Oosterlinck W, Lobel B, Jakse G, Malmström P-U, Stöckle M, Sternberg C. Guidelines on bladder cancer of the European Association of Urology. Eur Urol 2002; 41: 105–12.

47. Kristjansson A, Grubb A, Månsson W. Renal tubular dysfunction after urinary diversion. Scand J Urol Nephrol 1995; 29: 407–12.

Section 5

Treatment of regionally advanced and metastatic bladder cancer

23

Neoadjuvant chemotherapy in the treatment of muscle-invasive bladder cancer

Cora N Sternberg

Introduction

Bladder cancer is the second most common cancer of the genitourinary tract, with some 350,000 new cases worldwide,[1] in which one third are locally invasive or metastatic. There is a very high rate of early systemic dissemination. In patients with locally advanced bladder cancer infiltrating the musculature, 5-year survival is dependent upon pathologic stage, grade, and nodal status. As the stage advances, especially when there is cancer that extends outside of the bladder wall, the prognosis worsens. Local or metastatic failure is most often due to occult metastatic disease that was present at the time of initial diagnosis.

Cystectomy series

Most physicians consider cystectomy as the gold standard of treatment for localized muscle-invasive bladder cancer. This idea has been fortressed by the widespread practice of performing orthotopic bladder substitutions. Five-year survival after cystectomy in major published series in patients with muscle-invasive bladder cancer (P2–4) from the University of Padua, Memorial Sloan-Kettering Cancer Center (MSKCC), and the University of Southern California varies from 36% to 48%.[2–5] High-risk patients with pathologic stage pT3–4 and/or pN+ M0 bladder cancer have the poorest 5-year survival which is somewhere between 25% and 35%.

Neoadjuvant chemotherapy

Advantages and disadvantages

Neoadjuvant chemotherapy when given prior to cystectomy can reduce tumor volume, and can be effective in controlling metastatic disease when the volume of micrometastatic disease is small. Systemic chemotherapy is delivered early when the burden of metastatic disease is minimal. Patients may tolerate therapy better before they have received potentially debilitating local treatment with either surgery or radiation therapy (RT). Local therapy may also affect drug delivery by altering the blood supply to the tissues affected by the tumor.

Neoadjuvant chemotherapy was designed for patients with operable clinical stage cT2–4A muscle-invasive disease, and has been increasingly used with the intent of bladder preservation.[6] Neoadjuvant chemotherapy has the potential to deliver drugs at higher doses than in the adjuvant setting, and provides the opportunity to prospectively evaluate the response to chemotherapy. Toxicity is less than that seen in patients with metastatic disease, as subjects with localized disease usually have a better performance status.

Disadvantages to neoadjuvant chemotherapy are that patients treated with neoadjuvant chemotherapy are clinically staged which may lead to some difficulties in assessing response to therapy. A discrepancy between clinical and pathologic staging can be expected in some 30% of cases.[7,8] In addition, there is a delay in cystectomy or RT during the administration of neoadjuvant chemotherapy. This may be potentially harmful for those patients that do not respond to chemotherapy.

It is unknown whether three or four cycles of therapy are needed since this question has never been systematically evaluated. The mortality due to neoadjuvant chemotherapy can be assessed in two large cooperative group randomized trials. In the US Intergroup trial coordinated by the Southwest Oncology Group (SWOG), there were no deaths due to methotrexate, vinblastine, adriamycin, and cisplatin (MVAC) chemotherapy.[9] However, in the European Organisation for Research and Treatment of Cancer/Medical Research Council (EORTC/MRC) trial of neoadjuvant cisplatin, methotrexate, and vinblastine (CMV) chemotherapy, there was a 1% mortality rate due to CMV.[10]

Randomized trials

Neoadjuvant chemotherapy should theoretically have a similar benefit for patients whether they are definitively treated by cystectomy or by RT. In the US and in most of Europe, radical cystectomy is preferred for patients 70 years old or younger with a good performance status.

Several randomized trials, most of which have included cisplatin-based regimens, have been undertaken to investigate whether or not neoadjuvant chemotherapy improves survival. Older studies evaluated single agent cisplatin, but most recent trials have employed cisplatin-containing combination chemotherapy. These trials have been of modest size and have shown inconclusive results. Randomized trials in the literature can be found in Table 23.1.

Table 23.1 Randomized phase III trials of neoadjuvant chemotherapy: study group neoadjuvant arm versus standard arm patients' survival

Trial	Neoadjuvant arm	Standard arm	No. pts	Survival benefit
Aust/UK[66]	DDP/RT	RT	255	No difference
Canada/NCI[67]	DDP/RT or preop RT + Cyst	RT or preop RT + Cyst	99	No difference
Spain (CUETO)[68]	DDP/Cyst	Cyst	121	No difference
EORTC/MRC[10]	CMV/RT or Cyst	RT or Cyst	976	5.5% difference in favor of CMV
SWOG Intergroup[11]	MVAC/Cyst	Cyst	298	Benefit with MVAC
Italy (GUONE)[12]	MVAC/Cyst	Cyst	206	No difference
Italy (GISTV)[69]	MVEC/Cyst	Cyst	171	No difference
Genoa[70]	DDP/5FU/RT/Cyst	Cyst	104	No difference
Nordic 1[14]	ADM/DDP/RT/Cyst	RT/Cyst	311	No difference, 15% benefit with ADM + DDP in T3–4a
Nordic 2[15]	MTX/DDP/Cyst	Cyst	317	No difference
Abol-Enein[71]	CarboMV/Cyst	Cyst	194	Benefit with CarboMV

5FU, 5-fluorouracil; ADM, doxorubicin; CarboMV, carboplatin, methotrexate, vinblastine; CMV, cisplatin, methotrexate, vinblastine; Cyst, cystectomy; DDP or C, cisplatin; MTX, methotrexate; MVAC, methotrexate, vinblastine, adriamycin, cisplatin; MVEC, methotrexate, vinblastine, epirubicin, cisplatin; RT, cisplatin.

Results from the Intergroup trial conducted by the SWOG have been published in the *New England Journal of Medicine*.[9] Patients with cT2–4A were randomized between three cycles of neoadjuvant MVAC chemotherapy and cystectomy or cystectomy alone. Enrolment took place over an 11-year period at 126 institutions. Patients were stratified according to age (<65 years or ≥65 years) and stage (cT2 versus cT3 or cT4A). Of the 317 patients entered, 307 were eligible; 82% in the MVAC group and 81% in the surgery group actually underwent the planned cystectomy.

Median survival was 77 months in patients that received neoadjuvant MVAC as compared to 46 months in patients that underwent cystectomy alone. The results when initially presented were not statistically significant. The results at present do not show a statistically significant improvement in overall survival (p=0.06, two-sided testing). However, the size of the study has only limited potential to discern a clinically meaningful difference and as such does not rule out the relevance of this approach. There was a trend towards improved survival in favor of MVAC-treated patients. The estimated risk of death was reduced by 25% (hazard ratio 1.33).[11]

An almost identical trial to the SWOG study was performed by an Italian cooperative group (GUONE). In this trial, 206 patients were randomized in a 6.5-year period to neoadjuvant MVAC prior to cystectomy versus cystectomy alone.[12] No clear difference in survival was demonstrated. In fact, 3-year survival was 62% for the MVAC-treated patients and 68% for the cystectomy alone arm.

The EORTC/MRC trial, performed at the same time as the SWOG trial, is the largest neoadjuvant randomized trial in the literature.[10] In this trial, 976 patients from 106 institutions were accrued over a shorter period (5.5 years) than in the SWOG trial. Patients with transitional cell bladder cancer <7 cm in size that were cT2 (G3), cT3, or cT4A, N0, NX, M0, were randomized between three cycles of neoadjuvant CMV chemotherapy and cystectomy or cystectomy alone. Definitive local therapy was left up to the choice of the investigators and included cystectomy and RT. When published in 1999, there was a nonsignificant trend towards improvement in survival in patients on the CMV arm.[10] In a 2002 ASCO update, with follow-up of 7.4 years, the data reached statistical significance (p=0.048). There was a 5.5% benefit in favor of patients treated with CMV chemotherapy.[13] Survival at 5 years was 50% compared to 44%, and at 8 years was 43% as opposed to 37% in the CMV

arm. Although Hall concluded that there was no change in absolute benefit, patients treated with CMV had a consistent survival benefit that was maintained over time.

The Nordic Group, in their first randomized neoadjuvant trial, compared neoadjuvant adriamycin, cisplatin, and preoperative RT prior to cystectomy versus preoperative RT and cystectomy. In a subset analysis of patients with T3–4 disease, a 15% survival difference in favor of patients treated with chemoradiotherapy was seen.[14] These investigators were unable to confirm this survival advantage in a subsequent trial in which 317 patients were randomized between cystectomy or cystectomy preceded by methotrexate and cisplatin (without RT).[15] Nonetheless, when the two trials were combined in a subsequent analysis of 620 patients, the combined results were in favor of neoadjuvant chemotherapy.[16,17] The combined study results showed a hazard ratio (HR) of 0.80 (95% CI: 0.64–0.99) for overall survival in favor of neoadjuvant treatment. Survival was 56% at 5 years in the experimental group versus 48% in the control group, corresponding to an 8% absolute risk reduction after neoadjuvant chemotherapy. This was associated with a 20% reduction in the estimated risk of death.

What is the true value of neoadjuvant chemotherapy?[18] Although more than 3000 patients had been evaluated in neoadjuvant chemotherapy randomized trials, the real effect of neoadjuvant chemotherapy on survival was not clear. For this reason, two recent meta-analyses have combined the results of relevant randomized trials to obtain sufficient statistical power to reliably assess the value of neoadjuvant chemotherapy in invasive bladder cancer.[19,20]

The first meta-analysis was published by the MRC in *The Lancet*. Analysis of 10 neoadjuvant chemotherapy trials was performed, using individual patient data, which has many advantages in such an analysis.[21] Unfortunately, original data from the SWOG trial were not made available to the MRC.

Overall survival for the whole group and for a subgroup of patients treated with single agent cisplatin was not affected by neoadjuvant chemotherapy. In a subset of patients treated with cisplatin-containing combination chemotherapy, a 5% (p=0.17, 95% CI: 1–7%) difference in favor of neoadjuvant chemotherapy was demonstrated. This reflected a change in survival from 45% to 50%, also consistent with a 1% to 7% difference in survival. The majority of patients were from the EORTC/MRC trial, and thus the results are similar to the results in that trial.

The second meta-analysis was performed in Canada.[22] This analysis did not include individual patient data, but rather obtained data from a thorough literature search and use of published meta-analyses. Sixteen eligible randomized clinical trials were identified. Trials that employed concomitant chemotherapy and radiotherapy were excluded. Of a potential 3315 patients, 2605 patients provided suitable data for the meta-analysis of overall survival. Eight trials used cisplatin-based combination chemotherapy and the pooled HR was 0.87 (95% CI: 0.78–0.96, p=0.006), consistent with an absolute overall survival benefit of 6.5% (95% CI: 2–11%) from 50% to 56.5%. Mortality due to combination chemotherapy was 1.1%.

A third meta-analysis included individual patient data from the SWOG trial. Based on 11 trials and 3005 patients a survival benefit was found with platinum-based neo-adjuvant combination chemotherapy (HR=0.86, 95% CI 0.77–0.95, p=0.003); equivalent to a 5% absolute improvement in survival at 5 years. In addition, this was associated with a 9% absolute improvement in disease-free survival with combination chemotherapy (HR=0.78 95% CI 0.71–0.86, p <0.0001) at 5 years.[23]

It appears from these large meta-analyses of randomized trials that neoadjuvant cisplatin-based chemotherapy has some effect on improving overall survival in muscle-invasive bladder cancer, although the size of the effect is modest.

Combination chemotherapy can be administered safely without an adverse effect on the subsequent local therapy. These data are supported by the University of Texas M.D. Anderson Hospital trial of neoadjuvant and adjuvant MVAC chemotherapy,[24] the SWOG trial of neoadjuvant MVAC chemotherapy,[9] the EORTC/MRC trial of CMV neoadjuvant chemotherapy,[10] and our own data with neoadjuvant MVAC chemotherapy in Rome, Italy.[7]

Surgical factors were evaluated in 268 patients with muscle-invasive bladder cancer who underwent radical cystectomy in the SWOG Intergroup trial.[25] Cystectomies were performed by 106 surgeons in 109 institutions. Half of the patients received neoadjuvant MVAC. Five-year postcystectomy and local recurrence rates in all patients receiving cystectomy were 54% and 15%, respectively. Surgical variables associated with longer postcystectomy survival were negative margins (versus positive; HR, 0.37; p=0.0007), and ≥10 nodes removed (versus <10; HR, 0.51; p=0.0001). These associations did not differ by treatment arms (p>0.21 for all tests of interactions between treatment and surgical variables). Predictors of local recurrence were positive margins (versus negative; odds ratio [OR], 11.2; p=0.0001) and <10 nodes removed (versus ≥10; OR, 5.1; p=0.002). The quality of surgery was an independent prognostic factor for outcome after adjustment for pathologic factors and neoadjuvant chemotherapy.

Available data suggest that for 'average risk' cT2 patients, there is at best a modest benefit of adding chemotherapy to definitive local therapy (cystectomy or RT). Likewise, available studies suggest a much more substantial benefit for patients with high-risk disease, such as cT3b cancers.

Newer agents are being introduced into the neoadjuvant setting. The SWOG is evaluating neoadjuvant gemcitabine, paclitaxel, and carboplatin followed by observation or immediate cystectomy. Molecular markers, recurrence rates, and cystectomy-free survival are evaluated. At this time, however, an optimal chemotherapy regimen has not been identified, and newer regimens have not been tested in the context of randomized controlled trials in the neoadjuvant setting. Efforts to identify the patients most likely to benefit from neoadjuvant therapy are necessary. Furthermore, in cases where there are small differences in survival it is unfortunate that there are few data available on quality of life.

Bladder preservation

Although mortality rates with radical cystectomy have decreased by half since the 1990s, survival rates with surgery alone have remained steady, with 5-year survival rates of 66% for pathologic stage T2, 35% for T3, and 27% for T4 disease.[2,3,9,26–37] In addition, up to 15% of patients with muscle-invasive disease will have no pathologic residual disease at the time of cystectomy, indicating the potential curability of select patients with transurethral resection of bladder tumor (TURBT) alone. The risk of clinical understaging in 30% to 50% of patients,[38–40] the limited effectiveness of surgery alone, and the advent of more effective combination chemotherapy has led to a multidisciplinary approach to bladder preservation.

Since the advent of orthotopic bladder substitutions, many urologists prefer early cystectomy with the creation of a continent urinary neobladder. Surgery alone will be successful in only a limited percentage of patients, and bladder preservation can be a viable option to radical cystectomy in selected patients. Bladder preservation influences quality of life as it means less surgery, no need for a urinary diversion, and normal sexual function. From phase II trials, bladder preservation may be possible in selected patients that respond to neoadjuvant chemotherapy.[7,41,42] The question is, can we preserve the bladder and achieve the same survival as with radical cystectomy?

TURBT plays an important role in multimodality bladder preservation strategies, and it is difficult to interpret the contribution to survival of each component in a multimodality bladder-sparing approach. As restaging TURBT has not been performed as standard practice in all combined modality series, it is hard to know the impact that TURBT alone may have had on survival in most series. One would expect patients that have been rendered clinical p0 by either TURBT alone or TURBT plus chemotherapy prior to radiation or cystectomy to have better long-term survival,[43] and this has been demonstrated in several prospective series.[41,44–48] Clinical factors in these studies associated with a better chance of a complete clinical response to TURBT alone or TURBT plus chemotherapy, and thus better survival, are clinical stage (organ-confined), tumor size less than 3–5 cm, no hydronephrosis, no palpable mass, and unifocal disease,[21,22,25–29,31–38,49] although this has not been prospectively verified in a randomized trial.

Response to chemotherapy is another important prognostic factor.[6,7,9,13] However, this too may reflect patient selection, as it is possible that patients that do well have characteristics that would make them survive longer whether or not they were treated with chemotherapy. In the SWOG trial, the pT0 rate in MVAC patients was 38% as compared to 15% for patients that underwent cystectomy alone (p<0.001). The pT0 rate after CMV in the EORTC/MRC trial was similarly 33%. Likewise, after two cycles of neoadjuvant MVAC chemotherapy, the pT0 rate was 40% in the M.D. Anderson trial of neoadjuvant and adjuvant versus adjuvant MVAC.[24] The Canadian meta-analysis found that a major pathologic response was associated with improved overall survival in four trials.[20] Improved survival has clearly been shown in patients that become pT0 at cystectomy. These may be the same patients that would benefit from a bladder-preservation strategy.

In Rome, 104 patients with clinical T2–4 N0 M0 of the bladder were treated with three cycles of neoadjuvant MVAC[7] followed by clinical restaging (computed tomography scan, TURBT, and biopsies). At the TURBT following MVAC, 49 (49%) patients were T0. Responding patients were placed in a bladder preservation protocol and underwent TURBT alone or partial cystectomy following chemotherapy. Of the 52 patients that underwent TURBT alone, 13 had a partial cystectomy, and 39 had a radical cystectomy.

The median survival for the entire group was 7.49 years (95% CI: 4.86–10.0 years). Of the patients that had MVAC and TURBT alone, 60% were alive at a median follow-up of 56+ months (10–160+). Forty-four percent of the patients in this TURBT group maintained an intact bladder. Of the responding patients with monofocal lesions that underwent partial cystectomy, only one required salvage cystectomy, and 5-year survival was 69%.

Of note, in 77 patients that had downstaging to T0 or superficial disease, 5-year survival was 69%. This is in contrast to 5-year survival of only 26% in 27 patients that failed to respond and had muscle-invasive disease (T2 or greater) after chemotherapy. Additionally, the median survival for 27 elderly patients >70 years (median 73 years, range 70–82 years) was surprisingly long at 90 months (7.5 years). For elderly patients that underwent TURBT and partial cystectomy, 5-year survival was 67% with a median survival of 9 years; 47% preserved their bladders.

At MSKCC, 111 patients with T2–4 N0 M0 bladder cancer were treated with neoadjuvant MVAC. Downstaging was associated with improved survival. The 5-year survival rate was 54% for patients with downstaging versus 12% for those without downstaging.[50] Twenty-six patients underwent a partial cystectomy after neoadjuvant chemotherapy.[51] Of these 26 patients, 17 (65%) were alive beyond 5 years (median 6.9 years, range 4–8 years), including 14 (54%) with an intact, functioning bladder. Twelve patients (46%) developed bladder recurrences, which were invasive in five (19%) and superficial in seven (26%). Those patients without (p0) or noninvasive (pTis) tumor in their surgical specimens had a 5-year survival rate of 87%, compared with 30% in patients with residual invasive cancer.

Neoadjuvant MVAC chemotherapy permits bladder-sparing surgery in selected responding patients with invasive bladder cancer. The bladder remains at risk for new tumor development, but local recurrences can be treated successfully by local therapy or salvage cystectomy. Patients that undergo neoadjuvant chemotherapy and bladder preservation should be highly informed and willing to undergo frequent follow-up, multiple cystoscopies, and understand the possibility that cystectomy may become necessary.

Radiation therapy

Combining systemic chemotherapy with radiation therapy (RT) may preserve the bladder while sensitizing the tumor to radiation, while at the same time treating occult metastases. Trials of combined neoadjuvant chemotherapy and RT are shown in Table 23.2.

This approach has been used in the Radiation Therapy Oncology Group (RTOG) at the Massachusetts General Hospital,[42] and by investigators in Erlangen and Paris.[52,53]

Most patients undergo TURBT, followed by chemoradiation. They then have a restaging TURBT, and consolidative RT is given to responding patients and nonresponders under cystectomy. Five-year survivals between 42% and 63%, with organ preservation in approximately 40% of patients, have been reported. Selection criteria for chemoradiation are similar to those which predict a good prognosis after cystectomy. Patients with small T2–3 lesions without hydronephrosis who undergo a thorough TURBT tend to have the best results. Although survival is similar to that in contemporary cystectomy series, the combined morbidity of chemotherapy and RT can be significant. As in the case of neoadjuvant chemotherapy alone, patients should be highly motivated to preserve their bladders and understand the possible side effects of combined therapy.

Biologic and molecular approaches to muscle-invasive bladder cancer

Tumor formation and tumor progression are thought to result from an accumulation of several genetic alterations including the activation of oncogenes, loss of distinct chromosomal regions, and inactivation of tumor suppressor genes. Molecular markers are increasingly being used to predict survival and response to chemotherapy, with p53, pRb, and p21 being among the first evaluated as predictive markers in bladder cancer. In a landmark study, investigators at the University of Southern California found that patients with altered p53 had a markedly higher chance of recurrence than patients that had normal p53.[54] Furthermore, patients with tumors expressing alterations in both p53 and pRb had significantly increased rates of recurrence and decreased survival compared to patients without alterations in pRb and p53.[55,56] Although these results have been questioned,[57,58] evaluation of these markers is important as molecular markers may be able to determine the outcome of patients with locally advanced bladder cancer.

At MSKCC, p53 status was evaluated in 60 (54%) patients that had a complete clinical response (T0) to MVAC chemotherapy. Ten-year outcome was recorded and patients were stratified by p53 status, stage of the primary tumor (T2 versus T3), and type of

Table 23.2 Trials of combined chemotherapy and radiotherapy

Series	Year	No. pts	Chemotherapy	5-year survival (%)	5-year survival with intact bladder (%)
Radiation Therapy Oncology Group study 85-121[72]	1993	42	DDP	52	42
Radiation Therapy Oncology Group study 88-02[73]	1996	91	MCV + RT and DDP	62*	44
Radiation Therapy Oncology Group study 89-03[74]	1998	123	MCV + RT and DDP	48	36
University of Erlangen[52,75]	2001	199	DDP, or Carbo	52	41
University of Paris[53,76]	2001	120	DDP/5FU	63	
Massachusetts General[77]	2002	190	MCV or DDP/5FU	54	46

*Four-year survival data.
5FU, 5-fluorouracil; Carbo, carboplatin; DDP, cisplatin; MCV, methotrexate, cisplatin, vinblastine; RT, radiation therapy.

surgery (bladder sparing versus cystectomy).[59] These authors showed that in patients with stage T2 tumors that lacked detectable p53 and obtained a response to neoadjuvant chemotherapy, the bladder could be preserved for up to 10 years.

In a Spanish study, 82 patients with invasive bladder cancer treated on three different bladder-sparing studies were evaluated by immunohistochemistry (IHC) for p53, p21, and pRB expression.[60] Immunoreactivity for p53, p21, and pRB was observed in 47%, 52%, and 67% of patients, respectively. When combined expression of p53 and p21 was assessed, positive expression of both markers was a strong and unfavorable prognostic factor for survival for bladder preservation (p=0.006), disease-free survival (p=0.003), and overall survival (p=0.02). The authors concluded that, when simultaneously assessed, expression levels of p53 and p21 exhibited independent predictive value for long-term bladder preservation and survival in their patients treated with combined-modality therapy, and may be useful in selecting candidates for bladder-preserving treatments.

Two other recent studies have elucidated the role of these molecular markers in bladder cancer. At Baylor College of Medicine, IHC staining for p53, p21, pRB, and p16 was done on archival specimens from 80 patients that underwent bilateral pelvic lymphadenectomy and radical cystectomy for bladder cancer. The median follow-up was 101 months.[61] Alteration of each of the markers was independently associated with disease progression and disease-specific survival. When combined with pathologic prognostic factors such as lymph node positivity, the number of altered markers was associated with an increased risk of bladder cancer progression and mortality. P53 was the strongest molecular marker in this study, followed by p21, suggesting a more important role of the p53/p21 pathway in bladder cancer progression.

Another study from the University of Southern California sought to determine the predictive value of altered expression patterns of p53, p21, and pRb on progression of bladder cancer. P53, p21, and pRb expression was examined on archival radical cystectomy samples from 164 patients with invasive or high-grade recurrent superficial transitional cell carcinoma. The median follow-up was 8.6 years. Examined in combination after stratifying by stage, the authors concluded that the number of altered proteins significantly correlated with both time to progression and overall survival. This study again confirms that patients with bladder tumors with alterations in p53, p21, and pRb protein products are at high risk of recurrence and death.[62]

Other important markers such as BCL2, a protein fundamental in preventing apoptosis, are increasingly making their way into the clinic. In a small study from the UK, overexpression of BCL2 in patients receiving synchronous chemoradiotherapy was an independent indicator of poor survival in muscle-invasive bladder cancer.[63]

Most recently, microarray technology has permitted the study of expression of thousands of genes in tumor tissue. The new paradigm of treatment tailored to the individual patient could be realized in the very near future in bladder cancer patients where there are many opportunities to readily obtain tumor samples for microarray studies. Molecular profiling of samples should enable us to study the microevolution of tumors, to tailor existing treatment options, and to introduce new biologicals into the clinic.[64]

Conclusion

For muscle-invasive bladder cancer, neoadjuvant chemotherapy followed by radical cystectomy has become one of the new standards of care. Molecular prognostication is now being incorporated into the design of clinical trials. The p53 phenotype seems to be one of the most important molecular predictive factors for bladder cancer outcome and death in patients that undergo radical cystectomy. Determinations of molecular pathways are likely to become useful in the selection of candidates for bladder-preserving treatments. Clinical protocols based on the integration of conventional clinical and anatomic information with molecular approaches should be supported.[65]

References

1. Parkin DM, Pisani P, Ferlay J. Global cancer statistics. CA Cancer J Clin 1999; 49(81): 33–64.
2. Stein JP, Lieskovsky G, Cote R, et al. Radical cystectomy in the treatment of invasive bladder cancer: long-term results in 1,054 patients. J Clin Oncol 2001; 19(3): 666–75.
3. Dalbagni G, Genega E, Hashibe M, et al. Cystectomy for bladder cancer: a contemporary series. J Urol 2001; 165(4): 1111–16.
4. Bassi P, Ferrante GD, Piazza N, et al. Prognostic factors of outcome after radical cystectomy for bladder cancer: a retrospective study of a homogeneous patient cohort. J Urol 1999; 161(5): 1494–7.
5. Ghoneim MA, el-Mekresh MM, el-Baz MA, el-Attar IA, Ashamallah A. Radical cystectomy for carcinoma of the bladder: critical evaluation of the results in 1,026 cases. J Urol 1997; 158(2): 393–9.
6. Sternberg CN. Current perspectives in muscle-invasive bladder cancer. Eur J Cancer 2002; 38(4): 460–7.
7. Sternberg CN, Pansadoro V, Calabrò F, et al. Can patient selection for bladder preservation be based on response to chemotherapy? Cancer 2003; 97(7): 1644–52.
8. Herr HW, Scher HI. Surgery of invasive bladder cancer: is pathologic staging necessary? Semin Oncol 1990; 17: 590–7.
9. Grossman HB, Natale RB, Tangen CM, et al. Neoadjuvant chemotherapy plus cystectomy compared with cystectomy alone for locally advanced bladder cancer. N Engl J Med 2003; 349(9): 859–66.
10. International Collaboration of Trialists. Neoadjuvant cisplatin, methotrexate, and vinblastine chemotherapy for muscle-invasive bladder cancer: a randomised controlled trial. Lancet 1999; 354(9178): 533–40.
11. Grossman HB, Natale RB, Tangen CM, et al. Errata Corrige for: 'Neoadjuvant chemotherapy plus cystectomy compared with cystectomy alone for locally advanced bladder cancer' published in N Engl J Med 2003; 349(9): 859–866. N Engl J Med 2003; 349(9): 1880.
12. Bassi P, Pagano F, Pappagallo G, et al. Neoadjuvant M-VAC of invasive bladder cancer: The G.U.O.N.E. multicenter phase III trial. Eur Urol 1998; 33(Suppl 1): 142.
13. Hall RR. Updated results of a randomised controlled trial of neoadjuvant cisplatin (C), methotrexate (M) and vinblastine (V) chemotherapy for muscle-invasive bladder cancer. International Collaboration of Trialists of the MRC Advanced Bladder Cancer Group. Proc Annu Meet Am Soc Clin Oncol 2002; 21(1): 178a.
14. Malmstrom PU, Rintala E, Wahlqvist R, Hellstrom P, Hellsten S, Hannisdal E. Five year follow-up of a prospective trial of radical cystectomy and neoadjuvant chemotherapy. J Urol 1996; 155: 1903–6.
15. Sherif A, Rintala E, Mestad O, et al. Neoadjuvant cisplatin–methotrexate chemotherapy of invasive bladder cancer—Nordic cystectomy trial 2. Scand J Urol Nephrol 2002; 36(6): 419–25.
16. Sherif A, Rintala E, Mestad O, Nilsson J, Holmberg L, Nilsson S, Malmstrom PU. Neoadjuvant platinum based combination chemotherapy improves overall survival in patients with locally advanced bladder cancer. A meta-analysis of two Nordic collaborative studies of 620 patients. J Urol 2003; 169: 307.
17. Sherif A, Holmberg L, Rintala E, et al. Neoadjuvant cisplatinum based combination chemotherapy in patients with invasive bladder cancer: a

combined analysis of two Nordic studies. Nordic Urothelial Cancer Group. Eur Urol 2004; 45(3): 297–303.

18. Sternberg CN, Parmar MKB. Neoadjuvant chemotherapy is not (yet) standard treatment for muscle-invasive bladder cancer. J Clin Oncol 2001; 19(Suppl 1): 21S–6S.

19. Advanced Bladder Cancer Meta-analysis Collaboration. Neoadjuvant chemotherapy in invasive bladder cancer: a systematic review and meta-analysis. Lancet 2003; 361: 1927–34.

20. Winquist E, Kirchner TS, Segal R, Chin J, Lukka H. Genitourinary Cancer Disease Site Group of Cancer Care Ontario Program in Evidence-based Care Practice Guidelines Initiative. Neoadjuvant chemotherapy for transitional cell carcinoma of the bladder: a systematic review and meta-analysis. J Urol 2004; 171(2): 561–9.

21. Stewart LA, Clarke M. Practical methodology of meta-analyses (overviews) using updated individual patient data. Cochrane Working Group. Stat Med 2004; 124(19): 2057–79.

22. Winquist E, Kirchner TS, Segal R, Chin J, Lukka H. Neoadjuvant chemotherapy for transitional cell carcinoma of the bladder: a systematic review and meta-analysis. Genitourinary Cancer Disease Site Group, Cancer Care Ontario Program in Evidence-based Care Practice Guidelines Initiative. J Urol 2004; 171(2 Pt 1): 561–9.

23. Advanced Bladder Cancer (ABC) Meta-analysis Collaboration. Neoadjuvant Chemotherapy in Invasive Bladder Cancer: Update of a Systematic Review and Meta-Analysis of Individual Patient Data. European Urology; 2005; 48: 202–6.

24. Millikan R, Dinney C, Swanson D, et al. Integrated therapy for locally advanced bladder cancer: final report of a randomized trial of cystectomy plus adjuvant M-VAC versus cystectomy with both preoperative and postoperative M-VAC. J Clin Oncol 2001; 19: 4005–13.

25. Herr HW, Faulkner JR, Grossman HB, et al. Surgical factors influence bladder cancer outcomes: a cooperative group report. J Clin Oncol 2004; 22(14): 2781–9.

26. Ritchie JP, Skinner DG, Kaufman JJ. Radical cystectomy for carcinoma of the bladder: 16 years of experience. J Urol 1975; 113: 186–9.

27. Bredael JJ, Croker BP, Glenn JF. The curability of invasive bladder cancer treated by radical cystectomy. Eur Urol 1980; 6: 206–8.

28. Mathur VK, Krahn HP, Ramsey EW. Total cystectomy for bladder cancer. J Urol 1981; 125: 784–6.

29. Skinner DG, Lieskovsky G. Contemporary cystectomy with pelvic node dissection compared to preoperative radiation therapy plus cystectomy in the management of invasive bladder cancer. J Urol 1984; 131: 1069–72.

30. Montie JE, Straffon RA, Stewart BH. Radical cystectomy without radiation therapy for carcinoma of the bladder. J Urol 1984; 131: 477–82.

31. Giuliani L, Gilberti C, Martorrama G. Results of radical cystectomy for primary bladder cancer. Urology 1985; 26(3): 243–5.

32. Roehrborn CG, Sagalowsky AI, Peters PC. Long-term patient survival after cystectomy for regional metastatic transitional cell carcinoma of the bladder. J Urol 1991; 146: 36–9.

33. Pagano F, Bassi P, Galetti TP, et al. Results of contemporary radical cystectomy for invasive bladder cancer: a clinicopathological study with an emphasis on the inadequacy of the tumor, nodes and metastases classification. J Urol 1991; 145: 45–50.

34. Wishnow KI, Tenney DM. Will Rogers and the results of radical cystectomy for invasive bladder cancer. Urol Clin North Am 1991; 18: 529–37.

35. Waehre H, Ous S, Klevmark B, et al. A bladder cancer multi-institutional experience with total cystectomy for muscle-invasive bladder cancer. Cancer 1993; 72(10): 3044–51.

36. Vieweg J, Gschwend JE, Herr HW, et al. The impact of primary stage on survival in patients with lymph node positive bladder cancer. J Urol 1999; 161(1): 72–6.

37. Mardersbacher S, Hochreiter W, Burkhard F, et al. Radical cystectomy for bladder cancer today—a homogenous series without neoadjuvant therapy. J Clin Oncol 2003; 21(4): 690–6.

38. Frazier HA, Robertson JE, Dodge RK, Paulson DF. The value of pathologic factors in predicting cancer-specific survival among patients treated with radical cystectomy for transitional cell carcinoma of the bladder and prostate. Cancer 1993; 71: 3993–4001.

39. Amling CL, Thrasher JB, Frazier HA, Dodge RK, Robertson JE, Paulson DF. Radical cystectomy for stages Ta, Tis and T1 transitional cell carcinoma of the bladder. J Urol 1994; 151(1): 31–5.

40. Stein JP. Indications for early cystectomy. Semin Urol Oncol 2000; 18: 289–95.

41. Herr HW, Bajorin DF, Scher HI. Neoadjuvant chemotherapy and bladder sparing surgery for invasive bladder cancer: ten-year outcome. J Clin Oncol 1998; 16(4): 1298–301.

42. Shipley WU, Kaufman DS, Tester WJ, et al. Overview of bladder cancer trials in the Radiation Therapy Oncology Group. Cancer 2003; 97(8 Suppl): 2115–9.

43. Herr HW. Uncertainty and outcome of invasive bladder tumors. Urol Oncol 1996; 2: 92–5.

44. Hall RR, Newling DW, Ramsden PD, Richards B, Robinson MR, Smith PH. Treatment of invasive bladder cancer by local resection and high dose methotrexate. B J Urol 1984; 56: 668–72.

45. Thomas DJ, Roberts JT, Hall RR, Reading J. Radical transurethral resection and chemotherapy in the treatment of muscle-invasive bladder cancer: a long-term follow-up. Br J Urol 1999; 83: 432–7.

46. Angulo JC, Sanchez-Chapado M, Lopez JI, Flores N. Primary cisplatin, methotrexate and vinblastine aiming at bladder preservation in invasive bladder cancer: multivariate analysis on prognostic factors. J Urol 1996; 155(6): 1897–902.

47. Sternberg CN, Pansadoro V, Calabrò F, et al. Neoadjuvant chemotherapy and bladder preservation in locally advanced transitional cell carcinoma of the bladder. Ann Oncol 1999; 10(11): 1301–5.

48. De la Rosa F, Garcia-Carbonero R, Passas J, Rosino A, Lianes P, Paz-Ares L. Primary cisplatin, methotrexate and vinblastine chemotherapy with selective bladder preservation for muscle-invasive carcinoma of the bladder: long-term followup of a prospective study. J Urol 2002; 167: 2413–8.

49. Montie JE, Straffon RA, Stewart BH. Radical cystectomy without radiation therapy for carcinoma of the bladder. J Urol 1984; 131: 477–82.

50. Schultz PK, Herr HW, Zhang Z. Neoadjuvant chemotherapy for invasive bladder cancer: prognostic factors for survival of patients with M-VAC with 5 years follow-up. J Clin Oncol 1994; 12(7): 1394–401.

51. Herr HW, Scher HI. Neoadjuvant chemotherapy and partial cystectomy for invasive bladder cancer. J Clin Oncol 1994; 12(5): 975–80.

52. Sauer R, Birkenhake S, Kühn R, et al. Muscle-invasive bladder cancer: transurethral resection and radiochemotherapy as an organ-sparing treatment option. In Petrovich Z, Baert L, Brady LW (eds): Carcinoma of the Bladder. New York: Springer, 1998, pp 205–214.

53. Housset M, Dufour B, Maulard-Durdux C, Chretien Y, Mejean A. Concomitant fluorouracil (5-FU)-cisplatin (CDDP) and bifractionated split course radiation therapy (BSCRT) for invasive bladder cancer. Proc Am Soc Clin Oncol 1997; 16: 319A.

54. Esrig D, Elmajian D, Groshen S, et al. Accumulation of nuclear p53 and tumor progression in bladder. N Engl J Med 1994; 331(19): 1259–64.

55. Cote RJ, Esrig D, Groshen S, Jones PA, Skinner DG. p53 and treatment of bladder cancer. Nature 1997; 385(6612): 123–5.

56. Cote RJ, Dunn MD, Chatterjee SJ, et al. Elevated and absent pRb expression is associated with bladder cancer progression and has cooperative effects with p53. Cancer Res 1998; 58(6): 1090–4.

57. Williams SG, Gandour-Edwards R, Deitch AD, et al. Differences in gene expression in muscle-invasive bladder cancer: a comparison of Italian and American patients. Eur Urol 2001; 39(4): 430–7.

58. McShane LM, Aamodt R, Cordon-Cardo C, et al. Reproducibility of p53 immunohistochemistry in bladder tumors. National Cancer Institute, Bladder Tumor Marker Network. Clin Cancer Res 2000; 6(5): 1854–64.

59. Herr HW, Bajorin DF, Scher HI, Cordon-Cardo C, Reuter VE. Can p53 help select patients with invasive bladder cancer for bladder preservation? J Urol 1999; 161(1): 20–2.

60. Garcia del Muro X, Condom E, Vigues F, et al. p53 and p21 Expression levels predict organ preservation and survival in invasive bladder

carcinoma treated with a combined-modality approach. Cancer 2004; 100(9): 1859–67.

61. Shariat SF, Tokunaga H, Zhou J, et al. p53, p21, pRB, and p16 expression predict clinical outcome in cystectomy with bladder cancer. J Clin Oncol 2004; 22(6): 1014–24.

62. Chatterjee SJ, Datar R, Youssefzadeh D, et al. Combined effects of p53, p21, and pRb expression in the progression of bladder transitional cell carcinoma. J Clin Oncol 2004; 22(6): 1007–13.

63. Hussain SA, Ganesan R, Hiller L, et al. BCL2 expression predicts survival in patients receiving synchronous chemoradiotherapy in advanced transitional cell carcinoma of the bladder. Oncol Rep 2003; 10(3): 571–6.

64. Nawrocki S, Skacel T, Brodowicz T. From microarrays to new therapeutic approaches in bladder cancer. Pharmacogenomics 2003; 4(2): 179–89.

65. Cordon-Cardo C. p53 and RB: simple interesting correlates or tumor markers of critical predictive nature? J Clin Oncol 2004; 22(6): 975–7.

66. Wallace DM, Raghavan D, Kelly KA, et al. Neoadjuvant (pre-emptive) cisplatin therapy in invasive transitional cell carcinoma of the bladder. Br J Urol 1991; 67: 608–15.

67. Coppin CM, Gospodarowicz MK, James K, et al. Improved local control of invasive bladder cancer by concurrent cisplatin and preoperative or definitive radiation. The National Cancer Institute of Canada Clinical Trials Group. J Clin Oncol 1996; 14(11): 2901–7.

68. Martinez Pineiro JA, Gonzalez Martin M, Arocena F. Neoadjuvant cisplatin chemotherapy before radical cystectomy in invasive transitional cell carcinoma of the bladder: prospective randomized phase III study. J Urol 1995; 153: 964–73.

69. GISTV (Italian Bladder Cancer Study Group). Neoadjuvant treatment for locally advanced bladder cancer: a randomized prospective clinical trial. J Chemother 1996; 8: 345–6.

70. Orsatti M, Curotto A, Canobbio L. Alternating chemo-radiotherapy in bladder cancer: a conservative approach. Int J Radiat Oncol Biol Phys 1995; 33: 173–8.

71. Abol-Enein H, El-Makresh M, El-Baz M, Ghoneim M. Neoadjuvant chemotherapy in treatment of invasive transitional bladder cancer: a controlled, prospective randomised study. Br J Urol 1997; 80(Suppl 2):49.

72. Tester W, Porter A, Asbell S. Combined modality program with possible organ preservation for invasive bladder carcinoma: results of RTOG protocol 85-12. Int J Radiat Oncol Biol Phys 1993; 25: 783–90.

73. Tester W, Caplan R, Heaney J. Neoadjuvant combined modality program with selective organ preservation for invasive bladder cancer: results of Radiation Therapy Oncology Group phase II trial 88-02. J Clin Oncol 1996; 14(1): 119–26.

74. Shipley WU, Winter KA, Kaufman DS, et al. Phase III trial of neoadjuvant chemotherapy in patients with invasive bladder cancer treated with selective bladder preservation by combined radiation therapy and chemotherapy: initial results of Radiation Therapy Oncology Group 89-03. J Clin Oncol 1998; 16(11): 3576–83.

75. Sauer R, Rodel C. Biological selection for organ conservation. Eur J Cancer 2001; 37(Suppl 6): S286.

76. Durdux C, Housset M, Dufour B. Altered fractionation in chemoradiation for bladder cancer. Eur J Cancer 2001; 37(Suppl 6): S286.

77. Shipley WU, Kaufman DS, Zehr E, et al. Selective bladder preservation by combined modality protocol treatment: long-term outcomes of 190 patients with invasive bladder cancer. Urology 2002; 60(1): 62–67.

Adjuvant chemotherapy for invasive bladder cancer

James O Jin, Michelle Boyar, Daniel P Petrylak,
Walter M Stadler

Introduction

Approximately 15% to 20% of patients with bladder cancer presenting with locally invasive disease and 10% to 25% of patients with superficial disease will eventually develop muscle invasion. As discussed elsewhere in this book, the standard and most common definitive treatment for invasive bladder cancer is radical cystectomy. The 5-year disease-free survival rate is 50% to 80% for patients with muscle-invasive disease (pT2) and 20% to 50% for those with nonorgan-confined cancers (pT3–4).[1–8] For patients with node-positive disease, the 5-year disease-free survival rate is 7% to 36%.[2–8] Patients with metastatic bladder cancer can be treated with multi-agent chemotherapy, with high objective response rates and improved survival, but long-term (>5 year) survival is unusual.[9–11] Improved long-term survival has been demonstrated with adjuvant chemotherapy in other solid tumors, such as breast and colon cancer, in which high response rates with cytotoxic chemotherapy are observed in the metastatic setting. This is likely due to a greater sensitivity to chemotherapy of micrometastases present in patients destined for clinical metastatic disease than to the larger tumors present once metastatic disease is diagnosed.

The use of perioperative chemotherapy to improve survival for patients with locally advanced bladder cancer is thus theoretically attractive. Randomized data from trials utilizing neoadjuvant chemotherapy, as discussed in Chapter 63, lend further support to this concept. Unfortunately, these data suggest that the absolute survival advantage with neoadjuvant chemotherapy is only 10%. The value of exposing all patients to the toxicity of combination chemotherapy for such a modest effect is debatable. A major challenge is thus to identify patients most likely to benefit from perioperative chemotherapy as well as those that will not benefit and can at least avoid the chemotherapy toxicities.

In this context, adjuvant chemotherapy offers several advantages. First, definitive local therapy, for the large fraction of patients not benefiting from chemotherapy, is not delayed. There is some evidence that delay of cystectomy is clinically important.[12,13] Second, clinical staging of locally advanced bladder cancer is notoriously inaccurate (see Chapter 21), and cystectomy provides the definitive pathologic stage. This in turn provides the most useful information for the risk of recurrence. Under a traditional paradigm, patients with the highest risk of recurrence can then be offered chemotherapy.

It is important to recognize that offering chemotherapy to patients at the highest risk of recurrence is logical if the relative benefit of chemotherapy is the same in all patients. In other words, if chemotherapy provides a 30% improvement in relative survival, this translates into an improvement in absolute survival of 90% to 93% or 50% to 65%. Clinical studies of cytotoxic therapy in breast and colon cancer suggest that such an assumption is reasonable. On the other hand, it would be preferable to administer adjuvant chemotherapy only to patients whose tumors are sensitive to the chosen regimen. The improvements in understanding the molecular biology of bladder cancer and its therapeutic implications suggest that selection of patients for chemotherapy based on molecular markers may soon become a reality. In this context, adjuvant chemotherapy offers a further advantage over neoadjuvant therapy in that the heterogeneity of small specimens obtained by transurethral resection (TUR) is overcome by large pathologic specimens obtained at cystectomy. Thus, the molecular phenotypes of these patients can be more accurately assessed.

Completed clinical trials

Logothetis et al at the University of Texas M.D. Anderson Cancer Center first suggested a benefit for adjuvant chemotherapy in a retrospective study in 1988.[14] The study showed that cyclophosphamide, doxorubicin, and cisplatin (CISCA) chemotherapy prolonged the disease-free survival in patients with high-risk, invasive bladder cancer following cystectomy. Seventy-one patients with resected nodal metastases, extravesicular involvement of tumor, lymphatic/vascular permeation of the primary tumor, or pelvic visceral invasion received adjuvant CISCA chemotherapy. Sixty-two patients at a similar high risk for recurrence did not receive adjuvant CISCA chemotherapy because they refused, had medical contraindications, or were not referred for chemotherapy. An additional 206 patients that had none of these high-risk factors were not given adjuvant chemotherapy during the same study period. The 5-year disease-free survival was significantly better for high-risk patients that received adjuvant chemotherapy compared to those that did not (7% versus 37%, p = 0.00012), and was very similar to that of the low-risk patients (70%, p = 0.33). Although the findings are provocative, it is well recognized that multiple biases are introduced when patients and/or their physicians choose to undergo a potentially toxic therapy. In such a nonrandomized trial, it is unclear whether the differences in survival are due to the treatment received or to the selection process.

Since the 1990s, five randomized trials have been reported comparing adjuvant chemotherapy to observation after cystectomy (Table 24.1).[15–19] Skinner et al at the University of Southern California reported the first randomized trial in 1991.[15] Ninety-one patients with pT–4 or N+M0 transitional cell carcinoma (TCC) of the bladder

Table 24.1 Randomized trials of adjuvant chemotherapy

Investigator	Accrual year	No. pts	Chemotherapy	Survival benefit
Skinner et al[15]	1980–1988	91	CAP	Yes
Stockle et al[16]	1987–1991	49	MVAC or MEVC	Yes
Studer et al[18]	1984–1989	77	C	No
Bono et al[19]	1984–1987	83	CM	No
Freiha et al[17]	1986–1993	50	CMV	In relapse-free survival but not in overall survival

C, cisplatin; CAP, cyclophosphamide, doxorubicin, cisplatin; CM, cisplatin, methotrexate; CMV, cisplatin, methotrexate, vinblastine; MVAC, methotrexate, vinblastine, doxorubicin, cisplatin; MVEC, methotrexate, vinblastine, epirubicin, cisplatin.

were randomly assigned to four cycles of cisplatin, doxorubicin, and cyclophosphamide (CAP) or observation after radical cystectomy. This study demonstrated a significant 3-year disease-free survival (70% versus 46%, p = 0.0062) and median survival (4.4 versus 2.2 years, p = 0.0010) advantage for the adjuvant chemotherapy arm. This study has been heavily criticized for problems in its statistical design, as well as treatment employed. Only a small number of patients (91 of a total 498 eligible patients) were enrolled in the trial. This led to a small sample size, which rendered the study underpowered to detect any significant difference in survival. This once again raises the issue of bias in patient and physician selection and whether the results are applicable to the more general locally advanced bladder cancer population.

The statistical methodology used in this study has also been scrutinized, particularly the use of Wilcoxon statistics, which give more weight to early differences in survival. Although the authors report that all three nodal subgroups had a benefit from chemotherapy, closer analysis of patients with two or more nodes involved suggests that this particular subgroup fared worse than the observation group. The authors have also been criticized for drawing conclusions from subgroup analyses.

The chemotherapeutic regimen administered in the Skinner trial was not uniform. During the initial 3 years of the study, 17 patients received individualized chemotherapy based on a clonogenic assay, and 16 patients received cisplatin either as monotherapy or in combination with doxorubicin, cyclophosphamide, fluorouracil, vinblastine and bleomycin. Of the 44 patients randomized to chemotherapy, 11 subsequently elected not to be treated and 33 received one or more courses of chemotherapy.

Despite these inconsistencies, this was the first randomized clinical trial that suggested a role of adjuvant chemotherapy for invasive bladder cancer after radical cystectomy. The authors updated their results in 2001 after a median follow-up of 14 years.[20] There was a continued improvement in time-to-recurrence and survival in the chemotherapy group, although the difference in overall survival was not statistically significant. Data were also analyzed from 1054 patients at the University of Southern California treated with radical cystectomy, of which 255 (24%) received systemic chemotherapy either in the adjuvant or neoadjuvant setting in a nonrandomized fashion. Although the data were not presented, the investigators reported that only those patients with lymph node-positive disease had a significant benefit from adjuvant chemotherapy in terms of recurrence-free and overall survival.

The second randomized trial to assess the potential benefits of adjuvant chemotherapy following cystectomy was reported by Stockle et al at the University of Mainz, Germany, in 1992.[16] The initial design of this study was to recruit 100 patients powered to detect a 35%

improvement in the recurrence-free survival. Forty-nine patients with pT3B, PT4A, and/or pelvic lymph node involvement of TCC were initially enrolled and randomly assigned to observation or three cycles of methotrexate, vinblastine, and cisplatin plus either doxorubicin (MVAC) or epirubicin (MVEC) after radical cystectomy. This is the only randomized trial using a standard MVAC-type regimen. Interim analysis revealed a dramatic improvement in 3-year disease-free survival in the adjuvant chemotherapy arm (63% versus 13%, p=0.0015). The study also demonstrated the significant survival benefit in patients with node-positive disease. A survival benefit in the entire randomized population was demonstrated in later publications.[21] The trial was terminated prematurely after the results of interim analysis. Unfortunately, the early termination and small trial size mean that there remains a significant risk for lack of balance between the two arms for important but unmeasured prognostic factors. In addition, patients in the observation arm that developed metastatic disease were not offered chemotherapy. As such, this trial is inadequate to definitively demonstrate the survival benefit of adjuvant chemotherapy in the context of how these patients are treated today.

Freiha et al at Stanford University published data in 1996 from another small randomized trial of 50 patients with pT3–4 or node-positive TCC who received four cycles of cisplatin, methotrexate, and vinblastine (CMV) after cystectomy or cystectomy alone.[17] The adjuvant chemotherapy group had superior disease-free survival (median 37 versus 12 months, p=0.01). However, the study was terminated prematurely because of poor accrual and the significant disease-free survival found at the first interim analysis. Not surprisingly given the small study, an overall survival benefit was not observed.

Two other small, randomized trials failed to show a survival benefit from adjuvant chemotherapy[18,19] (see Table 24.1). However, the majority of patients enrolled in these studies had organ-confined disease (N0). Given the better baseline prognosis, the power to detect statistically significant survival benefit of adjuvant chemotherapy requires a larger number of patients. In addition, the chemotherapy regimen(s) used in these studies were considered less effective.

Methodologic problems in adjuvant trials

Three of the randomized studies suggest that adjuvant chemotherapy improves disease-free survival; however, interpretation of the data is difficult due to several methodologic problems common to these early trials.[15–17] These design problems are summarized below.

Sample size

In contrast to adjuvant chemotherapy trials performed in breast and colon cancer enrolling thousands of patients, small sample sizes and poor accrual rates have been a consistent problem in bladder cancer trials. Each of the randomized controlled trials of adjuvant chemotherapy following cystectomy reported to date has enrolled fewer than 100 patients. None of these studies was adequately powered to detect a small survival advantage in favor of adjuvant chemotherapy. A study designed to detect an improvement in 2-year survival of at least 10% (from 50% to 60%) would require an enrollment of 1000 patients. If the treatment effect to be detected is smaller, an even larger sample size is needed.

Several factors contribute to the poor accrual rates for bladder cancer trials. For example, bladder cancer is a less common entity than colon or breast cancer, making it difficult to enroll a large number of patients with muscle-invasive bladder cancer. In addition, patients that develop bladder cancer often have significant comorbid conditions related to age, smoking, and complications of the disease or local treatment, which can limit the administration and type of chemotherapy.

Treatment regimen

The published adjuvant treatment trials used a variety of chemotherapeutic regimens, most of which are no longer utilized for bladder cancer. Only one trial used MVAC, which has been shown to be more effective for metastatic bladder cancer than single-agent cisplatin or CISCA.[22,23] MVAC toxicity nevertheless remains a concern and may be one of the reasons that previous adjuvant trials have suffered from poor accrual. Gemcitabine, paclitaxel, and docetaxel all have promising single-agent activity in advanced TCC of the bladder.[24–32] The combination of gemcitabine and cisplatin has also been compared to MVAC in a phase III randomized trial.[33] Four hundred and five patients were randomly assigned to up to six cycles of gemcitabine and cisplatin or to MVAC. A similar response rate (49% versus 46%) and median survival (13.8 versus 14.8 months), but with fewer infectious complications and less mucositis, were observed in the gemcitabine and cisplatin arm. The trial was designed to detect a 20% improvement in survival, but the sample size was insufficient to detect true therapeutic equivalence. Although the lower toxicity of gemcitabine/cisplatin and the palliative nature of metastatic bladder cancer treatment has led to gemcitabine/cisplatin being accepted as a standard therapy in the metastatic setting, the lack of data for therapeutic equivalence, and the lack of data on gemcitabine/cisplatin in the adjuvant setting, make the use of this regimen in the adjuvant setting controversial.

Baseline renal insufficiency can limit the use of cisplatin in the adjuvant setting. This has led many practitioners to recommend or use taxanes and/or carboplatin, both of which can be administered more easily and safely in the setting of renal insufficiency.[34] The therapeutic equivalence of carboplatin compared to cisplatin remained a significant question. A randomized trial by the Hellenic Cooperative Oncology Group demonstrated improved toxicity of gemcitabine/carboplatin compared to gemcitabine/cisplatin, at the cost of a lower complete response rate in gemcitabine/carboplatin-treated patients.[35] A randomized trial of docetaxel/cisplatin versus MVAC in the metastatic setting demonstrated inferiority of the taxane regimen.[36] Thus, the use of carboplatin or taxane-based doublet therapy should be used in clinical trials, or if the patient is medically unfit to receive cisplatin-based therapy.

Pelvic lymph node dissection

Early studies of bladder cancer treated with total cystectomy found a significant decrease in local recurrence when pelvic lymphadenectomy was included.[2] The observation that pelvic nodal metastases could occur in the absence of distant metastatic spread further supported the rationale for including pelvic lymphadenectomy at the time of radical cystectomy, since the procedure can be curative for patients with a small volume of nodal disease. Retrospective studies have shown long-term survival of patients with grossly node-positive disease after pelvic lymph node dissection and radical cystectomy.[37] Bilateral pelvic iliac node dissection with en bloc radical and urinary diversion has been performed by Skinner and colleagues since 1971 on all patients undergoing radical cystectomy with the intent to cure. Preoperative clinical staging is often inaccurate, so a significant number of patients that appear to have localized tumors will have positive lymph nodes. Lymphadenectomy also enables accurate staging. Surgical technique, especially in regard to lymphadenectomy, introduces another variable into clinical trials of adjuvant chemotherapy. In the four randomized controlled trials, information regarding the technique used for lymphadenectomy is given in trials by Skinner[15] and Studer,[18] but no details are given in the Stockle[16] or Freiha[17] trials.

Timing of adjuvant therapy

The timing of chemotherapy is another variable that can affect outcome in an adjuvant therapy trial. In the Skinner trial,[15] chemotherapy began 6 weeks after cystectomy; the Studer trial[18] started chemotherapy within 8 weeks after cystectomy; Stockle and Freiha did not report when chemotherapy commenced.[16,17] Starting therapy too quickly after cystectomy can lead to poor tolerance of the treatment regimen with subsequent treatment delays and dose reductions, which may affect the overall outcome. Conversely, starting adjuvant therapy too late may abrogate some of the theoretical advantages to adjuvant treatment.

Ongoing adjuvant clinical trials

In order to address the deficits in previously published trials of adjuvant chemotherapy for bladder cancer, the European Organisation for Research and Treatment of Cancer (EORTC) has launched a large randomized clinical trial in which 660 patients with extravesical (pT3–4) or node-positive TCC will be randomly assigned either to immediate chemotherapy or to chemotherapy at the time of relapse. Given the above discussion on chemotherapy options, each participating institution can choose amongst MVAC, high-dose MVAC, or gemcitabine/cisplatin as the chemotherapeutic regimen to be used.

The Cancer and Leukemia Group B (CALGB), in collaboration with the Eastern Cooperative Oncology Group (ECOG), have taken a somewhat different approach. Taking into account both the reluctance of patients and physicians to participate in a 'no treatment' versus 'potentially toxic treatment' randomized study and the highly suggestive data noted above, these investigators have chosen to accept adjuvant therapy as the standard arm and a more aggressive approach as the experimental arm. The experimental arm is based on the Norton–Simon hypothesis in which a chemotherapy program of rapidly cycling sequential regimens is proposed to be more efficacious than a standard scheduled single regimen. Thus, 800 patients with extravesical (pT3–4) or node-positive TCC will be randomly assigned either to doxorubicin/gemcitabine followed by paclitaxel/cisplatin (sequenced doublet therapy), or to gemcitabine/cisplatin (conventional doublet therapy) after cystectomy. The choice of gemcitabine/cisplatin as the conventional arm was based on similar survival but less toxicity in a randomized trial versus MVAC in the metastatic setting. The sequential regimen is based on promising phase II data from investigators at the Memorial Sloan-Kettering Cancer Institute, who reported a much higher complete response to this regimen in the metastatic setting than expected in historical controls.

The final ongoing adjuvant study utilizes data on the molecular biology of bladder cancer. A number of studies have demonstrated that altered expression of p53, p21, pRB, and p16 act in cooperative or synergistic ways to promote bladder cancer progression.[38,39] Of these, p53 has been found to be the most consistent and strongest prognostic indicator[38] (see also Chapter 9). More importantly, investigators at the University of Southern California, using retrospective data from their randomized trial of adjuvant CISCA,[15] strongly suggested that patients with bladder tumors carrying p53 alterations are more likely to benefit from adjuvant chemotherapy than are patients with bladder tumors carrying a wild-type p53.[40] These observations have been supported by a number of laboratory studies, which demonstrate that p53 mutations confer sensitivity to DNA damaging agents such as cisplatin. These studies raise the intriguing possibility that p53 mutations not only define a population at high risk of recurrence, but also a population most likely to benefit from cisplatin-containing chemotherapy.

Thus, a multicenter, international randomized clinical trial testing this hypothesis has been initiated. Patients with organ-confined bladder cancers that carry a wild-type p53 have an overall good prognosis, with an estimated 5-year disease-free survival of 90%, and will be observed. Patients with organ-confined bladder cancer that carry an altered p53 have an approximately 40% 5-year disease-free survival and are predicted to benefit from chemotherapy.[41] Patients with p53 alterations will be randomly assigned to three cycles of MVAC or observation following their cystectomy. If this study is positive, it will define a molecularly-targeted therapy and usher in a new paradigm for bladder cancer treatment.

Conclusion

Despite the methodologic flaws of the early trials of adjuvant chemotherapy for bladder cancer, the combination of chemotherapy and surgery in high-risk patients does appear to confer a survival advantage, and many physicians are administering adjuvant chemotherapy outside a protocol setting for patients with a high risk of recurrence.[42,43] However, the role of adjuvant chemotherapy still needs to be clearly defined. The three large multicenter-randomized trials should further define the role of adjuvant chemotherapy in the management of muscle-invasive bladder cancer. Thus, patients should be encouraged to enter in these studies.

References

1. Wishnow KI, Levinson AK, Johnson DE, et al. Stage B (P2/3 A/N0) transitional cell carcinoma of bladder highly curable by radical cystectomy. Urology 1992; 39: 12–16.
2. Lerner SP, Skinner DG, Lieskovsky G, et al. The rationale for en bloc pelvic lymph node dissection for bladder cancer patients with nodal metastases: long-term results. J Urol 1993; 149: 758–64.
3. LaPlante M, Brice M III. The upper limits of hopeful application of radical cystectomy for vesical carcinoma: does nodal metastasis always indicate incurability? J Urol 1973; 109: 261–64.
4. Dretler SP, Ragsdale BD, Leadbetter WF. The value of pelvic lymphadenectomy in the surgical treatment of bladder cancer. J Urol 1973; 109: 414–16.
5. Smith JA Jr, Whitmore WF Jr. Regional lymph node metastasis from bladder cancer. J Urol 1981; 126: 591–3.
6. Skinner DG, Tift JP, Kaufman JJ. High dose, short course preoperative radiation therapy and immediate single stage radical cystectomy with pelvic node dissection in the management of bladder cancer. J Urol 1982; 127: 671–4.
7. Pagano F, Bassi P, Galetti TP, et al. Results of contemporary radical cystectomy for invasive bladder cancer: a clinicopathological study with an emphasis on the inadequacy of the tumor, nodes and metastases classification. J Urol 1991; 145(1): 45–50.
8. Schoenberg MP, Walsh PC, Breazeale DR, et al. Local recurrence and survival following nerve sparing radical cystoprostatectomy for bladder cancer: 10-year follow-up. J Urol 1996; 155(2): 490–94.
9. Loehrer P, Einhorn LH, Elson PJ, et al. A randomized comparison of cisplatin alone or in combination with methotrexate, vinblastine, and doxorubicin in patients with metastatic urothelial carcinoma: a Cooperative Group Study. J Clin Oncol 1992; 10: 1066–73.
10. Sternberg CN, Yagoda A, Scher HI, et al. Methotrexate, vinblastine, doxorubicin and cisplatinum for advanced transitional cell carcinoma of the urothelium: efficacy and patterns of response and relapse. Cancer 1989; 64: 2448–58.
11. Harker WG, Meyers FJ, Freiha FS, et al. Cisplatin, methotrexate, and vinblastine (CMV): an effective chemotherapy regimen for metastatic transitional cell carcinoma of the urinary tract. A Northern California Oncology Group study. J Clin Oncol 1985; 3: 1463–70.
12. Chang SS, Hassan JM, Cookson MS, et al. Delaying radical cystectomy for muscle invasive bladder cancer results in worse pathological stage. J Urol 2003; 170: 1085–87.
13. Sanchez-Ortiz RF, Huang WC, Mick R, et al. An interval longer than 12 weeks between the diagnosis of muscle invasion and cystectomy is associated with worse outcome in bladder carcinoma. J Urol 2003; 169(1): 110–15.
14. Logothetis C, Johnson D, Chong C, et al. Adjuvant cyclophosphamide, doxorubicin, and cisplatin chemotherapy for bladder cancer: an update. J Clin Oncol 1988; 6: 1590–96.
15. Skinner DG, Daniels JR, Russell CA, et al. The role of adjuvant chemotherapy following cystectomy for invasive bladder cancer: a prospective comparative trial. J Urol 1991; 145: 459–64.
16. Stockle M, Meyenburg W, Wellek S, et al. Advanced bladder cancer (stages pT3b, pT4a, pN1 and pN2): improved survival after radical cystectomy and 3 adjuvant cycles of chemotherapy. Results of a controlled prospective study. J Urol 1992; 148: 302–06.
17. Freiha F, Reese J, Torti F. A randomized trial of radical cystectomy versus radical cystectomy plus cisplatin, vinblastine and methotrexate chemotherapy for muscle-invasive bladder cancer. J Urol 1996; 155: 495–99.
18. Studer U, Bacchi M, Biederman C, et al. Adjuvant cisplatin chemotherapy following cystectomy for bladder cancer: results of a prospective randomized trial. J Urol 1994; 152: 81–4.
19. Bono AV, Benvenuti C, Reali L, et al. Adjuvant chemotherapy in advanced bladder cancer. Italian Uro-Oncologic Cooperative Group. Prog Clin Biol Res 1989; 303: 533–40.
20. Stein JP, Lieskovsky G, Cote R, et al. Radical cystectomy in the treatment of invasive bladder cancer: long-term results in 1,054 patients. J Clin Oncol 2001; 19(3): 666–75.
21. Stockle M, Meyenburg W, Wellek S, et al. Adjuvant polychemotherapy of nonorgan-confined bladder cancer after radical cystectomy revisited: long-term results of a controlled prospective study and further clinical experience. J Urol 1995; 153: 47–52.
22. Loehrer PJ Sr, Einhorn LH, Elson PJ, et al. A randomized comparison of cisplatin alone or in combination with methotrexate, vinblastine, and doxorubicin in patients with metastatic urothelial carcinoma: a cooperative group study. J Clin Oncol 1992; 10(7): 1066–73.

23. Logothetis CJ, Dexeus FH, Finn L, et al. A prospective randomized trial comparing MVAC and CISCA chemotherapy for patients with metastatic urothelial tumors. J Clin Oncol 1990; 8(6): 1050–55.
24. Lorusso V, Pollera CF, Antimi M, et al. A phase II study of gemcitabine in patients with transitional cell carcinoma of the urinary tract previously treated with platinum. Italian Co-operative Group on Bladder Cancer. Eur J Cancer 1998; 34: 1208–12.
25. Moore MJ, Tannock IF, Ernst DS, et al. Gemcitabine: a promising new agent in the treatment of advanced urothelial cancer. J Clin Oncol 1997; 15: 3441–45.
26. Stadler WM, Kuzel T, Roth B, et al. Phase II study of single-agent gemcitabine in previously untreated patients with metastatic urothelial cancer. J Clin Oncol 1997; 15: 3394–98.
27. Pollera CF, Ceribelli A, Crecco M, Calabresi F. Weekly gemcitabine in advanced bladder cancer: a preliminary report from a phase I study. Ann Oncol 1994; 5: 182–4.
28. Gebbia V, Testa A, Borsellino N, et al. Single agent 2',2'-difluorodeoxy-cytidine in the treatment of metastatic urothelial carcinoma: a phase II study. Clin Ter 1999; 150: 11–15.
29. Roth BJ, Dreicer R, Einhorn LH, et al. Significant activity of paclitaxel in advanced transitional-cell carcinoma of the urothelium: a phase II trial of the Eastern Cooperative Oncology Group. J Clin Oncol 1994; 12: 2264–70.
30. Dreicer R, Gustin DM, See WA, Williams RD. Paclitaxel in advanced urothelial carcinoma: its role in patients with renal insufficiency and as salvage therapy. J Urol 1996; 156: 1606–08.
31. McCaffrey JA, Hilton S, Mazumdar M, et al. Phase II trial of docetaxel in patients with advanced or metastatic transitional-cell carcinoma. J Clin Oncol 1997; 15(5): 1853–57.
32. de Wit R, Kruit WH, Stoter G, et al. Docetaxel (Taxotere): an active agent in metastatic urothelial cancer: results of a phase II study in non-chemotherapy-pretreated patients. Br J Cancer 1998; 78: 1342–45.
33. von der Masse H, Hansen SW, Roberts JT, et al. Gemcitabine and cisplatin versus methotrexate, vinblastine, doxorubicin, and cisplatin in advanced or metastatic bladder cancer: results of a large, randomized, multinational, multicenter, phase III study. J Clin Oncol 2000; 18: 306–77.
34. Bamias A, Deliveliotis Ch, Aravantinos G, et al. Hellenic Cooperative Oncology Group. Adjuvant chemotherapy with paclitaxel and carboplatin in patients with advanced bladder cancer: a study by the Hellenic Cooperative Oncology Group. J Urol. 2004; 171(4): 1467–70.
35. Carteni G, Dogliotti L, Crucitta E, et al. Phase II randomised trial of gemcitabine plus cisplatin and gemcitabine plus carboplatin in patients with advanced or metastatic transitional cell carcinoma of the urothelium [abstract]. Proc Am Soc Clin Oncol 2003; 22: 384, Abstract 1543.
36. Bamias A, Aravantinos G, Bafaloukos D, et al. Docetaxel plus cisplatin versus MVAC in advanced urothelial carcinoma: a multicenter, randomized phase III study conducted by the Hellenic Cooperative Oncology Group [abstract]. Proc Am Soc Clin Oncol 2003; 22: 384, Abstract 1541.
37. Herr HW, Donat SM. Outcome of patients with grossly node positive bladder cancer after pelvic lymph node dissection and radical cystectomy. J Urol 2001; 16562–64.
38. Chatterjee SJ, Datar R, Youssefzadeh D, et al. Combined effects of p53, p21, and pRb expression in the progression of bladder transitional cell carcinoma. J Clin Oncol 2004; 22(6): 1007–13.
39. Shariat SF, Tokunaga H, Zhou J, et al. p53, p21, pRB, and p16 expression predict clinical outcome in cystectomy with bladder cancer. J Clin Oncol 2004; 22(6): 1014–24.
40. Cote R, Esrig D, Groshen S, et al. p53 and the treatment of bladder cancer. Nature 1997; 385: 123–25.
41. Esrig D, Elmajian D, Groshen S, et al. Accumulation of nuclear p53 and tumor progression in bladder cancer. N Engl J Med 1994; 331(19): 1259–64.
42. Crawford ED, Wood DP, Petrylak DP, et al. Southwest Oncology Group studies in bladder cancer. Cancer 2003; 97(Suppl 8): 2099–108.
43. Small EJ, Halabi S, Dalbagni G, et al. Overview of bladder cancer trials in the cancer and leukemia Group B. Cancer 2003; 97(Suppl 8): 2090–98.

25

Treatment of metastatic cancer

Avishay Sella, Joaquim Bellmunt

Introduction

Transitional cell carcinoma (TCC) of the bladder is the fifth most common solid malignancy in the United States. It is diagnosed in approximately 57,400 patients and results in more than 12,500 deaths annually.[1] The standard treatment for invasive bladder cancer is radical cystectomy, whereas patients with metastatic or locally advanced urothelial cancer are usually treated with systemic chemotherapy. Notable advances have been developed during the last 20 years in the chemotherapeutic management of patients with advanced urothelial tumors.

Single agents and MVAC era

Studies in the 1970s identified the chemosensitivity of urothelial cancer to several agents: cisplatin, methotrexate, adriamycin, vinblastine, and 5-fluorouracil (5FU) were shown to be the most active.[2] Although these earlier trials led to a response rate of only 10% to 30% when used in monotherapy and with limited duration of responses, they established the foundation for combination chemotherapeutic trials which characterized the 1980s.[3] These trials were mainly cisplatin-based combination regimens such as cisplatin/methotrexate/vinblastine (CMV), cisplatin/adriamycin/cyclophosphamide (CISCA), and methotrexate/vinblastine/adriamycin/cisplatin (MVAC).[4–6] These combinations were reported initially as single-institution phase II studies with objective response rates as high as 65% to 75%, with approximately 20% to 35% of cases achieving complete remission (CR), and median survival periods increasing from 3–4 months to 12–14 months.[3–7]

As a consequence, it became apparent that cisplatin was an essential component of combination chemotherapy regimens for patients with adequate renal function. A randomized study conducted in the UK comparing methotrexate and vinblastine (MV) with CMV demonstrated an absolute improvement in 1-year survival of 13% with the treatment containing cisplatin (29% for CMV and 16% for MV). The median survival for CMV was significantly longer than that for MV: 7 months compared with 4.5 months.[8] This study demonstrated the significant survival impact of cisplatin and has helped to justify the routine use of cisplatin-based combination chemotherapy. In addition, as more experience was gained with MVAC, it emerged as the preferred cisplatin-based combination therapy (Table 25.1).[9–13] In randomized trials, MVAC produced a modest, though significant, survival benefit when compared with cisplatin as a single agent, CISCA, or carboplatin-based regimens.[11,13,14] The tumor origin did not have an impact on response to MVAC.[2] Patients with CR appeared to gain survival benefits, and prognosis for those with nodal disease appeared more favorable.[2,9] Patients with nontransitional-cell histology and poor performance status had a poor prognosis and were unlikely to benefit significantly from MVAC chemotherapy.[15] In addition, long-term survival was low, with only 3.7% of patients experiencing more than 6 years of disease-free survival.[9,11–15]

Due to the toxicity that was reported with MVAC, with up to 25% incidence of neutropenic fever, 50% grade 2–3 stomatitis, and 3% drug-related mortality, the incorporation of granulocyte colony-stimulating factor (G-CSF) or granulocyte-macrophage colony-stimulating factor (GM-CSF) was added to the schedule. This was done both in an effort to reduce toxicity and to increase the dose density of the combination since, in the majority of patients, cycles were delivered every 5 weeks instead of every 4 weeks.[9–13] With the simultaneous use of G-CSF or GM-CSF, these toxicities can be reduced, allowing more patients to receive the dose originally planned in the conventional MVAC treatment, and even an intensified MVAC schedule. Unfortunately, dose intensification of the MVAC regimen has not translated into a clinical benefit in terms of improved survival.[16–22] A recent phase III study by the European Organisation for Research and Treatment of Cancer (EORTC), comparing classical MVAC to a high dose (HD) MVAC regimen every 2 weeks with G-CSF support, revealed significant differences in terms of complete response and overall response rates in favor of the HD-MVAC arm (25% and 72%, respectively), compared with the standard MVAC arm (11% and 58%, respectively). However, there was no statistically significant difference between the two treatment arms in terms of the primary endpoint: overall survival with a median survival of 15.5 months for the HD-MVAC arm and 14.1 months for the standard MVAC arm.[23]

The dismal long-term survival with the classical MVAC combination has led to the search for new treatment approaches aiming to improve outcome and treatment tolerance. Throughout the years, many phase III trials have evaluated new combinations, such as gemcitabine/cisplatin, carboplatin/paclitaxel, docetaxel/cisplatin, and interferon-α/5-fluorouracil/cisplatin. Unfortunately, in all of these randomized trials, the new regimens have failed to demonstrate superiority in terms of overall survival when compared with the classical MVAC.[22,24–26]

The experience of using MVAC chemotherapy has enabled the establishment of several prognostic factors that predict the benefits of chemotherapy. Investigators from the Memorial Sloan-Kettering Cancer Center (MSKCC) determined that two factors had an independent prognosis: Karnofsky performance status (KPS) less than 80%, and visceral (lung, liver, or bone) metastasis. Three risk categories were established on the basis of KPS and the presence or absence of visceral metastases. Median survival times for patients who had zero, one, or two risk factors were 33, 13.4, and 9.3 months,

Table 25.1 Early global experience with MVAC

Lead author	No. pts	Response rate (%)	Complete response (%)	Median survival (months)
Sternberg[9]	121	72	36	13.4
Tannock[10]	30	40	13	10.0
Logothetis[11]	55	65	35	11.0
Boutan-Laroze[12]	67	57	57	13.0
Loehrer[13]	120	38	38	12.5

Table 25.2 Risk factors in metastatic bladder cancer

	MVAC	Paclitaxel/gemcitabine/cisplatin
No. risk factors	Median survival (months)	Median survival (months)
0	33.0	32.8
1	13.4	18.0
2	9.3	10.6

Risk factors: Presence of visceral metastases, Karnofsky performance status <80%.

respectively (p = 0.0001) (Table 25.2). Based on these data, it is clearly demonstrated that the median survival time of patient cohorts could vary from 9 to 26 months simply by altering the proportion of patients from different risk categories. This explains the divergent reported outcomes reported from different trials. Similar findings regarding prognostic factors, risk categories, and survival have been seen when using the triple combination of paclitaxel/cisplatin/gemcitabine reported by the Spanish Group (SOGUG).[27,28]

New active agents and combinations: single agents and doublets

The efforts to improve the outcome of patients with metastatic TCC have focused on the identification of new drugs with single-agent activity and on their incorporation into platinum-based combination regimens.

Paclitaxel

Paclitaxel emerged initially as one of the effective single-agent drugs (Table 25.3).[29–34] The paclitaxel/carboplatin combination rapidly found its way into routine clinical practice because of its modest toxicity profile.[29–34] However, a randomized phase III study comparing the doublet with MVAC, conducted by the Eastern Cooperative Oncology Group (ECOG), was closed prematurely due to poor accrual when the limited efficacy of the doublet paclitaxel/carboplatin seen in several phase II trials became apparent.[25] It is not possible to interpret the results of this study because it failed to reach its accrual goal.

Gemcitabine

Gemcitabine also revealed activity in locally advanced and metastatic urothelial cell cancer. Complete responses were noted even in

patients previously treated with cisplatin.[35–38] In view of the synergistic effects between cisplatin and gemcitabine and the mild toxicity profile of gemcitabine, the two-drug combination of gemcitabine and cisplatin was soon evaluated.[39] Initial studies produced results similar to those with MVAC (Table 25.4).[35–42] Based on these results, a large randomized trial in which the MVAC regimen was compared with the combination of gemcitabine and cisplatin (GC), both delivered every 4 weeks, was conducted. The study was designed to demonstrate a 4-month improvement in survival benefit with GC. The two treatment arms turned out to be very similar in terms of median survival (13.8 months for GC and 14.8 months for MVAC), time to progression (7.4 months in both arms), and overall response rate (46% and 49%, respectively). Fewer patients on GC than on MVAC had grade 3/4 neutropenia (71% versus 82%, respectively), neutropenic fever (2% versus 14%), grade 3/4 mucositis (1% versus 22%), and hospital admissions (9 admissions for a total of 33 days versus 49 admissions for a total of 272 days). The toxic death rate was 1% with GC and 3% with MVAC. More GC than MVAC patients had grade 3/4 anemia and thrombocytopenia. One limitation of this large randomized study was that the better safety and tolerability of GC was not reflected in the quality of life (QoL) results.[43] Although this trial was not designed to show the equivalence of the two regimens, many researchers have interpreted the results as showing therapeutic noninferiority and determined that any difference in survival was unlikely to be sufficiently large to offset the improvement in toxicity with GC.[26]

In an attempt to improve the thrombocytopenic toxicity profile of GC which occurred around day 15, small phase II trials have evaluated a 3-week program of GC in which cisplatin is given either concomitantly on day 1, or fractionated, and gemcitabine on days 1 and 8, recycling on day 21. This alteration did not modify the response rate. The indications of a better toxicity profile and fewer treatment delays will have to be confirmed in larger trials.[44,45]

Docetaxel

Docetaxel has demonstrated activity in chemotherapy-naive patients (31% response rate) and previously treated patients (13.3% response rate).[46,47] Although phase II studies of two-drug combinations of docetaxel with cisplatin (DC) have shown activity in untreated patients with response rates that are similar to MVAC, a recent randomized study reported by the Hellenic Group has shown inferior activity of the cisplatin/docetaxel combination compared to classical MVAC. Although this study was designed to detect a survival advantage for DC, the investigators instead observed that survival was inferior for patients treated with DC. Because performance status was not used in this trial as a prospective stratification variable, the treatment arms were not appropriately balanced. After adjusting for prognostic factors, difference in time to progression (TTP) remained significant (hazard ratio [HR] 1.61, p = 0.005), whereas the survival difference was nonsignificant at the 5% level (HR 1.31, p = 0.089).[22]

Table 25.3 Paclitaxel in advanced urothelial cancer

Lead author	Year	Other therapy	Taxol (mg/m²)	Response rate (%)	Prior therapy
Tu[29]	1995	Methotrexate, cisplatin	200 + G-CSF	40	Yes
Roth[30]	1994	Ifosfamide	250 + G-CSF	42	No
Sweeney[31]	1999	Ifosfamide	135 + G-CSF	23	Yes
Vaughn[32]	1997	Carboplatin	200	64	No
Zielinski[33]	1998	Carboplatin	175	65	No
Redman[34]	1998	Carboplatin	200	52	No

G-CSF, granulocyte colony-stimulating factor.

Table 25.4 Gemcitabine in advanced urothelial cancer

Lead author	Year	Prior therapy	Response rate (%)	Gemcitabine (mg/m²) weekly × 3 q 4 weeks	Cisplatin (mg/m²)
Pollera[35]	1994	Yes	27	Above 1000	
Stadler[36]	1997	No	28	1200	
Moore[37]	1997	No	24	1200	
Lorusso[38]	1998	Yes	23	1200	
Von der Masse[40]	1999	No	42	1000	35
Moore[41]	1999	No	57	1000	70
Kaufman[42]	2000	No	41	1000	100, 75

Gallium nitrate and Ifosfamide

Gallium nitrate has activity as a single agent in the treatment of advanced bladder cancer, including activity in heavily pretreated patients. Partial responses were observed in 4 of 23 patients (17.4%) that received 350 mg/m²/d or more for 5 days by continuous intravenous infusion.[48] Likewise, ifosfamide was evaluated in previously treated patients in whom it produced a 20% objective response rate. However, administration of ifosfamide at 1500 mg/m² with MESNA 750 mg/m²/d for 5 days every 3 weeks resulted in significant renal and central nervous system toxicity.[49] The clinical activity obtained by combining ifosfamide with etoposide (14% response rate), paclitaxel (15% response rate in previously treated patients, 30.7% response rate in chemotherapy-naive patients), CMV (62.5% response rate), or vinblastine/gallium (44% response rate) is not justified in view of the significant toxicity.[50–53] To date, doublet ifosfamide-based regimens have no role in the routine therapy of advanced urothelial tumors.

Carboplatin

Carboplatin exerted limited clinical activity as a single agent.[54] Carboplatin-based combinations were reported in the 1990s. The combination of carboplatin with methotrexate and vinblastine (carbo-MV and M-CAVI) have shown response rates of 30% to 40% and a median survival of 8–10 months. These results are inferior to those obtained with MVAC. Two underpowered, randomized studies also suggested that carboplatin-based chemotherapy had suboptimal efficacy.[55,56] Similarly, cisplatin also seems to be more effective than carboplatin when combined with gemcitabine. In another underpowered randomized phase II trial, a response rate of 66% was achieved in patients treated with cisplatin/gemcitabine as compared with a response rate of only 35% with carboplatin/gemcitabine.[57]

Lobaplatin and oxaliplatin

Lobaplatin, a third-generation platinum complex, demonstrated a 10% response rate in previously treated patients.[58] Oxaliplatin monotherapy has shown minimal activity in previously treated patients, but it is feasible to combine this with gemcitabine, with encouraging preliminary data in patients unfit for cisplatin.[59–61]

Antifolate compounds

With regard to antifolate compounds, de Wit et al reported a response rate of 17% for trimetrexate in patients who had received prior chemotherapy.[62] Piritrexim, an oral second-generation antimetabolite, was tested in two studies. As a single agent in chemotherapy-naive patients, it demonstrated a 38% response rate, whereas in previously treated patients, partial response (PR) was obtained only at a rate of 23%.[63] This compound is now being evaluated with gemcitabine.[64]

Pemetrexed, a novel multitargeted antifolate (MTA) that inhibits multiple folate-dependent enzymes, achieved a 33% response rate in 22 chemonaive patients; however, there were two drug-related deaths.[65] It was also active in previously treated patients. A recent phase II trial as second line therapy (including relapses after adjuvant or neoadjuvant therapy) achieved an overall response rate of 27.7% (13 out of 47), with three patients obtaining CR. Of the responders, six were enrolled with prior adjuvant therapy within 12 months. Overall survival was 9.8 months.[66] A confirmatory second line trial is now planned.

Vinflunine

Vinflunine is a new synthetically designed vinca alkaloid that has been recently studied in second line bladder cancer after platinum failure.

Due to the reported activity of 16% response rate and a median survival of 6 months, a phase III second line multinational trial is presently ongoing, comparing this drug with best supportive care followed by treatment upon progression.[67,68]

Irinotecan

Witte et al reported a response rate of 10% with irinotecan in patients that had previously received chemotherapy.[69] This agent is now being studied with gemcitabine in a phase II trial and as a single agent in the regimens of patients previously treated with a platinum-containing agent (Southwest Oncology Group).[70]

Nonplatinum-based regimens

Both gemcitabine and the taxanes have been extensively evaluated in single-drug studies. In view of their toxicity profile, particularly the lack of nephrotoxicity, it is not surprising that multiple studies have been performed with this combination (Table 25.5).[71–79] Response ranges from 0% to 60% have been reported. This variability reflects diversity in patient prognostic factors and the effect of prior chemotherapy—lower responses when the combination was given for active disease, and higher when the combination was given after an adjuvant/neoadjuvant approach.[71–73,76–78]

Unfit patients

Most of the phase II and large phase III trials include patients with normal renal function and good performance status. Unfortunately, since this disease may interfere with kidney function, and often involves the elderly, many patients do not 'fit' with these good criteria.

Various strategies have been considered to avoid this problem, including modulation of cisplatin's nephrotoxicity by using nephroprotective agents, modifying the scheduling of cisplatin, using less cisplatin-intense regimens, or substituting carboplatin for cisplatin.[80] The emergence of active nontoxic agents enabled the design of other approaches for these patients. The ECOG reported on a 20.6% response rate with the combination of paclitaxel/carboplatin.[81] With gemcitabine-based regimens the response rates were gemcitabine/epirubicin, 46%; gemcitabine/vinorelbine, 47.6%; and gemcitabine/carboplatin, 44%.[82–84] This later trial was a dose-finding study with the combination of gemcitabine and carboplatin, and it was evaluated in clearly predefined 'unfit' bladder cancer patients: performance status >2 and/or creatinine clearance less than 60 ml/min. Using this combination, investigators reported a median time survival of 14.4 months in the 16 patients that were ineligible for a cisplatin-based regimen ('unfit' patient population). The preliminary results found on this phase II trial using the carboplatin/gemcitabine doublet prompted an EORTC randomized phase II/III trial (EORTC protocol 30986) comparing carboplatin/gemcitabine with M-CAVI in patients ineligible for cisplatin-based chemotherapy. This trial is presently ongoing.

It is important to mention that chronologic age should not exclude patients from the potential benefit of conventional cisplatin-based therapy, because elderly patients with adequate renal function tolerate conventional platinum-based chemotherapy as well as younger patients and may benefit equally.[85,86]

Future directions

Several approaches are being investigated to improve the dismal outcome of advanced transitional cell carcinoma patients.[9,11–15,87] These approaches include the search for molecular treatment-response predicting markers, management of minimal/microscopic residual disease, dose-dense sequential approaches, incorporation of triple combination regimens, and targeted therapies.

Table 25.5 Gemcitabine/taxanes combination therapy in urothelial cancer

Lead author	Gemcitabine	Paclitaxe	Docetaxel	Pts with prior therapy	No. pts	Response rate (%)	Median survival (months)
Sternberg[71]	2000–3000 D 1 q 14 days	150 D 1 q 14 days		41	41	60	14.4
Kaufman[72]	3000 D 1 q 14 days	150 D 1 q 14 days		6	37	19	
Meluch[73]	1000 D 1, 8, 15 q 21 days	200 D 1 q 21 days		15	54	54	14.4
Parameswaran[74]	1000 D 1, 8, 15 q 28 days	110 D 1 q 28 days			23	61	
Srinivas[75]	1000 D 1, 15 q 28 days	110 D 1, 15 q 28 days			17	65	7.5
Garcia Del Muro[76]	2000 D 1 q 14 days		65 D 1 q 14 days	10	39	56	
Friedland[77]	1000 D 1, 8 q 21 days		75 D 1 q 21 days	7	41	32	68% 1 year survival
Dreicer[78]	800 D 1, 8 q 21 days		40 D 1, 8 q 21 days	25	25	20	
Gitlitz[79]	800 D 1, 8, 15 q 28 days		60–80 D 1 q 28 days		27	33	12

Molecular treatment-response predicting markers

Alterations in p53 and pRb occur in approximately 50% and 35%, respectively, of bladder cancers and have been reported to correlate with high grade and stage.[88–90] There are conflicting reports regarding the relationship between chemosensitivity and p53, and several authors suggest that altered expression of p53 may be associated with resistance to MVAC, although others suggest the contrary. Paclitaxel can induce apoptosis, using p53 independent pathways.[91,92] Some studies have shown that the metastatic potential of bladder cancer correlates with the expression of several genes that regulate proliferation (EGFR) and angiogenesis (bFGF, VEGF, MMP9, and interleukin 8). Inhibition of the epidermal growth factor receptor type I pathway, either by physical receptor blockade, as with the monoclonal antibody IMC225, or with the tyrosine kinase inhibitor ZD1839, leads to demonstrable antitumor effects in animal models. Adding paclitaxel to EGFR-directed therapy produced a synergistic biologic effect on xenographs.[93,94] At present, none of the molecular markers has entered into routine clinical practice. Prospective studies of chemotherapy selection based on molecular markers are needed.

Residual disease postchemotherapy

It is important to distinguish between 'minimal residual disease' after chemotherapy in patients who achieved a complete response to therapy (= microscopic), and radiographically detected minimal residual disease (= macroscopic), representing a good clinical PR to the treatment.

Regarding minimal residual disease postchemotherapy, researchers at the University of Texas M.D. Anderson Cancer Center have designed a phase II trial in which patients that have responded to initial cytotoxic chemotherapy are randomized to treatment with either docetaxel alone, or a combination of docetaxel and ZD1839 (Iressa). The objectives of this trial are to compare the proportion of patients free from progression 9 months after the start of consolidation therapy, testing the hypothesis that the antiproliferative, and especially the antiangiogenic, effects of concomitant docetaxel and Iressa will inhibit progression of residual disease following maximal response (complete response) to front-line chemotherapy.[94]

The postchemotherapy surgical resection of macroscopic residual disease could be a reasonable approach for some selected patients with small volume residual disease after chemotherapy. Patients that benefited most from this approach were those with a major response to chemotherapy, initially tumor confined to pelvic, bladder, regional lymph nodes, or with a solitary metastatic site. Postchemotherapy surgical resection of residual cancer extends the median survival of these patients to 31–37 months, and may result in disease-free survival in some patients that would otherwise die of disease.[95–97]

Salvage therapy

Patients whose disease recurs following their initial chemotherapy are destined to die. Objective remission rates up to 30% have been reported with treatment based on paclitaxel, ifosfamide, gemcitabine,

trimetrexate, piritrexim, pemetrexed, and vinflunine after cisplatinum-based therapy.[29–31,35,38,49,62,63,65–73,76–78]

There are limited data regarding salvage therapy following MVAC and no data after gemcitabine/cisplatin. Since patients that relapse after MVAC (particularly if there was a 3–6 months' progression-free survival following the previous platinum-based chemotherapy) have responded again to the earlier same regimen, it could be suggested that their exposure again to gemcitabine/cisplatin after long-term disease-free progression (more than 6–12 months) could be a reasonable option. However, no definitive data exist in the literature.[98]

Until now, second line bladder cancer therapy is an unmet medical need with no data favoring monotherapy, polychemotherapy, or alternating therapy.[99] An alternative approach to identify early treatment failures has been suggested, with an early switch of therapy if there is not an at least 40% tumor reduction (the so-called 'play-the-winner-and-drop-the-loser' strategy). This not-yet-proved methodology is used to select one best treatment, or a best pair of treatments, as a two-stage strategy out of four different treatments.[100]

Dose-dense approach

Based on the results obtained with the ITP[101] combination of ifosfamide, paclitaxel, and cisplatin, and on concepts derived from kinetic models studied in breast cancer, investigators from MSKCC have developed the concept of dose-dense sequential chemotherapy in bladder cancer using the two-drug regimen of doxorubicin and gemcitabine (AG), followed by the three-drug ITP regimen. In a phase I study with 15 patients, AG was well tolerated at all dose levels, and no grade 3 or 4 myelosuppression was observed.[102] In a phase II trial in 21 patients, the overall response rate reported was 86%. However, toxicity was significant. ITP increased the response seen after AG in six patients. This suggests noncross resistance for the two regimens. The same approach is being evaluated in patients with impaired renal function using AG, but followed by paclitaxel and carboplatin.[103]

Triplet combinations

Several triple combinations have been studies in urothelial cancer patients. Bajorin et al have reported the activity of the ITP combination.[101] They demonstrated a response rate of 68% and a median survival in the range of 20 months, which was reported initially as a 50% increment in survival compared historically to the original MVAC series. Taking in consideration the significant activity of paclitaxel and gemcitabine, either alone or in combination with cisplatin, their different mechanism of action, and their nonoverlapping toxicities, the Spanish Group (SOGUG) studied the feasibility of adding paclitaxel to the doublet of gemcitabine/cisplatin in a phase I/II trial. In 58 patients, an overall response rate of 78% was observed with a median survival time of 24 months for the phase I segment of the trial and 15.6 months for the phase II part of the study.[104] A similar triplet was also evaluated using carboplatin. Investigators at Wayne State University, Detroit, incorporated gemcitabine in the carboplatin/paclitaxel combination in a phase II trial with 49 previously untreated patients with advanced urothelial malignancy and normal renal function. Of the 47 patients assessable for response, 15 obtained a CR and 15 obtained a PR, for an overall response rate of 68%. The median survival was 14.7 months.[105] Other triplets reported to date are presented in Table 25.6.[106–113] A large global international study comparing cisplatin/gemcitabine/paclitaxel with the conventional GC doublet has now been closed to patient accrual (with 610 patients). This trial will shed light on the role of the triplets in the management of advanced urothelial tumors. Whether or not we can improve survival with the newer triplet regimen will depend upon the results of this phase III trial.

Targeted therapy

The family of epidermal growth factor receptors is among the most studied growth factor receptors in bladder cancer[114] and several anti-EGFR strategies have been tested in urothelial patients. The activity of gefitinib (Iressa) has been analyzed in a recent phase II trial conducted by the Southwest Oncology Group in chemorefractory TCC of the bladder, with very limited results. Twenty-nine patients whose disease progressed after one chemotherapy regimen were treated

with gefitinib and, of these, only one had a partial response. The estimated median progression-free survival was only 1.7 months.[115] Combination with gemcitabine/cisplatin resulted in excessive toxicity, and two patients died because of neutropenic infections. The toxicity was attributed to the fixed dose rate infusion of gemcitabine used in this Cancer and Leukemia Group B (CALGB) trial. The study is ongoing using the standard gemcitabine mode of administration.[116] As mentioned above, a trial combining docetaxel and Iressa for minimal residual disease following chemotherapy is also being conducted.[94]

The Her2/neu oncogene is another member of the epidermal growth factor receptor family. Its overexpression results in increased cell proliferation and an increase in metastatic potential. The Her2/neu oncogene contribution to the malignant phenotype of the cell is consistent with the high rates of expression in poorly differentiated tumors and with a poorer prognosis in breast cancer. Her2/neu is also overexpressed in bladder cancer. Overexpression was detected by immunohistochemistry in 28% of the primary tumors and in 53% of metastatic lymph nodes. Overexpression in the primary tumors consistently predicts overexpression in distant or regional metastasis, although some Her2/neu-negative primary tumors may show overexpression in their corresponding metastasis.[115] No prognostic implication was demonstrated in these bladder cancer patients. Discordant results regarding overexpression have been published, related to the diversity of the techniques used for the assays.[117] There are also conflicting results regarding gene amplification in these overexpressed Her2/neu tumors, ranging between 7% and 95%. The low amplification suggests that mechanisms other than gene amplification may account for the observed high protein overexpression.[118–120]

Preclinical and clinical data have shown marked enhancement of the antitumor activity of chemotherapy when combined with the monoclonal antibody against Her2/neu trastuzumab.[121] Thus, Hussain et al recently combined trastuzumab with the carboplatin/paclitaxel/gemcitabine triplet for patients with overexpressed Her2/neu and reported a 61% objective response rate in patients with advanced urothelial cancer.[122] It is too soon to define the role of Her2/neu blockage with chemotherapy. The response rate appears to be similar to the results obtained with cisplatin-based triplets (see Table 25.6).[29,78,92,104–110,112–113,118]

GW572016 is an oral, reversible, dual inhibitor of ErbB1 and ErbB2 receptors that has also been tested in second line urothelial cancer. All patients that were included in this trial had confirmed expression of ErbB1 and/or ErbB2 (1+, 2+ or 3+ by immunohistochemistry). However, limited numbers of patients included were finally eligible for response evaluation, with only 10% being partial responders. Only one response was confirmed at 8 weeks.[123]

Several other strategies have been designed to target other elements involved in the activation of the cascade of biochemical and physiologic responses of the mitogenic signal transduction pathways. Preliminary results of the oral SCH66336 (a farnesyl protein transferase inhibitor) have indicated limited activity in previously treated patients with advanced/metastatic urothelial tract tumors.[124] Although this compound will not be further developed due to the inactivity seen in other indications, a study by the Early Clinical Study Group (ECSG) of the EORTC with the combination of SCH663366 and gemcitabine as second line in patients with advanced urothelial tract tumors revealed a 38.2 % encouraging response rate.[125]

Some clinical activity has been reported with several other compounds such as the histone deacetylase inhibitors.[126] In addition, cyclooxygenase 2 (COX2) might also be a therapeutic target in urothelial tumors. Although its expression had conflicting correlation with

Table 25.6 Triplet combination chemotherapy in urothelial cancer

Agents	No. pts with prior therapy	No. pts	Response rate (%)	Median survival time (months)
Cisplatin[104] Paclitaxel Gemcitabine	None	58	77.6	15.8
Cisplatin[106] Paclitaxel Gemcitabine	None	29	52	10.7
Cisplatin[107] Paclitaxel Gemcitabine	None	15	66.6	13.5
Cisplatin[108] Paclitaxel Ifosfamide	None	44	68	20
Cisplatin[29] Paclitaxel Methotrexate	21	25	40	
Cisplatin[109] Docetaxel Epirubicin	None	30	66.7	14.5
Carboplatin[105] Paclitaxel Gemcitabine	None	47	68	14.7
Carboplatin[110] Paclitaxel Gemcitabine	None	26	47.6	7.1
Carboplatin[78] Paclitaxel Gemcitabine	None	15	53	
Carboplatin[112] Docetaxel Gemcitabine	6	13	38	
Carboplatin[92] Paclitaxel Methotrexate Gemcitabine[113]	None	32	56	15.5
Paclitaxel Methotrexate	None	20	45	18

Table 25.7 Published abstracts on urothelial cancer in the *Proceedings of the American Society of Clinical Oncology* (ASCO)

ASCO	Phase II		Phase III		Unfit	Elderly	Salvage	Total
	No.	No. pts	No.	No. pts	No. pts	No. pts	No. pts	No. pts
2000	10	293	1	263	42		48	556
2001	8	193				27	15	193
2002	7	186			27	23	11	186
2003	7	276	2	309		25	49	585
2004	7	279			36		103	279

tumor grade or stage, in a subgroup of 62 patients that received chemotherapy, strong COX2 expression significantly correlated with poor overall survival.[127] Targeted therapy is discussed in more detail in Chapter 67.

Conclusion

A review of abstracts published over the last 5 years (Table 25.7) indicates that most of the clinical activity in this relatively small patient population focuses on small phase II trials in various phases of the disease, many of which will never mature for routine clinical use. At the present time, the cisplatin/gemcitabine (CG) combination in a phase III trial has been demonstrated to be a valuable alternative to the classical MVAC regimen with similar efficacy and survival probabilities, but with the benefit of less toxicity.

Other new double and triple combinations have yet to define their activity in phase III trials. To date, there are no randomized data to show that any of these new regimens improve patient survival as compared with either MVAC or CG. Strategies have been developed to minimize toxicity in patients that are 'unfit', 'elderly', or have 'compromised renal function'. Clinical trials should be designed to clearly distinguish among these three groups of patients. Outside a clinical trial, M-CAVI, carboplatin/gemcitabine, CBDCA/paclitaxel, gemcitabine/taxane or monotherapy with gemcitabine, CBDCA or a taxane could be used in 'unfit' patients in an individual basis. The new era of targeted therapy is being incorporated in the management of urothelial cancer with the hope of improving patient management in the not too distant future.

References

1. http://www.cancer.org/downloads/STT/CAFF2003PWSecured.pdf
2. Yagoda A. Chemotherapy of urothelial tract tumors. Cancer 1987; 60: 574–85.
3. Raghavan D, Shipley WU, Garnick MB, et al. The biology and management of bladder cancer. N Engl J Med 1990; 322: 1129–38.
4. Harker WG, Meyers FJ, Freiha FS, et al. Cisplatin, methotrexate, and vinblastine (CMV): an effective chemotherapy regimen for metastatic transitional cell carcinoma of the urinary tract. A Northern California Oncology Group study. J Clin Oncol 1985; 3: 1463–70.
5. Logothetis CJ, Dexeus FH, Chong C, et al. Cisplatin, cyclophosphamide and doxorubicin chemotherapy for unresectable urothelial tumors: the M.D. Anderson experience. J Urol 1989; 141: 33–37.
6. Sternberg CN, Yagoda A, Scher HI, et al. Preliminary results of M-VAC (methotrexate, vinblastine, doxorubicin and cisplatin) for transitional cell carcinoma of the urothelium. J Urol 1985; 133: 403–07.
7. Yagoda A. The role of cisplatin-based chemotherapy in advanced urothelial tract cancer. Semin Oncol 1989; 16(4 Suppl 6): 98–104.
8. Mead GM, Russell M, Clark P, et al. A randomized trial comparing methotrexate and vinblastine (MV) with cisplatin, methotrexate and vinblastine (CMV) in advanced transitional cell carcinoma: results and a report on prognostic factors in a Medical Research Council study. MRC Advanced Bladder Cancer Working Party. Br J Cancer 1998; 78: 1067–75.
9. Sternberg CN, Yagoda A, Scher HI, et al. Methotrexate, vinblastine, and cisplatin for advanced transitional cell carcinoma of the urothelium. Efficacy and patterns of response and relapse. Cancer 1989; 64: 2448–58.
10. Tannock I, Gospodarowicz M, Connolly J, Jewett M. M-VAC (methotrexate, vinblastine, doxorubicin and cisplatin) chemotherapy for transitional cell carcinoma: the Princess Margaret Hospital experience. J Urol 1989; 142(2 Pt 1): 289–92.
11. Logothetis CJ, Dexeus FH, Finn L, et al. A prospective randomized trial comparing MVAC and CISCA chemotherapy for patients with metastatic urothelial tumors. J Clin Oncol 1990; 8: 1050–5.
12. Boutan-Laroze A, Mahjoubi M, Droz JP, et al. M-VAC (methotrexate, vinblastine, doxorubicin and cisplatin) for advanced carcinoma of the bladder. The French Federation of Cancer Centers experience. Eur J Cancer 1991; 27: 1690–94.
13. Loehrer PJ Sr, Einhorn LH, Elson PJ, et al. A randomized comparison of cisplatin alone or in combination with methotrexate, vinblastine, and doxorubicin in patients with metastatic urothelial carcinoma: a cooperative group study. J Clin Oncol 1992; 10: 1066–73.
14. Bellmunt J, Ribas A, Eres N, et al. Carboplatin-based versus cisplatin-based chemotherapy in the treatment of surgically incurable advanced bladder carcinoma. Cancer 1997; 80: 1966–72.
15. Saxman SB, Propert KJ, Einhorn LH, et al. Long-term follow-up of a phase III intergroup study of cisplatin alone or in combination with methotrexate, vinblastine, and doxorubicin in patients with metastatic urothelial carcinoma: a cooperative group study. J Clin Oncol 1997; 15: 2564–69.
16. Gabrilove JL, Jakubowski A, Scher H, et al. Effect of granulocyte colony-stimulating factor on neutropenia and associated morbidity due to chemotherapy for transitional-cell carcinoma of the urothelium. N Engl J Med 1988; 318: 1414–22.
17. Moore MJ, Iscoe N, Tannock IF. A phase II study of methotrexate, vinblastine, doxorubicin and cisplatin plus recombinant human granulocyte-macrophage colony stimulating factors in patients with advanced transitional cell carcinoma. J Urol 1993; 150: 1131–34.
18. Loehrer PJ Sr, Elson P, Dreicer R, et al. Escalated dosages of methotrexate, vinblastine, doxorubicin, and cisplatin plus recombinant human granulocyte colony-stimulating factor in advanced urothelial carcinoma: an Eastern Cooperative Oncology Group trial. J Clin Oncol 1994; 12: 483–88.
19. Seidman AD, Scher HI, Gabrilove JL, et al. Dose-intensification of MVAC with recombinant granulocyte colony-stimulating factor as initial therapy in advanced urothelial cancer. J Clin Oncol 1993; 11: 408–14.
20. Scher HI, Geller NL, Curley T, Tao Y. Effect of relative cumulative dose-intensity on survival of patients with urothelial cancer treated with M-VAC. J Clin Oncol 1993; 11(3): 400–07.

21. Logothetis CJ, Finn LD, Smith T, et al. Escalated MVAC with or without recombinant human granulocyte-macrophage colony-stimulating factor for the initial treatment of advanced malignant urothelial tumors: results of a randomized trial. J Clin Oncol 1995; 13(9): 2272–7.

22. Bamias A, Aravantinos G, Deliveliotis C, et al. Docetaxel and cisplatin with granulocyte colony-stimulating factor (G-CSF) versus MVAC with G-CSF in advanced urothelial carcinoma: a multicenter, randomized, phase III study from the Hellenic Cooperative Oncology Group. J Clin Oncol 2004; 22: 220–28.

23. Sternberg CN, de Mulder PH, Schornagel JH, et al. European Organisation for Research and Treatment of Cancer Genitourinary Tract Cancer Cooperative Group. Randomized phase III trial of high-dose-intensity methotrexate, vinblastine, doxorubicin, and cisplatin (MVAC) chemotherapy and recombinant human granulocyte colony-stimulating factor versus classic MVAC in advanced urothelial tract tumors: European Organisation for Research and Treatment of Cancer Protocol no. 30924. J Clin Oncol 2001; 19: 2638–46.

24. Siefker-Radtke AO, Millikan RE, Tu SM, et al. Phase III trial of fluorouracil, interferon alpha-2b, and cisplatin versus methotrexate, vinblastine, doxorubicin, and cisplatin in metastatic or unresectable urothelial cancer. J Clin Oncol 2002; 20: 1361–67.

25. Dreicer R, Manola J, Roth BJ, et al. Phase III trial of methotrexate, vinblastine, doxorubicin, and cisplatin versus carboplatin and paclitaxel in patients with advanced carcinoma of the urothelium. Cancer 2004; 100: 1639–45.

26. von der Maase H, Hansen SW, Roberts JT, et al. Gemcitabine and cisplatin versus methotrexate, vinblastine, doxorubicin, and cisplatin in advanced or metastatic bladder cancer: results of a large, randomized, multinational, multicenter, phase III study. J Clin Oncol 2000; 18: 3068–77.

27. Bajorin DF, Dodd PM, Mazumdar M, et al. Long-term survival in metastatic transitional-cell carcinoma and prognostic factors predicting outcome of therapy. J Clin Oncol 1999; 17: 3173–81.

28. Bellmunt J, Albanell J, Paz-Ares L, et al. Pretreatment prognostic factors for survival in patients with advanced urothelial tumors treated in a phase I/II trial with paclitaxel, cisplatin, and gemcitabine. Cancer 2002; 95: 751–7.

29. Tu SM, Hossan E, Amato R, Kilbourn R, Logothetis CJ. Paclitaxel, cisplatin and methotrexate combination chemotherapy is active in the treatment of refractory urothelial malignancies. J Urol 1995; 154: 1719–22.

30. Roth BJ, Dreicer R, Einhorn LH, et al. Significant activity of paclitaxel in advanced transitional-cell carcinoma of the urothelium: a phase II trial of the Eastern Cooperative Oncology Group. J Clin Oncol 1994; 12: 2264–70.

31. Sweeney CJ, Williams SD, Finch DE, et al. A phase II study of paclitaxel and ifosfamide for patients with advanced refractory carcinoma of the urothelium. Cancer 1999; 86: 514–8.

32. Vaughn DJ, Malkowicz SB, Zoltick B, et al. Phase I trial of paclitaxel/carboplatin in advanced carcinoma of the urothelium. Semin Oncol 1997; 24(1 Suppl 2): S2–47, S2–50.

33. Zielinski CC, Schnack B, Grbovic M, et al. Paclitaxel and carboplatin in patients with metastatic urothelial cancer: results of a phase II trial. Br J Cancer 1998; 78: 370–374.

34. Redman BG, Smith DC, Flaherty L, Du W, Hussain M. Phase II trial of paclitaxel and carboplatin in the treatment of advanced urothelial carcinoma. J Clin Oncol 1998; 16: 1844–48.

35. Pollera CF, Ceribelli A, Crecco M, Calabresi F. Weekly gemcitabine in advanced bladder cancer: a preliminary report from a phase I study. Ann Oncol 1994; 5: 182–4.

36. Stadler WM, Kuzel T, Roth B, Raghavan D, Dorr FA. Phase II study of single-agent gemcitabine in previously untreated patients with metastatic urothelial cancer. J Clin Oncol 1997; 15: 3394–98.

37. Moore MJ, Tannock IF, Ernst DS, Huan S, Murray N. Gemcitabine: a promising new agent in the treatment of advanced urothelial cancer. J Clin Oncol 1997; 15: 3441–45.

38. Lorusso V, Pollera CF, Antimi M, et al. A phase II study of gemcitabine in patients with transitional cell carcinoma of the urinary tract previously treated with platinum: Italian Cooperative Group on Bladder Cancer. Eur J Cancer 1998; 34: 1208–12.

39. Van Moorsel CJ, Veerman G, Vermorken JB, et al. Mechanisms of synergism between gemcitabine and cisplatin. Source Adv Exp Med Biol 1998; 431: 581–85.

40. Von der Maase H, Andersen L, Crino L, Weinknecht S, Dogliotti L. Weekly gemcitabine and cisplatin combination therapy in patients with transitional cell carcinoma of the urothelium: a phase II clinical trial. Ann Oncol 1999; 10: 1461–65.

41. Moore MJ, Winquist EW, Murray N, et al. Gemcitabine plus cisplatin, an active regimen in advanced urothelial cancer: a phase II trial of the National Cancer Institute of Canada Clinical Trials Group. J Clin Oncol 1999; 17: 286–2881.

42. Kaufman D, Raghavan D, Carducci M, et al. Phase II trial of gemcitabine plus cisplatin in patients with metastatic urothelial cancer. J Clin Oncol 2000; 18: 1921–27.

43. Lehmann J, Retz M, Stockle M. Is there standard chemotherapy for metastatic bladder cancer? Quality of life and medical resources utilization based on largest to date randomized trial. Crit Rev Oncol Hematol 2003; 47: 171–9.

44. Hussain SA, Stocken DD, Riley P, et al. A phase I/II study of gemcitabine and fractionated cisplatin in an outpatient setting using a 21-day schedule in patients with advanced and metastatic bladder cancer. Br J Cancer 2004; 91: 844–849.

45. Wilson JJ, Winquist E, Dorreen M, et al. A phase II trial of gemcitabine plus day 1 cisplatin given on a 21 day schedule in patients with advanced unresectable or metastatic bladder cancer. Proc Am Soc Clin Oncol 2002; 21: 151b.

46. McCaffrey JA, Hilton S, Mazumdar M, et al. Phase II trial of docetaxel in patients with advanced or metastatic transitional-cell carcinoma. J Clin Oncol 1997; 15: 1853–57.

47. de Wit R, Kruit WH, Stoter G, et al. Docetaxel (Taxotere): an active agent in metastatic urothelial cancer; results of a phase II study in non-chemotherapy-pretreated patients. Br J Cancer 1998; 78: 1342–45.

48. Seidman AD, Scher HI, Heinemann MH, et al. Continuous infusion gallium nitrate for patients with advanced refractory urothelial tract tumors. Cancer 1991; 68: 2561–65.

49. Witte RS, Elson P, Bono B, et al. Eastern Cooperative Oncology Group phase II trial of ifosfamide in the treatment of previously treated advanced urothelial carcinoma. J Clin Oncol 1997; 15: 589–589.

50. Sweeney CJ, Williams SD, Finch DE, et al. A phase II study of paclitaxel and ifosfamide for patients with advanced refractory carcinoma of the urothelium. Cancer 1999; 86: 514–8.

51. Muller M, Heicappell R, Steiner U, Goessl C, Miller K. Side effects of chemotherapy for advanced urothelial carcinoma with etoposide and ifosfamide. Urol Int 1997; 59: 248–51.

52. Kyriakakis Z, Dimopoulos MA, Kostakopoulos A, et al. Cisplatin, ifosfamide, methotrexate and vinblastine combination chemotherapy for metastatic urothelial cancer. J Urol 1997; 158: 408–11.

53. Dreicer R, Propert KJ, Roth BJ, Einhorn LH, Loehrer PJ. Vinblastine, ifosfamide, and gallium nitrate—an active new regimen in patients with advanced carcinoma of the urothelium. A phase II trial of the Eastern Cooperative Oncology Group (E5892). Cancer 1997; 79: 110–4.

54. Raabe NK, Fossa SD, Paro G. Phase II study of carboplatin in locally advanced and metastatic transitional cell carcinoma of the urinary bladder. Br J Urol 1989; 646: 604–07.

55. Petrioli R, Frediani B, Manganelli A, et al. Comparison between a cisplatin-containing regimen and a carboplatin-containing regimen for recurrent or metastatic bladder cancer patients. A randomized phase II study. Cancer 1996; 77: 344–51.

56. Bellmunt J, Ribas A, Eres N, et al. Carboplatin–based versus cisplatin-based chemotherapy in the treatment of surgically incurable advanced bladder carcinoma. Cancer 1997; 80: 1966–72.

57. Carteni G, Dogliotti L, Crucitta E, et al. Phase II randomized trial of gemcitabine plus cisplatin (GP) and gemcitabine plus carboplatin (GC) in patients (pts) with advanced or metastatic transitional cell carcinoma of the urothelium (TCCU). Proc Am Soc Clin Oncol 2003; 22: A1543.

58. De Mulder P, Sternberg CN, Fossa S, et al. Lobaplatin in advanced urothelial tract tumors (EORTC 30931). Proc Am Soc Clin Oncol 1997; 16: A1158.

59. Moore MJ, Winquist E, Vokes EE, Hirte H, Hoving H, Stadler WM. Phase II study of oxaliplatin in patients with inoperable, locally advanced or metastatic transitional cell carcinoma of the urothelial tract (TCC) who have received prior chemotherapy. Proc Am Soc Clin Oncol 2003; 22: 408 (Abstract 1638).

60. Culine S, Rebillard X, Iborra F, et al. Gemcitabine and oxaliplatin in advanced transitional cell carcinoma of the urothelium: a pilot study. Anticancer Res 2003; 23: 1903–06.

61. Font A, Esteban E, Carles J, et al. Gemcitabine and oxaliplatin combination: a multicenter phase II trial in unfit patients with locally advanced or metastatic urothelial cancer. Proc Am Soc Clin Oncol 2004; 22: A4544.

62. de Wit R, Kaye SB, Roberts JT, et al. Oral piritrexim, an effective treatment for metastatic urothelial cancer. Br J Cancer 1993; 67: 388–90.

63. Khorsand M, Lange J, Feun L, et al. Phase II trial of oral piritrexim in advanced, previously treated transitional cell cancer of bladder. Invest New Drugs 1997; 15: 157–63.

64. Dreicer R, Roth B, Wilding G. Perspectives in bladder cancer, supplement to Cancer. Overview of advanced urothelial cancer trials of the Eastern Cooperative Oncology Group. Cancer 2003; 97(Suppl 8): 2109–114.

65. Paz-Ares L, Tabernero J, Moyano A, et al. A phase II of the multitargeted antifolate, MTA (LY231514), in patients with advanced transitional cell carcinoma of the bladder. Proc Am Soc Clin Oncol 1998; 17: A1307.

66. Sweeney C, Roth BJ, Kaufman DS, Nicol SJ. Phase II study of pemetrexed (pem) for second-line treatment of transitional cell cancer (tcc) of the bladder. Proc Am Soc Clin Oncol 2003; 22: A1653.

67. Bui B, Theodore C, Culine S, et al. Preliminary results of a phase II study testing intravenous (iv) vinflunine (VFL) as second line therapy in patients with advanced transitional cell cancer (TCC) of the bladder. Proc Am Soc Clin Oncol 2003; 22: A1571.

68. www.cancerbacup.org.uk

69. Witte RS, Propert KJ, Burch B, et al. An ECOG phase II trial topotecan (T) in previously treated advanced urothelial carcinoma (UC). Proc Annu Meet Am Soc Clin Oncol 1997; 16: A115.

70. www.ClinicalTrials.gov

71. Sternberg CN, Calabro F, Pizzocaro G, et al. Chemotherapy with an every-2-week regimen of gemcitabine and paclitaxel in patients with transitional cell carcinoma who have received prior cisplatin-based therapy. Cancer 2001; 92(12): 2993–98.

72. Kaufman D, Stadler W, Carducci M, et al. Gemcitabine and paclitaxel every two weeks: a multicenter phase II trial in locally advanced or metastatic urothelial cancer. Proc Am Soc Clin Oncol 2000; 19: A1341.

73. Meluch AA, Greco FA, Burris HA 3rd, et al. Paclitaxel and gemcitabine chemotherapy for advanced transitional-cell carcinoma of the urothelial tract: a phase II trial of the Minnie pearl cancer research network. J Clin Oncol 2001; 19: 3018–24.

74. Parameswaran R, Fisch MJ, Rafat H, et al. A Hoosier Oncology Group phase II study of weekly paclitaxel and gemcitabine in advanced transitional cell carcinoma (TCC) of the bladder. Proc Am Soc Clin Oncol 2001; 20: A798.

75. Srinivas S, Guardino AE. Gemcitabine and paclitaxel chemotherapy effective for good risk advanced urothelial malignancies. Proc Am Soc Clin Oncol 2004; 23: A4675.

76. Garcia Del Muro X, Marcuello E, Mellado B, et al. Phase II multicenter study of docetaxel plus gemcitabine as first-line treatment in advanced urothelial cancer. Proc Am Soc Clin Oncol 2003; 22: A1643.

77. Friedland D, Gregurich MA, Belt R, et al. Phase II evaluation of docetaxel plus gemcitabine in patients with advanced unresectable urothelial cancer. Proc Am Soc Clin Oncol 2002; 21: A2427.

78. Dreicer R, Manola J, Schneider DJ, et al. Phase II trial of gemcitabine and docetaxel in patients with advanced carcinoma of the urothelium: a trial of the Eastern Cooperative Oncology Group. Cancer 2003; 97: 2743–47.

79. Gitlitz BJ, Baker C, Chapman Y, et al. A phase II study of gemcitabine and docetaxel therapy in patients with advanced urothelial carcinoma. Cancer 2003; 98: 1863–69.

80. Chestera JD, Halla GD, Forsterb M, Protheroeb AS. Systemic chemotherapy for patients with bladder cancer—current controversies and future directions. Cancer Treat Rev 2004; 30: 343–58.

81. Vaughn D, Dreicer R, Manola J, et al. E2896 paclitaxel/carboplatin in advanced urothelial carcinoma and renal insufficiency: a phase II trial of the Eastern Cooperative Group. Proc Am Soc Clin Oncol 2000; 19: A343.

82. Neri B, Di Cello V, Biscione S, et al. Phase II evaluation of gemcitabine (GEM) and epirubicin (EPI) in advanced bladder cancer. Proc Am Soc Clin Oncol 2000; 19: A1380.

83. Turkolmez K, Beduk Y, Baltaci S, Gogus CA, Gogus O. Gemcitabine plus vinorelbine chemotherapy in patients with advanced bladder carcinoma who are medically unsuitable for or who have failed cisplatin-based chemotherapy. Eur Urol 2003; 44: 682–6.

84. Bellmunt J, de Wit R, Albanell J, Baselga J. A feasibility study of carboplatin with fixed dose of gemcitabine in 'unfit' patients with advanced bladder cancer. Eur J Cancer 2001; 37: 2212–15.

85. Sella A, Logothetis CJ, Dexeus FH, Amato R, Finn L, Fitz K. Cisplatin combination chemotherapy for elderly patients with urothelial tumours. Br J Urol 1991; 67: 603–7.

86. Bamias A, Efstathiou E, Hamilos G, et al. Outcome of elderly patients following platinum-based chemotherapy for advanced urothelial cancer. Proc Am Soc Clin Oncol 2004; 22: A4542.

87. Stadler WM, Hayden A, von der Maase H, et al. Long-term survival in phase II trials of gemcitabine plus cisplatin for advanced transitional cell cancer. Urol Oncol 2002; 7: 153–7.

88. Esrig D, Elmajian D, Groshen S, et al. Accumulation of nuclear p53 and tumor progression in bladder cancer. N Engl J Med 1994; 331: 1259–64.

89. Chatterjee SJ, Datar R, Youssefzadeh D, et al. Combined effects of p53, p21, and pRb expression in the progression of bladder transitional cell carcinoma. J Clin Oncol 2004; 22: 1007–13.

90. Slaton JW, Benedict WF, Dinney CP. P53 in bladder cancer: mechanism of action, prognostic value, and target for therapy. Urology 2001; 57: 852–59.

91. Sarkis AS, Bajorin DF, Reuter VE, et al. Prognostic value of p53 nuclear overexpression in patients with invasive bladder cancer treated with neoadjuvant MVAC. J Clin Oncol 1995; 13: 1384–90.

92. Edelman MJ, Meyers FJ, Miller TR, et al. Phase I/II study of paclitaxel, carboplatin, and methotrexate in advanced transitional cell carcinoma: a well-tolerated regimen with activity independent of p53 mutation. Urology 2000; 55: 521–25.

93. Highshaw RA, McConkey DJ, Dinney CP. Integrating basic science and clinical research in bladder cancer: update from the first bladder Specialized Program of Research Excellence (SPORE). Curr Opin Urol 2004; 14: 295–300.

94. Inoue K, Slaton JW, Perrotte P, et al. Paclitaxel enhances the effects of the anti-epidermal growth factor receptor monoclonal antibody ImClone C225 in mice with metastatic human bladder transitional cell carcinoma. Clin Cancer Res 2000; 6: 4874–84.

95. Herr HW, Donat SM, Bajorin DF. Post-chemotherapy surgery in patients with unresectable or regionally metastatic bladder cancer. J Urol 2001; 165: 811–14.

96. Siefker-Radtke AO, Walsh GL, Pisters LL, et al. Is there a role for surgery in the management of metastatic urothelial cancer? The M.D. Anderson experience. J Urol 2004; 171: 145–8.

97. Miller RS, Freiha FS, Reese JH, et al. Cisplatin, methotrexate and vinblastine plus surgical restaging for patients with advanced transitional cell carcinoma of the urothelium. J Urol 1993; 150: 65–69.

98. Kattan J, Culine S, Theodore C, Droz JP. Second-line M-VAC therapy in patients previously treated with the M-VAC regimen for metastatic urothelial cancer. Ann Oncol 1993; 4: 793–94.

99. Tu SM, Millikan RE, Pagliaro LC, et al. Treatment of refractory urothelial carcinoma with alternating paclitaxel, methotrexate, cisplatin (TMP) and 5-fluorouracil, α-interferon, cisplatin (FAP) Urol Oncol 2003; 21: 342–48.

100. Siefker-Radtke AO, Thall PF, Tannir NM, et al. Implementation of a novel statistical design to evaluate successive treatment courses for metastatic transitional cell carcinoma. A phase II trial at the M.D. Anderson Cancer Center. Proc Am Soc Clin Oncol 2004; 22: A4543.

101. Bajorin DF, McCaffrey JA, Dodd PM, et al. Ifosfamide, paclitaxel, and cisplatin for patients with advanced transitional cell carcinoma of the urothelial tract. Final report of a phase II trial evaluating two dosing schedules. Cancer 2000; 88: 1671–8.

102. Dodd PM, McCaffrey JA, Hilton S, et al. Phase I evaluation of sequential doxorubicin gemcitabine then ifosfamide paclitaxel cisplatin for patients with unresectable or metastatic transitional-cell carcinoma of the urothelial tract. J Clin Oncol 2000; 18: 840–46.

103. Novick S, Higgins G, Hilton S, et al. Phase I/II sequential doxorubicin plus gemcitabine followed by paclitaxel plus carboplatin in patients with transitional cell carcinoma and impaired renal function. Proc Am Soc Clin Oncol 2000; 19: A1423.

104. Bellmunt J, Guillem V, Paz-Ares L, et al. Phase I/II study of paclitaxel, cisplatin, and gemcitabine in advanced transitional-cell carcinoma of the urothelium. J Clin Oncol 2000; 18: 3247–55.

105. Hussain M, Vaishampayan U, Du W, Redman B, Smith DC. Combination carboplatin, paclitaxel and gemcitabine is an active treatment for advanced urothelial carcinoma. J Clin Oncol 2001; 19: 2527–33.

106. Clark PE, Stindt D, Hall MC, et al. Phase II trial of gemcitabine, paclitaxel, and cisplatin in advanced transitional cell carcinoma. Proc Am Soc Clin Oncol 2004; 22: A4610.

107. Hogan F, Lamm D, Schunn G, Kandzari S. Cisplatin (C), gemcitabine (G), and paclitaxel (P) for 50 poor-risk patients (pts) with advanced intra-pelvic (M0) or metastatic (M1) urothelial cancer. Proc Am Soc Clin Oncol 2003; 21: A1703.

108. Bajorin DF, McCaffrey JA, Dodd PM, et al. Ifosfamide, paclitaxel and cisplatin for patients with advanced transitional cell carcinoma of the urothelial tract: final report of a phase II trial evaluating two dosing schedules. Cancer 2000; 88: 1671–78.

109. Pectasides D, Visvikis A, Aspropotamitis A, et al. Chemotherapy with cisplatin, epirubicin and docetaxel in transitional cell urothelial cancer. Phase II trial. Eur J Cancer 2000; 36: 74–79.

110. Chahine GY, Kattan G, Farhat FS, et al. The weekly triplet: gemcitabine, carboplatin and paclitaxel as first line therapy for advanced urothelial cancer. ASCO Annual Meeting Proceedings (Post-Meeting Edition). J Clin Oncol 2004; 22(Suppl 14): 4704.

111. DiPaola RS, Rubin E, Toppmeyer D, et al. Gemcitabine combined with sequential paclitaxel and carboplatin in patients with urothelial cancers and other advanced malignancies. Med Sci Monit 2003; 9: I5–11.

112. Elizabeth H, Owen C, Shelton G, et al. Phase I/II study of docetaxel, gemcitabine, carboplatin in poor prognosis and previously treated patients with urothelial carcinoma. Proc Am Soc Clin Oncol 2000; 19: A1376.

113. Law LY, Primo NL, Meyers FJ, et al. Platinum free combination chemotherapy in locally advanced and metastatic transitional cell carcinoma: phase I/II trial of gemcitabine, paclitaxel, methotrexate. Proc Am Soc Clin Oncol 2001; 20: A767.

114. Mchugh LA, Leyshon Griffiths TR, Kriajevska M, Symonds RP, Mellon JK. Tyrosine kinase inhibitors of the epidermal growth factor receptor as adjuncts to systemic chemotherapy for muscle-invasive bladder cancer. Urology 2004; 63: 619–24.

115. Petrylak D, Faulkner JR, Van Veldhuizen PJ, Mansukhani M, Crawford ED. Evaluation of ZD1839 for advanced transitional cell carcinoma (TCC) of the urothelium: a Southwest Oncology Group Trial. Proc Am Soc Clin Oncol 2003; 22: A1619.

116. Philips G, Halabi S, Sanford B, Bajorin D, Small E. Phase II trial of cisplatin (C), fixed-dose rate gemcitabine (G) and gefitinib for advanced transitional cell carcinoma (TCC) of the urothelial tract: preliminary results of CALGB 90102. Proc Am Soc Clin Oncol 2004; 23: A4540.

117. Jimenez RE, Hussain M, Bianco FJ Jr, et al. Her-2/neu overexpression in muscle-invasive urothelial carcinoma of the bladder: prognostic significance and comparative analysis in primary and metastatic tumors. Clin Cancer Res 2001; 7: 2440–2447.

118. de Pinieux G, Colin D, Vincent-Salomon A, et al. Confrontation of immunohistochemistry and fluorescent in situ hybridization for the assessment of HER-2/neu(c-erbb-2) status in urothelial carcinoma. Virchows Arch 2004; 444: 415–9.

119. Latifa Z, Wattersa AD, Dunna I, et al. HER2/neu gene amplification and protein overexpression in G3 pT2 transitional cell carcinoma of the bladder: a role for anti-HER2 therapy? Eur J Cancer 2004; 40: 56–63.

120. Piccart M. Closing remarks and treatment guidelines. Eur J Cancer 2001; 37: 30–33.

121. Slamon DJ, Leyland-Jones B, Shak S, et al. Use of chemotherapy plus a monoclonal antibody against HER2 for metastatic breast cancer that overexpresses HER2. N Engl J Med 2001; 344: 783–92.

122. Hussain M, Smith DC, Vaishampayan U, et al. Trastuzumab (T), paclitaxel (P), carboplatin (C) and gemcitabine (G) in patients with advanced urothelial cancer and overexpression of HER-2 (NCI study #198). Proc Am Soc Clin Oncol 2003; 22: A1568.

123. Machiels J-P, Wülfing C, Richel DJ, et al. A single arm, multicenter, open-label phase II study of orally administered GW572016 as single-agent, second-line treatment of patients with locally advanced or metastatic transitional cell carcinoma of the urothelial tract. Interim analysis. Proc Am Soc Clin Oncol 2004; 23: A4615.

124. Winquist E, Moore MJ, Chi K, et al. NCIC CTG IND.128: a phase II study of a farnesyl transferase inhibitor (SCH 66336) in patients with unresectable or metastatic transitional cell carcinoma of the urothelial tract failing prior chemotherapy. Proc Am Soc Clin Oncol 2001; 20: A785.

125. Theodore C, Geoffrois L, Vermorken JB, et al. A phase II multicentre study of SCH66336 in combination with gemcitabine as second line treatment in patients with advanced/metastatic urothelial tract tumor. Proc Am Soc Clin Oncol 2003; 22: A1667.

126. Kelly WK, Richon VM, O'Connor O, et al. Phase I clinical trial of histone deacetylase inhibitor: suberoylanilide hydroxamic acid administered intravenously. Clin Cancer Res 2003; 9: 3578–88.

127. Wulfinga C, Eltzeb E, von Struenseea D, et al. Cyclooxygenase-2 expression in bladder cancer: correlation with poor outcome after chemotherapy. Eur Urol 2004; 45: 46–52.

INDEX

Notes: Please note that as the subject of this book is bladder cancer, all entries refer to this disease unless otherwise stated. Also entries followed by 'f' and 't' refer to figures and tables/boxed material respectively.

Abbreviations: To save space in the index, the following abbreviations have been used: BCG–bacillus Calmette–Guérin; MVAC–methotrexate/vinblastine/adriamycin/cisplatin combined chemotherapy; TURBT–transurethral resection of bladder tumor

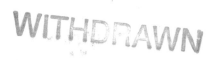